This book describes the underlying mechanisms and pathophysiological processes which relate to various childhood injuries, and brings together experimental and empirical data which bear on the rational management of injury in childhood. It also deals with the wider issues of service organisation and rehabilitation. The book describes the commonest causes and types of injury encountered in the young, including trauma, head injury, near drowning and burns. It also deals with essential aspects of effective management of injury in the hospital including trauma scoring, life support and nutritional support. It is intended for trainees and consultants in paediatrics, paediatric surgery, accident and emergency, anaesthesia and intensive care, and it will also serve as a source book for medical and non-medical researchers.

INJURY IN THE YOUNG

INJURY IN THE YOUNG

Edited by

M. P. WARD PLATT

Royal Victoria Infirmary
Newcastle upon Tyne, UK

R. A. LITTLE

North Western Injury Research Unit
Manchester, UK

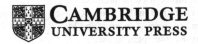

CAMBRIDGE UNIVERSITY PRESS
Cambridge, New York, Melbourne, Madrid, Cape Town, Singapore, São Paulo

Cambridge University Press
The Edinburgh Building, Cambridge CB2 8RU, UK

Published in the United States of America by Cambridge University Press, New York

www.cambridge.org
Information on this title: www.cambridge.org/9780521481175

First published 1998
This digitally printed version 2007

A catalogue record for this publication is available from the British Library

Library of Congress Cataloguing in Publication data
Injury in the young / edited by M. P. Ward Platt and R. A. Little.
  p. cm.
ISBN 0 521 48117 1 (hardback)
1. Children – Wounds and injuries.   I. Platt, M. P. Ward (Martin Peter
Ward), 1954– .   II. Little, R. A. (Rod A.)
[DNLM: 1. Wounds and Injuries – in infancy & childhood.   2. Wounds
and Injuries – therapy.   WO 700 I586 1998]
RD93.5.C4I65   1998
617.1′0083 – dc21   97-11815 CIP
for Library of Congress

ISBN 978-0-521-48117-5 hardback
ISBN 978-0-521-03737-2 paperback

Contents

Contributors

J. G. Andrew
Department of Orthopaedic Surgery
Hope Hospital
Salford M6 8HD, UK

C. M. Bannister
Booth Hall Children's Hospital
Manchester M9 2AA, UK

R. M. Bingham
The Hospital for Sick Children
London WC1N 3JH, UK

D. Bohn
Department of Critical Care
The Hospital for Sick Children
Toronto, Canada M50 1X8

C. Childs
Burns Unit
Booth Hall Children's Hospital
Manchester M2 9AA, UK

M. Crouchman
Variety Club Childrens Hospital
Kings College Hospital
London SE5 9RS, UK

P. Edwards
Department of Child Health
University of Newcastle upon Tyne
Newcastle, UK

J. Grigg
Department of Child Health
Leicester Royal Infirmary NHS Trust,
Leicester, UK

J. Harris
Centre for Social Ethics and Policy
University of Manchester
Manchester M13, UK

D. N. Herndon
Shriners Burns Institute
Texas 77550, USA

S. Jarvis
Gateshead Health Authority
Gateshead NE8 3EP, UK

R. A. Little
North Western Injury Research Centre
University of Manchester
Manchester M13 9PT, UK

M. J. Muller
Shriners Burns Institute
Texas 77550, USA

B. M. Phillips
Alder Hey Children's Hospital
Liverpool L12 2AP, UK

G. S. Samra
The Hospital for Sick Children
London WC1N 3JH, UK

P. M. Sharples
Royal Hospital for Sick Children
Bristol B52 8BJ, UK

M. P. Ward Platt
Royal Victoria Infirmary
Newcastle upon Tyne NE1 4LP, UK

B. Wright
Accident and Emergency Department
Leeds General Hospital
Leeds LS1 3EX, UK

Editors' Preface

The purpose of the book is to bring together current knowledge about injury in childhood. While there are many books, and a large literature, which address the epidemiology of childhood injury, and textbooks to which doctors can refer when in need of guidance about management of injuries, we believe there has not yet been a book which brings together the science of injury responses and injury management in relation to children.

We have asked our contributors to review experimental and empirical data which influence the rational management of injury in childhood. Because management of injury in its widest sense has to relate to the organisation of pre-hospital services and emergency rooms, and because the needs of children are different to those of adults, we have also included material on organisational issues, and on the management of families when a child cannot be saved. We all start, unashamedly, from the assumption that knowledge acquired in adults cannot readily be extrapolated to the young.

There is no doubt that in recent years there has been a huge advance in our knowledge of injuries in childhood, although publication of this work is scattered across a wide variety of journals and clinical disciplines as can be seen from the reference lists in all the chapters. Other trends have been in evidence as well. Advanced life support courses have become established, both for trauma and specifically for paediatrics. Efforts have been made to improve pre-hospital care, for instance by training ambulance paramedics. Cars are safer, both for the occupants and for pedestrians struck by them. Local councils continue to increase traffic calming schemes and car-free shopping streets. Probably all of these initiatives have contributed to the steady decline in the death toll from childhood injuries. This begs the question: what is the role of hospital care in improving outcome for childhood injury? Can we have any confidence that in understanding the pathophysiology of injury, we can develop new and more effective therapeutic strategies?

To try to answer this, the UK Major Trauma Outcome Study has recently published data from children and young adults who were alive on arrival at hospital (Roberts, Campbell, Hollis & Yates (1996) *British Medical Journal* **313**: 1239–1241). In a large cohort of seriously injured young people (Injury Severity Score at least 16), they were able to demonstrate a progressive and continuous reduction in death rates from 1989 to 1995 even when corrected for Injury Severity Score, Revised Trauma Score, and age. They went on to suggest on the basis of some plausible assumptions, that 'the proportion of deaths that might have been averted by improved hospital care is about 8%'.

No one would quarrel with the notion that prevention is best, least of all the clinicians and researchers who grapple with injury, but children will continue to get hurt, sometimes seriously, and we owe it to them to give the best possible care. That there is room for improvement is clear, and that mortality can be further reduced seems very likely. The challenge also lies in improving survival without merely creating a disproportionate burden of disability, and this will be fertile ground for further research. We are optimistic, therefore, that a scientific approach to understanding injury in children is crucial to improving their care and their outcome.

This book is intended to be of value both to researchers and clinicians. It is not intended to be a textbook of paediatric trauma or to be of immediate use in a clinical situation. We hope that it will be read and reflected upon by those who conduct any kind of injury research; consultants and specialist trainees in paediatrics and paediatric surgery, anaesthesia and intensive care, accident and emergency, and trauma surgery; and any clincian who works with acutely injured children.

M. P. Ward Platt and R. A. Little

1

The epidemiology of trauma involving children

S. JARVIS and P. EDWARDS

Injury is disruption to the structure or function of the human organism resulting from exposure to excessive or deficient energy, regardless of intent (Baker *et al.*, 1992). Traumatic injury is associated with acute transfer of environmental energy to the body in quantities beyond the ordinary limits of homeostasis to the point where the integrity of the organism is breached. This energy may be mechanical, chemical, thermal, electrical or through pressure waves (trauma therefore excludes suffocation/drowning and poisoning injury).

There is no clear minimum energy transfer or degree of 'injury' to define where for instance a bruise, graze, sprain or scald might result. There are methods, however, to categorise the severity of traumatic injury which are intended to be related to this original energy transfer, but which are usually calibrated by their ability to predict case fatality (e.g. Injury Severity Score, ISS (Baker *et al.*, 1976), Revised Trauma Score (Champion *et al.*, 1989), Combination = TRISS). These injury severity scales are among a number developed for rapid field triage, for casemix standardisation in trauma care resource use/outcome studies, or as prognostic indications during intensive treatment (MacKenzie, 1984). More recently the ISS has been used to disaggregate incident cases in epidemiological studies (Walsh *et al.*, 1996).

An important element in the future development of such injury severity scales will be their recalibration by the ability to predict non-fatal outcomes such as short-term impairment or longer term functional incapacity (Chapter 14).

For practical purposes, the epidemiology of traumatic injury in childhood has to be based on the records of those children who have died of a trauma related cause, or who have been admitted to hospital for such a reason. These forms of case definition do not necessarily relate to particular severities of injury, but there are unfortunately no routine sources of data from which one might extract the epidemiology of non-fatal injuries at any objective level of severity.

Causes of trauma

The origins of traumatic injuries in childhood are principally unintentional 'accidents' or from therapeutic surgical operations. A relatively small number are the result of intentional injuries (Office of Population Censuses and Surveys, 1995).

The principal cause of fatal traumatic injury is road traffic accidents – mostly children suffering blunt trauma as pedestrians. For non-fatal traumatic unintentional injury in childhood the principal cause is 'falls', without further definition (Walsh *et al.*, 1996).

This picture varies with nationality. For instance in the USA (Fingerhut *et al.*, 1993) not only are injury mortality rates in childhood at least twice those in the UK but also some causes of traumatic injury are much more common. Among 1 to 14-year-olds in the USA, injury from firearms and stabbing cause up to 20% of trauma deaths (less than 1% in England and Wales); also a much lower proportion are described as unintentional (82% child trauma deaths in the USA compared with 98% in England and Wales).

Types of injury

At all ages in childhood it can be seen that the majority of fatal injuries are as a result of head injuries (Table 1.1), either with or without fractures and associated internal injuries (OPCS, 1995; various years). For children under 5 years old, non-traumatic categories of injury become particularly significant, e.g. poisoning, suffocation and inhalation of foreign bodies. Burns are the next commonest single cause of injury fatalities, again rather commoner in children under 5 years of age.

Injuries which are of sufficient severity to lead to admission to hospital are something like 100–200 times commoner than fatalities from the same causes (Table 1.2) (Department of Health, 1995). The cumulative rate of such admissions in childhood mean that about 1–2% of children are admitted to hospital with injuries each year.

Trends in injury mortality and morbidity

Over the last 30 years or so injury mortality rates have roughly halved. This fall has been steeper for some types of injuries than others (Figure 1.1), thus deaths from burns have shown a relatively shallow decline (Figure 1.1a), while those from fractures have shown steeper falls (Figure 1.1b). Mortality from intracranial trauma has had an intermediate trend (Figure 1.1c). When we come to look at changes in the rates of non-fatal injuries as judged by hospital admission rates there is little evidence that these have changed in line with mortality. On the contrary, over the last 30 years there has been a tendency for hospital admission rates for injuries to have increased, although there is little detail about the trends for individual types of injury (Jarvis *et al.*, 1995). This might suggest that changes in mortality over time are caused by improvements in survival rather than prevention of potentially fatal injury but there is actually little evidence to clarify this. Indeed it seems that the rate of hospital admissions for injury is itself a poor indication of non-fatal injury frequency (see section on injury severity below).

Injury rates by personal characteristics

For virtually all types of traumatic injury there is a considerable excess of boys over girls. This is at least partly due to differences in rates of exposure to hazards rather than necessarily attributable to more risky behaviour in hazardous situations. There are also very steep gradients in the rates of traumatic injury by social deprivation/social class (Roberts, 1997). These gradients are steeper than for any other cause of death in childhood and the explanation is again partly associated with differences in exposure to potential hazards for injury (e.g. road traffic) (Towner *et al.*, 1994). Once non-traumatic causes of death are excluded then it is clear that there is a rise in mortality rates from traumatic injury as children get older (Walsh & Jarvis, 1992). This increased rate of trauma with age is also reflected in hospital admission data when injury severity is taken into account (see later). Otherwise there are no characteristics by which we might reliably identify any substantial group of children at high risk of injury (Jarvis *et al.*, 1995).

Injury rates by severity of injury

There are no sources of routine data where fatal or non-fatal injuries are enumerated by severity. Studies of inpatient and Emergency Room attendance data in the North East of England (Walsh *et al.*, 1996) show that apparent changes in the frequency of non-fatal injuries as judged by admission rates over time can be misleading and are probably more related to changes in admission threshold for minor injuries. Similarly, there are important effects on this admission threshold from other factors, such as young age in children and poor social circumstances. These biases can disguise the fact that non-fatal injuries are actually commoner as children get older and can exaggerate the excess frequency of non-fatal injuries among children from socially deprived areas. Furthermore, a large fraction of these minor injuries which lead to 'discretionary' short-term admission for observations is made up of particular types of injury, namely minor head injuries and suspected poisonings.

When attention is confined to those children admitted to hospital with injuries of

Table 1.1. *Childhood mortality by diagnostic H list: England and Wales*

H47–H56	ICD9	Injury and poisoning	Rate per 100 000 (years 1988–92 aggregated)			
			Male		Female	
			0–4	5–14	0–4	5–14
H470	800–804	Fractures of skull and face	1.80	2.94	1.32	1.48
H471–6	805–829	Fractures: other	0.32	0.52	0.19	0.21
H48	830–848	Dislocations, sprains and strains	0.01	0.05	0.04	0.02
H49	850–869, 950–957	Intracranial and internal injuries including nerves	2.69	2.91	1.65	1.25
H50	870–904	Open wounds and injury to blood vessels	0.09	0.13	0.11	0.07
H51	930–939	Effects of foreign body entering through orifice	1.20	0.13	0.66	0.07
H52	940–949	Burns	0.70	0.24	0.60	0.15
H53	960–989	Poisonings and toxic effects	1.80	0.55	1.64	0.57
H54	996–999	Complications of medical and surgical care	0.06	0.02	0.05	0.03
H55	910–929,958,959, 990–995	Other injuries, early complications of trauma	2.69	1.46	1.49	0.32
H56	905–909	Late effects of injuries, poisonings, toxic effects and other external causes	0.08	0.05	0.01	0.02
		Total mortality rate	11.45	9.01	7.76	4.18
		Approximate number of deaths per annum	198	287	128	126

Table 1.2. *Childhood inpatient cases by diagnostic H list (1993–94): England*

H47–H56	ICD9	Injury and poisoning	Rate per 100 000 children (mid year 1993)			
			Male		Female	
			0–4	5–14	0–4	5–14
H470	800–804	Fractures of skull and face	76.0	73.3	60.3	31.7
H471–6	805–829	Fractures: other	256.7	625.3	188.6	355.2
H48	830–848	Dislocations, sprains and strains	8.1	30.6	7.1	19.5
H49	850–869, 950–957	Intracranial and internal injuries including nerves	346.7	322.5	283.6	157.0
H50	870–904	Open wounds and injury to blood vessels	214.4	146.6	153.8	80.2
H51	930–939	Effects of foreign body entering through orifice	121.5	38.6	119.5	31.7
H52	940–949	Burns	138.9	22.7	94.8	10.2
H53	960–989	Poisonings and toxic effects	385.4	62.3	319.7	145.3
H54	996–999	Complications of medical and surgical care	88.3	61.5	55.5	48.6
H55	910–929, 958, 959, 990–995	Other injuries, early complications of trauma	142.0	123.0	111.1	71.5
H56	905–909	Late effects of injuries, poisonings, toxic effects and other external causes	4.5	8.9	2.8	6.7
		Total admission rate	1782.5	1515.5	1396.7	957.8
		Total admissions: number of cases	29640	47672	22092	28532

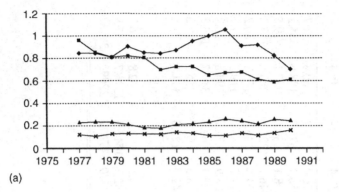

(a)

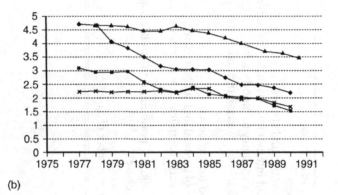

(b)

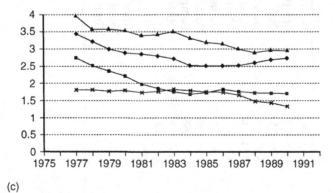

(c)

Figure 1.1. Trends in childhood mortality rates in England and Wales 1975–92. (a) Burns; (b) fractures; (c) intracranial and internal injuries including nerves. ♦: M0–4; ■: F0–4; ▲: M5–14; ×: F5–14. Rates per 100 000 per year.

ISS of 4 or greater the majority have fractures of long bones. Moreover, this form of trauma is under-represented by inpatient data, as some three-quarters of long bone fractures are actually managed on an outpatient basis and do not appear in inpatient records (Walsh *et al.*, 1996). Of these fractures with an ISS of 4 or greater, about three-quarters are of the upper limb. The remainder are divided between lower leg and skull fractures in the ratio 2:1.

Trauma during therapeutic operations

As well as those forms of trauma associated with injury, either intentional or unintentional, there is also a large number of children who are deliberately subject to trauma while under anaesthesia during therapeutic operations. In England, there are some 400 000 children operated on each year under the age of 15 years (Department of Health, 1995). Only about one in 20 of these operations, however, involves significant trauma, i.e. with a Surgical Stress Score of more than 5 (Anand & Aynsley-Green, 1988). Furthermore, half of these 22 000 more serious operations are made up of appendectomies and urethral repairs where there is considerable variation in the trauma inflicted. Table 1.3 details the distribution of the 10 000 or so more severe surgical operations undergone by children under 15 years of age in England each year. This represents a rate of about 1 per 1000 children per annum. It will be noted that something like one-quarter of these more serious operations are for congenital heart disease and a further 7% for congenital dislocation of the hip. It is unlikely that the overall rate of operations will change over time or show much variation by social class or other personal characteristics. The detailed pattern of operative trauma does vary, however, as some techniques become less invasive (patent ductus arteriosus (PDA) corrections) and others become feasible (switch operation for transposition) (Chapter 9).

Conclusions

The most common type of relatively severe trauma (ISS equal to or more than 4) suffered by children in the UK is long bone fracture (affecting about 2% of children each year). Of these, about one-quarter are admitted to hospital where they form a substantial fraction of the 1–2% of children admitted to hospital each year with injury. The principal cause of such injury is a 'fall', without further detail.

For injuries of greater severity, head injuries either with or without fracture, assume much greater significance and are the principal type of fatal injuries. Such injuries are most frequently the result of pedestrian road traffic accidents. The next commonest type of severe traumatic injury, primarily in young children, is burns and scalds.

Table 1.3. *Childhood major surgery cases by principal operation (1993–94): England*

Chapter (OPCS4)	3-digit OPCS4R	Rate per 100000 children	
		0–4	5–14
Nervous system	A01, A02, A10	4.3	2.8
Respiratory tract	E54, E55, E57, E59, E61	3.4	0.7
Upper digestive tract	G05, G07, G09–10, G23–24, G29, G31, G35–38, G48, G49, G51, G53, G57–58, G61, G63, G67, G69–72, G74, G76–78, G82	43.7	6.0
Lower digestive tract: appendix	H01–03	13.6	181.4
Lower digestive tract: other	H05–H13, H15, H17, H30–H34, H46–47	21.8	3.9
Other abdominal organs: principally digestive	J01, J03–J05, J18, J29, J31, J37, J57, J69–72	3.9	3.9
Heart	K01–14, K19–26, K28, K31–K34, K37, K40, K52–55	38.6	6.8
Arteries and veins	L02, L06–L12, L19, L21, L23–25, L33, L38, L46, L51, L77	26.3	2.2
Urinary: repair of urethra	M73	62.5	8.6
Urinary: other	M01–M08, M18–M21, M23–25, M35–41, M51–52, M55, M72, M75	31.7	11.3
Upper female genital tract	Q07, Q09, Q22–23, Q32, Q43–44, Q47	0.8	1.8
Soft tissue	T03, T15–16, T33–37, T39–41	6.8	2.8
Bones and joints of skull and spine	V01–03, V27–29, V31, V33–34	5.3	2.6
Miscellaneous operations	X22	13.2	4.1
Total rate		275.8	238.9
Total rate excluding appendix and urethra		199.8	48.9
Number excluding appendix and urethra		6859	3181

These sources of traumatic injury are commoner among boys, increase in frequency with age and the most serious trauma is much more frequent among the socially deprived.

Surgical operations associated with a relatively large amount of trauma occur with less than one-twentieth the frequency of fractures.

References

Anand, K. J. S. & Aynsley-Green, A. (1988). Measuring the severity of surgical stress in newborn infants. *Journal of Pediatric Surgery*, **23**, 297–305.

Baker, S., O'Neill, B., Gibsburn, M. & Guohua, L. (1992). *The Injury Fact Book*, 2nd edn. Oxford: Oxford University Press, pp. 344.

Baker, S., O'Neill, B. & Haddow, W. (1976). The Injury Severity Score: a method for describing patients with multiple injuries and evaluating emergency care. *Journal of Trauma*, **14**, 187.

Champion, S., Sacco, W. & Copes, W. (1989). A revision of the Trauma Score. *Journal of Trauma*, **29**, 623.

Department of Health (DoH). (1995). *Hospital Episode Statistics*, vol. 1, *Finished Consultant Episodes by Diagnosis, Operation and Speciality. England: Financial Year 1993–4.* London: HMSO.

Fingerhut, L. A., Annest, J. L., Baker, S. P., Kochanek, K. D. & McLoughlin, E. (1996). Injury mortality among children and teenagers in the United States, 1993. *Injury Prevention*, **2**, 93–4.

Jarvis, S., Towner, E. & Walsh, S. (1995). Accidents. In *The Health of Our Children*, ed. B. Botting, p. 95. *Decennial supplement.* London: HMSO.

MacKenzie, E. J. (1984). Injury Severity Scales: overview and directions for future research. *American Journal of Emergency Medicine*, **2**, 537–549.

Office of Population Censuses and Surveys (OPCS). (1995). *1993 Mortality statistics: cause. England and Wales (series DH2)*. London: HMSO.

Office of Population Censuses and Surveys (OPCS). *Mortality statistics: childhood. England and Wales (series DH6)*. London, HMSO – various years.

Roberts, I. (1997). Cause specific social class mortality differentials for child injury and poisoning in England and Wales. *Journal of Epidemiology and Community Health*, **51**, 334–335.

Towner, E., Jarvis, S., Walsh, S. & Aynsley-Green, A. (1994). Measuring exposure to injury risk in schoolchildren aged 11–14. *British Medical Journal*, **308**, 449.

Walsh, S. S. & Jarvis, S. N. (1992). Measuring the frequency of 'severe' accidental injury in childhood. *Journal of Epidemiology and Community Health*, **46**, 26–32.

Walsh, S., Jarvis, S., Towner, E., Aynsley-Green, A. (1996). Annual incidence of unintentional injury among 54 000 children. *Injury Prevention*, **2**, 16.

2
Emergency room requirements for children

B. M. PHILLIPS

Definition

In the USA and Canada the hospital department designated for receiving acutely ill or injured children is known as the Emergency Room: in the UK we are more familiar with the terminology 'Accident and Emergency department', although the term Emergency department alone is becoming more common. This chapter will look at the needs of children in the emergency department with particular reference to trauma.

Background: children in Emergency departments

Data identified by the Charity Action for Sick Children (Action for Sick Children, 1994) shows the following in the UK:

> One-third of all patients seen in Accident and Emergency departments are children.
>
> Approximately 3 million children per year attend Accident and Emergency and for many this is their first experience of hospital.
>
> Children are more likely to be admitted to hospital as an emergency than in a planned way.
>
> More than half the admissions of under 5 year olds into hospital are emergencies.

In the UK most emergency care is given to children in general Accident and Emergency departments which treat all age groups. There are nine specialist consultant-led paediatric Accident and Emergency departments in the UK and three in Eire. These departments are a teaching, training and research resource for the surrounding area and are recommended in the Joint Statement on Children's Attendances at Accident and Emergency produced in 1988 by the British Paediatric Association, the British

Association of Paediatric Surgeons and the Casualty Surgeons Assocation (now the British Association for Accident and Emergency Medicine) (British Paediatric Association, British Association of Paediatric Surgeons, Casualty Surgeons Association, 1988). An update of this document is in preparation.

In the rest of Europe, Accident and Emergency medicine has not yet widely developed as a specialty, but in the USA, Canada and to a lesser extent Australia, paediatric emergency medicine is a well-developed speciality. In large conurbations the 'Emergency Room' usually offers primary care at all levels to the children of that area.

Requirements for children in the Emergency departments

In looking at children's requirements we need to address two broad aspects. The first is the clinical problems with which children present and the second is the special needs of children (and their families) attending an Emergency department.

Clinical problems

Cardiopulmonary resuscitation

Overall, the outcome from cardiac arrest in childhood is significantly worse than that in adults (Orlowski, 1984). The difference in outcome is the result of a difference in the pathogenesis of cardiac arrest between children and adults. In children the arrest is rarely primarily of cardiac origin but usually secondary to pulmonary, circulatory or neurological dysfunction, all of which may obtain in the child suffering from major trauma. By the time the heart stops in a child suffering from a life-threatening injury, other organs have usually undergone such a severe period of anoxia or ischaemia that recovery is impossible. There is evidence that resuscitation skills are not always of the highest standard in our Health Services (Tunstall-Pedoe *et al.*, 1992) so training and audit is an urgent requirement in this area.

Major trauma

Trauma is the leading cause of death in children over the age of 1 year in the developed world. A number of studies both from the UK and from the USA have shown that a significant number of trauma deaths are preventable (Royal College of Surgeons of England, 1988; Sharples *et al.*, 1990) and this has led to the institution of improved training for doctors managing trauma both in adults and in children with the development of courses such as Advanced Trauma Life Support and Advanced Paediatric Life Support (UK).

The seriously ill child

Although trauma is the commonest presenting complaint of a child attending an Emergency department, there are a significant minority who have acute illness. In fact, there are more children who present with serious illness than do with major trauma. There are two significant themes underlying acute serious illness in childhood. The first is infection. Life-threatening diseases are often infection related, although these are decreasing through immunisation programmes. Recovery is potentially excellent given appropriate resuscitation and the correct choice of antibiotic drugs. A second and more complex theme underlying the seriously ill child in the Emergency department is that of congenital abnormalities. As we are improving our techniques of care, more and more children with complex congenital problems are surviving for longer periods and even into adult life. This means that children presenting to an Emergency department with either illness or trauma may have a significant underlying congenital problem such as cystic fibrosis, an inborn error of metabolism, congenital heart disease or neurological impairment. There is also an increasing number of survivors of neonatal intensive care. All of these children are likely to have a varying degree of decreased physiological reserve when acutely ill or injured.

There are a number of other categories of presenting problems in children in Emergency departments. These include the 'inappropriate attender', a discussion of which is not relevant for this text, children brought in dead, and children who may have been abused.

Special needs of children and families attending the Emergency department

Child attenders at an Emergency department cover a wide range of age and development; therefore, a wide range of differing facilities both for accommodation and treatment are required. Facilities for changing and feeding are needed for very young infants; pre-school children have need of a safe, stimulating play area. Older children require books or videos suitable for their age group and teenagers may need a much greater degree of privacy. Physical facilities including toilet facilities must be appropriate for wheelchair users.

It is often thought that because children are smaller than adults they need a smaller space in the Emergency department. A moment's consideration makes it clear that this is not the case. A child attending the Emergency department is accompanied by at least one adult and often other siblings with attendant push chairs and prams, leading to a greater requirement for space in waiting and consultation areas.

Within the general Emergency department there should be audiovisual separation of children and adults. It is sensible for all age groups to use a common reception area, but triage, consultation, waiting and treatment rooms should be designated for either adults or children. The exception is possibly the resuscitation rooms. As child resuscitations are much less common than adults and there may be a limited number of personnel with advanced life support skills available at any one time, it is generally considered acceptable to have a paediatric resuscitation bay in the general resuscitation room, ensuring the maximal use of experienced personnel. Dedicated equipment and facilities for children as detailed below will of course be needed in this area.

While managing a child in the Emergency department, with either significant or minor injury, parental involvement is of high priority. There are often difficulties in assessing a frightened child. The presence of a familiar carer such as a parent or grandparent will do much to both reassure the child and to facilitate examination and treatment. The parent or carer should stay with the child during triage, assessment, investigations (such as X-ray) and treatment. In some cases it is appropriate for the carer to be present in the resuscitation room, especially if the child is a frequent hospital attender. More usually the parent of the unconscious child will find refuge in the parent's room or 'quiet room' which should be a dedicated room set aside for the families of seriously ill or injured patients. It should be close to the major area of the Emergency department and should have an outside telephone.

As mentioned above, it can be very difficult to assess the degree of pain experienced by a child. Wherever possible pain prevention is a priority and this includes splinting injured limbs and keeping movement to a minimum. It is often the case that the severity of pain in a child, especially a very young one, is not recognised. This failing should be addressed with appropriate training of staff and protocols for pain relief in differing circumstances agreed.

Training of staff is at least as important as the physical facilities of the Emergency department for children. There should be a registered sick children's trained nurse on every shift in a general Accident and Emergency department and in a specialist paediatric Accident and Emergency department all nurses should have children's training. Again in a general Emergency department, other staff such as medical support staff, social workers, etc. will require children's training if this has not already been included in their general training requirements. A Play Specialist can be an extremely useful resource both to the children and to other staff members in creating an awareness of children's needs. As far as emergency life support training is concerned, medical staff should have undertaken an Advanced Life Support Course such as the APLS and nurses a course such as Paediatric Advanced Life Support (PALS) or the Advanced Paediatric Life Support Nursing Course (APLSNC). All of these courses give guidance on the recognition and immediate management of life-threatening illness and injury in infancy and childhood.

Physical requirements for an Emergency department

In this area I will especially highlight the requirements for the injured child.

Triage room

Triage is the key initial activity in an Emergency department. It is usually carried out by nursing staff and includes an assessment of the patient's illness or injury so that prioritisation of treatment can occur. Severity is triaged into three categories.

1. Emergency: immediate treatment.
2. Urgent: treatment within 5–15 minutes.
3. Non-urgent: treatment may wait.

Especially in the category 3 patient, re-assessment is necessary during the waiting period (which should be less than 2 hours) as the patients' conditions may change over this time. It is important that the triage room is situated within easy access and line of observation to the departmental entrances so that assessment of the patient is not delayed. The room should contain monitoring and measuring equipment so that in addition to the nurse's clinical observations a record of the patient's temperature, pulse, respiration, blood pressure, oxygen saturation, coma scale, etc. can be made and documented.

Resuscitation room

In a general Emergency department it is usual practice to have one resuscitation bay specifically for children. In a very large department a separate resuscitation room may be appropriate. In a paediatric Emergency department a single resuscitation room is usually sufficient, although there is a need in addition for two to three high dependency spaces which are conveniently placed together in one room. These should also be equipped to resuscitation standards in the event of more than one resuscitative effort occurring at the same time or in the event of a major incident. The recommended size of the resuscitation room is 30–35 sq. metres and 50 sq. metres for the three bay high dependency room. Both the resuscitation room and high dependency room must be fully equipped with piped air, oxygen and suction and with paediatric monitoring and resuscitation equipment.

One of the problems in the management of the acutely ill or injured child is the calculation of drug doses. There are a number of commercially available charts, e.g. the Oakley Chart (Oakley, 1988), which should be prominently displayed in the resuscitation room so that equipment and drugs may be appropriately selected for the child's age. An alternative method is the Broselow tape which is used to relate equipment size and drug dose to the child's length (Luten *et al.*, 1992). In addition, trauma scoring and coma scoring charts should be prominently displayed in the resuscitation areas.

There should be an X-ray gantry in the resuscitation and high dependency areas for radiographs for the seriously injured patient and the Emergency department should have easy access to the main Radiography, Ultrasonography and Computerised Tomography departments.

Tables 2.1 to 2.3 detail the equipment, drugs and monitors required for children in the Resuscitation room.

Reception, waiting and play areas

For the patients triaged at level 3, some waiting will be required. The patient's details are documented at the Reception area which should hold the computerised record system. Computerised records are of vital importance in the management of injured children as they can be used both for audit of quality and appropriateness of care and, also, after liaison with community groups and colleagues for the promotion of accident prevention activities.

Waiting and play areas

The waiting and play areas in the Emergency department should be informal. Ideally the department should have a Play Therapist to organise and supervise play. Play reduces anxiety in an unfamiliar situation as children express themselves through play. Cooperation of distressed children can be more easily secured if they are distracted by playing and if, when examined or undergoing procedures, the element of play is introduced. The Play Therapist can both organise material and train other departmental members in this approach to the injured child. A combined waiting and play area of 60–80 sq. metres should be sufficient for a department of 30 000 child attendances. In the waiting and play areas, the role of the Emergency department as a health care information source should not be forgotten. Information leaflets and videos of suitable health educational value can be helpful to supplement the role of the departmental staff in promoting health as well as treating illness and injury for minor and treatment areas. Less seriously injured patients will be examined and treated in the minor area. A 'surgery' type office with couch and chairs is suitable for the Emergency Doctor to examine and diagnose minor injury problems. The treatment area should be used to perform only minor treatments for children. These will include plastering of undisplaced fractures and suturing, gluing or steri-stripping of

Table 2.1. *Resuscitation room equipment*

Airway and spine control
Oropharyngeal airway sizes 000, 00, 0, 1, 2, 3
Endotracheal tube sizes 2.5–7.5 mm uncuffed
Laryngoscopes:
    a. straight paediatric blade
    b. curved paediatric blade
    c. curved adult blade
McGill's forceps: paediatric and adult size
Yankauer's sucker: paediatric and adult size
Soft suction catheters 2.5 to 16 French gauge
Needle cricothyrotomy set
Hard cervical collars: baby 'no neck' to adult size
Sand bags and tape
Paediatric and adult spinal boards

Breathing
Oxygen masks: infant to adult sizes with reservoir
Self-inflating bag with reservoir:
    a. 240 ml infant size
    b. 500 ml child size
    c. 1600 ml adult size
Face masks:
    a. infant – circular 01, 1, 2
    b. child – anatomical 2, 3
    c. adult – anatomical 4, 5
Catheter mounts and connectors
Ayre's T piece
Chest drains French gauge 8 to 24 with insertion set

Circulation
Intravenous access requirements:
    a. Intravenous cannulae 18 to 25 gauge
    b. Intraosseous infusion needles 16 to 18 gauge
    c. Graduated burette
    d. Intravenous giving sets
    e. Syringes 1 to 50 ml
    f. Intravenous drip monitoring device
    g. Cut down set
    h. ECG monitor and defibrillator with adult and paediatric paddles
    i. Non-invasive blood pressure monitor with infant and child size cuffs
    j. Pulse oximeter with infant and child size probes
    k. Capnometer with infant and child sized probes

ECG: electrocardiogram.

Table 2.2. *Fluids for the resuscitation room*

Sodium chloride 0.9%
Hartman's solution
Ringer's lactate
Dextrose 4% and 0.18% saline
Dextrose 5%, 10%, 20%
An artificial colloid, e.g. Haemaccel
Naturally occurring colloid, e.g. 4.5% human albumin
Mannitol 10%, 20%

superficial wounds. If children should require a general anaesthetic for manipulation or major wound repair, then this should be undertaken in a properly equipped theatre with an anaesthetist who has had suitable paediatric training. The management of children possibly abused is often carried out in a busy Emergency department. This is not always an appropriate place and an ideal situation is to have a specialised unit in close proximity to the Emergency department. Such a unit would have facilities for awaiting examination and treatment in addition to facilities for video recording of child interviews, with safe storage of the resulting videos under the supervision of the Child Protection Unit of the local police force.

Observation ward

There is an increasing trend to avoid hospital admission for children where at all possible. This is based on the perception that the best place for a child to be treated is within their own home and by an awareness of the risks of cross infection on wards. There is often, however, a need for a short period of observation following mild to moderate trauma and this can be appropriately carried out in an Emergency department observation bed. Suitable candidates for admissions to such an observation bed would include children who have had a moderate head injury or required manipulation of a fracture under an anaesthetic. Three to five beds would be a reasonable number to provide for a department with 30 000 child attendees; however, it must be remembered that if children are to stay in observations beds that facilities for accompanying parents must be arranged.

Table 2.3. *Drugs for the resuscitation room*

Drug	Presentation
Adenosine	3 mg/ml injection
Adrenaline	1:10 000 minijet
	1:1000 ampoules
Alprostadil	0.5 mg/ml ampoules
Aminophylline	25 mg/ml ampoules
Amiodarone	50 mg/ml ampoules
Amoxycillin	250 mg powder
Atropine	100 μg/ml minijet
Benzyl penicillin	600 mg ampoules
Bupivacaine	2.5 mg/ml ampoules
Calcium gluconate	10% ampoules
Calcium chloride	10% ampoules
Cefotaxime	500 mg, 1 g, 2 g ampoules
Ceftazidime	500 mg, 1 g, 2 g ampoules
Cefuroxime	250 mg, 750 mg, 1.5 g ampoules
Chlorpheniramine	25 mg/ml ampoules
Clonazepam	1 mg/ml ampoules
Desferrioxamine	500 mg ampoules
Dexamethasone	4 mg in 1 ml ampoules
Diazemuls	5 mg/ml ampoules
Diazepam	5 mg/ml ampoules
Digoxin	100 μg/ml ampoules
Dobutamine	250 mg ampoules
Dopamine	40 mg/ml ampoules
Flecainide	10 mg/ml ampoules
Flucloxacillin	250 to 500 mg ampoules
Flumazenil	100 μg/ml ampoules
Frusemide	10 mg/ml ampoules
Gentamicin	10 mg/ml ampoules
Hydrocortisone	100 mg ampoules
Ipratropium bromide	250 μg/ml nebuliser solution
Isoprenaline	20 μg/ml minijet
Labetalol	5 mg/ml ampoules
Lignocaine	20 mg/ml minijet
Morphine	2.5 mg/ml ampoules
Naloxone	20 μg/ml ampoules
Paraldehyde	rectal solution
Phenobarbitone	30 mg/ml ampoules
Phenytoin	50 mg/ml ampoules
Potassium chloride	15% solution
Prednisolone tablets	5 μg
Propranolol injection	1 mg/ml ampoules
Salbutamol nebules	2.5 mg in 2.5 ml, 5 mg in 5 ml
Sodium bicarbonate	8.4% minijet
Verapamil	2.5 mg/ml ampoules

Operational requirements

In the management of a child with major trauma a dedicated trauma team approach has been shown to improve outcome (Ramenofsky *et al.*, 1984). The trauma team should consist of the following:

General/Paediatric Surgeon
Anaesthetist
Emergency Physician
Emergency Room Nurses
Orthopaedic, Vascular, Cardiothoracic and Neurosurgical expertise is included as appropriate.

References

Action for Sick Children (1994).

Advanced Life Support Group (1993). Advanced paediatric life support – the practical approach. *British Medical Journal.*

British Paediatric Association (1988). British Association of Paediatric Surgeons, Casualty Surgeons Association. Joint statement on children's attendances at accidant and emergency departments. London: British Paediatric Association.

Luten, R. C., Wears, R. L., Broselow, J. *et al.* (1992). Length-based endotracheal tube and emergency equipment selection in pediatrics. *Annals of Emergency Medicine*, **2**, 900–4.

Oakley, P. A. (1988). Inaccuracy and delay in decision making in paediatric resuscitation and a proposed reference chart to reduce error. *British Medical Journal*, **297**, 817–19.

Orlowski, J. P. (1984). The effectiveness of pediatric cardiopulmonary resuscitation. *American Journal of Diseases of Childhood*, **138**, 1097.

Ramenofsky, M. L., Luterman, A., Quindlen, E. *et al.* (1984). Maximal survival in pediatric trauma; the ideal system. *Journal of Trauma*, **24**, 818–23.

Royal College of Surgeons of England (1988). Report of the working party on the management of patients with major injury. London: Royal College of Surgeons of England.

Sharples, P. M. *et al.* (1990). Avoidable factors contributing to death in children with head injury. *British Medical Journal*, **300**, 87–91,

Tunstall-Pedoe, H., Bailey, L., Chamberlain, D. A., *et al.* (1992). Survey of 3765 cardiopulmonary resuscitations in British hospitals (the BRESUS study): methods and overall results. *British Medical Journal*, **304**, 1347–51.

3

Child deaths in Accident and Emergency

B. WRIGHT

Introduction

Beginning to deal with the death of a child, particularly after the body has been traumatised, can be overwhelming both for parents and carers. In recent years, more has been written about this catastrophic experience from the parents', siblings' and family's viewpoint. Much less is written about the trauma team's experience. Ahmedzai (1982) highlighted how doctors in training are unsupported and 'out on a limb', and how they are neglected by consultants when caring for dying patients.

This chapter will review work on caring for everyone involved in the death of a child, particularly when this is sudden and traumatic.

You may ask why we need actively to intervene at all. For thousands of years the human race has dealt with death. Bereavement is listed in the Holmes and Rahe Social Readjustment Rating Scale (1967) as the most stressful life event. The significance of the loss of a child produces the strongest pain (Sanders, 1980) and the most widespread reactions. Raphael (1985: 229) focused on the reason for this:

> a child is many things: a part of the self, and of the loved partner; a representation of the generations past; the genes of the forebears; the hope of the future; a source of love, pleasure, even narcissistic delight; a tie or a burden; and sometimes a symbol of the worst parts of self and others.

As children grow they become persons in their own right, evoking both positive and negative feelings as they interact with individuals and the family and society. These ambivalent feelings are carried into the grief, introducing major problems into this complex process. The death does not fit in with the natural order of things. Rando (1985) demonstrated that parents feel it is unnatural that the child pre-deceases them. The role of providing for, guiding and doing things for the child is central to a parent's identity. A bereaved parent has feelings of helplessness, failure and guilt.

The death of a child will have major consequences for the health and well-being of the bereaved. Parkes (1975) identified the determinants of an unfavourable outcome.

Sudden death, death following a short illness and death preceded by little warning all have serious implications for the recovery process. Sanders (1983) showed that where the death is sudden, signs of intense bereavement reactions and physical ill health were more evident and difficult to disengage from. The value of reassuring and reaffirming by health workers, from the moment of impact through ongoing support, was seen as an important contribution to healing the grief (Rogers & Reich, 1988).

The role of anticipatory grief, in helping people to cope with the grief process, has been challenged, and there is a suggestion that it has been conceptually confused with forewarning of loss. Fulton & Gottesman (1980) comment that forewarning of loss says nothing about whether anticipatory grief will follow. They conclude that it is not simply the presence of anticipatory grief, or the length of time involved, that determines its usefulness; it is rather the manner in which it is experienced and responded to by those concerned. Therefore, even if we have a short time to prepare parents for the death, they may not be able to accept or assimilate the information. It is not unusual for parents, despite some preparation for 'bad news', to protest and say 'You never said he would die'.

On the child's arrival in the Accident and Emergency department

Major difficulties arise in caring for the distressed parents. Some parents/relatives will have been present when the accident occurred and, at the scene or in the ambulance, will have witnessed their child being actively resuscitated. It may be difficult to separate them from the child as the child enters the resuscitation area.

Parental distress is increased by separation from their child (Renner, 1991). The main issue for them, particularly if the child dies, is that they failed the child by not being there at his or her death. Many doctors believe there is no reason why relatives should not watch resuscitation (Whitlock *et al.*, 1994). It should be noted that the medical staff able to cope with this are usually senior, well-experienced doctors. Others suggest that it produces too much anxiety for junior doctors, and that often an invasive procedure is involved which would cause unreasonable distress for the relatives (Schilling, 1994).

A study from the Foote hospital surveyed 47 family members present during a resuscitation (Hanson & Strawser, 1992). Of those surveyed, 76% felt their adjustment to the death was made easier by their presence in the room. Thirty respondents (64%) felt that their presence was beneficial to the dying person. Many were sure the dying person had heard them express their love and goodbyes.

This is important as far as healing the grief is concerned (Parkes, 1975). Another study (Doyle *et al.*, 1987) concluded that there appears to be no reason for continuing policies which exclude family members. This paper talks about it being an option, which highlights giving relatives a choice.

A relatives' room

A study of 100 suddenly bereaved relatives (Wright, 1991) demonstrated how much relatives valued the privacy of a room where they could wait and meet with other relatives. The availability of essential facilities such as a telephone, refreshments and toilets nearby, and the room being well-decorated and furnished, were important.

The aim is to engender privacy without creating a sense of isolation. Many respondents described themselves as being 'frightened' if left alone too long. While department design may be outside the remit of most of us, it would help if relatives viewing the deceased did not have to walk through public areas.

Waiting for long periods, and not being given periodical access to the child, should be avoided as both will have a detrimenal effect on the grieving process if the child dies (Raphael, 1986). This work emphasises the importance of the immediate care on the long-term grief process.

Breaking bad news

A study of the parents of critically ill children admitted to hospital was able, later, to clarify their needs at the time (Farrell & Frost, 1992). Although the information they received was distressing and traumatic, there was an overwhelming need to know that it was correct and honest. Frequently, the person communicating the bad news feels they have done it badly. Communication is a dynamic, complex, continuous series of reciprocal events, through which messages are exchanged. It is difficult for the message to be perceived and assimilated, and powerful feelings interfere with the process. To complicate matters even further, the encounter is often between strangers. We all fear the unknown, and anything can happen. While some responses are expected, a wide range of human feelings can emerge. In a study of responses that incapacitate the worker (Wright, 1991), it was found that some responses, such as withdrawal, denial and anger, disempowered the bearer of the message. Strong feelings of ineffectiveness and being at a loss as to which direction to follow were experienced.

A training package for junior doctors (British Medical Association 1992) showed how the doctor breaking the bad news can feel he or she made a complete mess of it. The package goes on to stress that training, mentorship and support are essential.

Initially, the recipient of the news may experience shock, disbelief and an inability to accept the loss. These characteristics are all part of the normal grieving process. At the time the bad news is given, all these feelings may be experienced at once. Lindemann (1944), a major theorist on acute grief, described how this was compounded by waves of somatic distress lasting 20–60 minutes. These are experienced as decreased muscular power, a feeling of emptiness in the stomach, tightness of the throat, choking, shortness of breath, sighing, perspiring, flushed face and finally exhaustion or fainting.

It is easy for the bearer of the bad news to feel that by saying what they did, they have inflicted intense pain on the recipient. The news of the death should be given by a doctor and nurse or nurses. In a large group of people with diverse needs, one or two members of staff could be overwhelmed by the disorder and distress. While a nurse who has cared for the relatives just prior to the death is capable of giving the bad news, relatives value talking to the doctor involved in the care. In a study (Wright, 1993) in which relatives discussed their needs at the time the bad news was given, they frequently stated that if the doctor present did not see them 'he may have had something to hide'.

Some of the immediate anger I have witnessed has been when a doctor has taken a long time, often giving a lot of detailed information, before getting round to breaking the news. More detailed clinical information can be given after the news of the child's death. Euphemisms are to be avoided – words such as 'dead' or 'died' are unequivocal.

If siblings or other children are present, it is best that they are informed of the death by a parent or close relative. If they are too distressed or ill to do so, Accident and Emergency staff must be prepared to take on the role.

Children cope well with honest, short, clear explanations (Grollman, 1992). Severe distress witnessed in surviving adults is less disturbing than isolating the child or withholding information. Children must be allowed to scream or cry, be silent or protest, and not to have these feelings explained away (Couldrick, 1988). They are often told they must be brave and that now they have to look after mummy and daddy. This is inappropriate and can be damaging, as it imposes upon them an interolable burden (McGuinness 1988). Because of their own grief, parents are often at a loss as to how to cope with other siblings, and they value some guidance on how to care for them. Some children, for example, may be very active, or they may want to be alone or may appear to respond inappropriately. Parents should be advised that this is not unusual and does not mean the child does not care.

The report on good practice from the British Association of Accident and Emergency Medicine and the Royal College of Nurses Joint Working Party also advises that a suddenly bereaved child may (with the parents' consent) need some extra support. It suggests that the general practitioner, health visitor and school nurse are informed of the death.

Many schools regret a lack of information which prevents more care being given in school. The special needs of grieving children are emphasised by Raphael (1985) whose studies demonstrate how childhood grief, if not dealt with well, will cause serious emotional distress in later adult life, particularly when facing another life crisis.

Viewing the body

This area of care produces the greatest regrets in bereaved parents. Usually they regret they did not see their child's body. Not only is this a clear focus for regret, it will also have a strong influence on the grieving process. Intervention by Accident and Emergency staff will have a significant impact on the parents' grief response (Parrish *et al.*, 1987). Most parents who viewed their dead child's body in this study agreed that, though painful, viewing did create a strong sense of the reality of the death. The decision to view did not appear to have any relation to cause of death (medical as against traumatic). It is presumed that reducing the number of people with regrets would have a positive influence on staff intervention (Holland & Rogich, 1980). Staff should avoid referring to the deceased in terms of 'the body' or 'it', because this is upsetting and is later viewed as insensitive (Dubin & Sarnoff, 1986).

While it may be easier to avoid the issue, staff should deal proactively with the question of whether children present should view the dead child's body. If asked by the family whether a child should do so, a neutral position should be taken, and a discussion on the merits of doing so should take place. It is an area where the family could be in conflict, often holding opposite views.

Wright (1991) demonstrated how the family will value the help of the objective, uninvolved outsider (i.e. hospital staff) at this time, in helping them arrive at a decision.

If the child's body is damaged the bereaved should be informed, but this should not prevent them spending time with the deceased (Cassem, 1978). Staff should clean and make the child's body as presentable as possible.

A study of 81 parents whose child had died suddenly reported that nearly all of them wished to spend time with the dead child, even when the body was mutilated (Finlay & Dallimore, 1991). Of the 81, 49 felt they had not been given enough time with the child, particularly when the death had been caused by a road traffic accident. Subsequently, two of the parents in this study remained angry that they had been actively dissuaded from seeing their child's body. Several expressed regret that they were not allowed to hold, wash, or touch the child after death.

This study also indicated that 68% of these parents had not been approached about organ donation. Of this group, 59% wished they had been approached, which suggests that the option of organ donation may help rather than hinder the parents' grief process.

Most of these studies stress the importance of the parents knowing they can return and spend time with the dead child. Many have other family members or friends with whom they wish to return to the child.

Written information given on leaving about who to contact for further information is valued. Further information about ongoing help and support is also important. Lack of more formal support from community services has been criticised (Rostron, 1981).

Lundin (1984) reported an increased psychiatric morbidity in a sample of relatives after sudden unexpected deaths. All the indications are that most parents will benefit from some ongoing counselling, and from access to the health care staff involved at the time of their child's death.

Care and support for staff involved

It is important that we consider how the team encountering the sudden death of a child will begin to cope themselves with the distress it may have caused. Listening to a colleague's story of the details of the incident may sound a simple response; its value should not be underestimated. It is a well-used and caring response. Self-disclosure is involved here, and the teller will need to trust the listener because glimpses of 'the person' behind the teller's role will be revealed (Wright, 1992). How the story is told and heard, and how the story teller hears his or her own story, is examined in other work on coping with stressful incidents (McKechnie, 1993). The process helps to clarify and identify difficulties, and often alters the teller's perception of the event. Defusing or demobilising the critical incident for the staff is now more clearly defined (Wright, 1993).

Defusion

Defusion may best be described as a short type of crisis intervention. Its aim is to make a critical incident less harmful, a critical incident being any situation faced by the Accident and Emergency team that causes them to feel strong emotional reactions. These feelings could potentially interfere with their ability to function at the time or later.

Defusing helps to restore control and provides immediate support and assistance. It should reduce tension, focus on strengths and skills and help staff to regain emotional control. This focus on skills helps to ensure a return to normal functioning and to start the recovery process. A return to cognitive functioning enables the person to think rather than to react.

The facilitator maintains a low profile and mostly provides the right conditions for the defusing to occur. This will usually be to send all (if possible), or as many people as possible who were involved in the incident, for a tea or coffee break. They will then, naturally and spontaneously, go over the details of the event. They take charge of the level of emotional ventilation and take it where they went to, then return to normal functioning.

Most nurses will recognise how the report or handover of a shift is used to defuse. Although the whole shift is to be reported on, or a group of patients in a certain order, any critical incident will receive immediate attention. Details of other events, or other information, will not be shared until the whole story has been told.

Any attempts made to curtail disclosure of a critical incident will cause it to emerge later. Time and attention given to those involved will, on the other hand, allow the incident to be laid to rest or ended more appropriately.

Demobilisation

Demobilisation provides the staff with a structure to end a span of duty. While most people will end a shift together, remember that some, because of the workload, will leave at a different time. Their needs should not be ignored.

Large-scale incidents benefit most from this approach. A room will be needed to hold large numbers of staff. Ideally the group should be multidisciplinary. These people should be expected to remain no more than 15 minutes, and this time should be part of their working span of duty.

The team leader should have up to date, accurate information about the whole event from its beginning to the present time. There is no room for rumours or guesswork. Everyone should be ordered to attend the demobilisation; it is not just for the vulnerable or sensitive or those who think they need it. It is for the whole team and it should be made clear that it is an issue for the whole team. It is designated to facilitate an end to a stressful working period.

The aims of the demobilisation are:

1. To regain emotional control and cognitive functioning, and to reduce tension.
2. To focus on strengths and skills, to re-evaluate the incident and receive some factual information.
3. To begin the recovery process and leave behind some of the stress.
4. To begin to be educated by the incident.

The process of demobilisation is begun by saying, for example:

> At 1340 hours today a school bus collided with a truck on the M1, resulting in six seriously injured children...

All available information is then given as to services concerned, types of casualties and personnel involved. Different members of staff will have worked in different aspects of the incident but not have been in the whole. For this reason, information about the whole event will be useful.

For staff, this complete picture reduces the possibility of unanswered questions before they leave the hospital. The difference between a demobilisation and a defusing is that although they have similar aims the demobilisation is clearly time-limited and focused. On this occasion, staff are told that anyone may seek and will be given further help if they have further difficulties about the event.

At the end of the demobilisation the opportunity should be used to thank everyone for their valuable contribution to a difficult and demanding event. They are then given permission to leave, hopefully with reliable information about the event and a better overall perception of the incident.

The focus of demobilisation is primarily on cognitive functioning rather than on emotional ventilation. If demobilisation is a positive event, staff are more likely to return for debriefing if they think this is necessary. Assuring them that this was an abnormal event will be more likely to help them seek further support if needed.

Some Accident and Emergency departments have set up critical incident stress debriefing teams, which include all the emergency services involved. They feel that this explores the incident more thoroughly. In my experience, this approach is more difficult to expedite and may prevent a team demobilisation occurring at all.

Critical incident stress debriefing (CISD)

This is a more formal type of debriefing and should ideally be carried out by someone with a knowledge of counselling skills. Formal debriefings occur 24–48 hours after the event and should be a short, well-focused type of intervention. I prefer to use the three 1-hour session format and for all three sessions to be completed within 10 days.

Session 1

After introductions, rules about confidentiality should be explained. This confirms that no information about the debriefing will be disclosed to anyone. The client is then asked to give a factual account of the whole incident and his part in it. This first session involves mostly factual information, but asks the client for a detailed account.

Session 2

Return to the incident and begin the story again, but ask about some of the sounds, smells, visual images and things he felt. Ask questions about feelings:

> How did you feel when it was happening?
> How has it left you feeling?
> Have you ever felt like this before?

These questions are intended to help the client to get nearer some of the distress of the incident. This often includes feelings of frustration, helplessness, fear, guilt, anger and ambivalence at being involved. There may be a major focus on what appears to be a trivial aspect of the incident. The client will often apologise for this.

This whole session should allow some of the more disturbing aspects of the incident to be explored.

Session 3

This final session is used to teach something about stress, the emphasis being on the normal and the natural. Common physical symptoms will be identified and these symptoms connected to an abnormal experience. The last session is often called the re-entry phase because it is working towards normal function and 'closing-off' the incident. Any outstanding issues are dealt with and loose ends tied up.

A plan of action may be discussed, i.e. what the client would do differently next time in a similar incident. Questions highlighting the educational aspects of the event are useful in this final session:

> What have you learnt about yourself?
> How will this influence your work in future incidents?

This type of approach to debriefing a critical incident will be short term if the only problem presented concerns the incident. If the event returns the client to a previous life crisis, a much longer period of counselling will be required as CISD is aimed solely at reducing stress reactions and returning quickly to normal functioning. Some would question its effectiveness in group settings (Kleber & Brom, 1992), as people are often reluctant to participate in intervention programmes. My experience is that CISD is more likely to be accepted if offered on an individual basis, and for those whom defusing and demobilisation did not offer enough to enable them to disengage from the incident.

Work on Post-Traumatic Stress Disorder suggests that critical care staff are capable of suffering from it (Chandler, 1993). This paper emphasises that we need to create healing enrivonments for ourselves as well as for the patients and their families.

Departmental policies which address these issues make a clear statement that it is the department's philosophy to care for its staff, and that it acknowledges the difficulty of the work. This philosophy should apply to any department dealing with the death of a child.

Increasingly, time and thought are being given to the education of medical staff in this area of work. The literature suggests that while a formally structured teaching centred approach is useful, other methods should be incorporated (Knowles, 1990). The need to emphasise interpersonal skills, self-awareness and reflection is also demonstrated.

The literature reviewed highlights that despite our feelings of helplessness, that we have done little to help bereaved parents, much is achieved at the time of the impact of death. This care will be valued if we respond appropriately, with knowledge and sensitivity. This care will also influence the ongoing healing process.

References

Ahmedjai, S. (1982). Dying in hospital: the resident's viewpoint. *British Medical Journal*, **285**, 712–14.

British Medical Association (1992). *A Stressful Shift*. London, BMA Board of Science & Education.

Cassem, N. H. (1978). Treating the person confronting death. In *The Harvard Guide to Modern Psychiatry*, Nicholi, A. M. (ed.). Massachusetts: Bellknap Press of Harvard University Press.

Chandler, E. (1993). Can post-traumatic stress disorder be prevented? *Journal of Accident & Emergency Nursing*, **1**, 87–91.

Couldrick (1988). *Grief and Bereavement: Understanding Children*. London: Sobell.

Couldrick, A. (1994). What do we tell the children? *Professional Nurse*, **9**, 506.

Doyle, C., Post, H., Burney, R. E., Maino, J., Keefe, M. & Rhee, K. J. (1987). Family participation during resuscitation: an option. *Annals of Emergency Medicine*, **16**, 673–5.

Dubin, W. R. & Sarnoff, J. R. (1986). Sudden and unexpected death: interventions with the survivors. *Annals of Emergency Medicine*, **15**, 54–7.

Farrell, M. F. & Frost, C. (1992). The most important needs of parents of critically ill children: parents' perception. *Journal of Intensive Care & Critical Care Nursing*, **8**, 130–9.

Finlay, I. & Dallimore, D. (1991). Your child is dead. *British Medical Journal*, **302**, 1524–5.

Fulton, R. & Gottesman, D. J. (1980). Anticipatory grief: a psychosocial concept reconsidered. *British Journal of Psychiatry*, **137**, 45–54.

Grollman, E. A. (1992). *Talking About Death*. Boston: Beacon.

Hanson, C. & Strawser, D. (1992). Family presence during cardio-pulmonary resuscitation. *Journal of Emergency Nursing*, **18**, 104–6.

Holland, J. & Rogich, S. (1980). Dealing with death in the emergency room. *Health and Social Work*, **5**.

Holmes, T. H. & Rahe, R. H. (1967). The Social Readjustment Rating Scale. *Journal of Psychosomatic Research*, **11**, 213–18.

Kleber, R. J. & Brom, D. (1992). *Coping with Trauma*. Amsterdam: Swetz & Zetlinger.

Knowles, M. I. (1990). *The Adult Learner: a Neglected Species*, 3rd edn. Texas: Gulf.

Lindemann, E. (1944). Symptomatology and management of acute grief. *American Journal of Psychiatry*, **101**, 141–8.

Lundin, T. (1984). Morbidity following sudden and unexpected bereavement. *British Journal of Psychiatry*, **144**, 84–8.

McGuinness, S. (1988). Sudden death in the emergency department. In *Management and Practice in Emergency Nursing*, B. Wright (ed.) London: Chapman and Hall.

McKechnie, R. (1993). Earwitness to disaster. *Journal of Accident & Emergency Nursing*, **3**, 149–53.

Parkes, C. M. (1975). Determinants of outcome following bereavement. *Omega (Journal of Death & Dying)*, **6**, 303–23.

Parrish, G. A., Holden, K. S. & Skiendzielewski, J. J. (1987). Emergency department experience with sudden death: a survey of survivors. *Annals of Emergency Medicine*, **16**, 792–6.

Rando, T. A. (1985). Bereaved parents: particular difficulties, unique factors and treament issues. *Social Work*, **30**, 19–23.

Raphael, B. (1985). *The Anatomy of Bereavement: a Handbook for the Caring Professions*. London: Hutchinson.

Raphael, B. (1986). *When Disaster Strikes*. London: Hutchinson.

Renner, S. (1991). I desperately needed to see my son. *British Medical Journal*, **30**, 56.

Rogers, M. P. and Reich, P. (1988). On the health consequences of bereavement. *New England Journal of Medicine*, **319**, 510–11.

Rostron, J. (1981). The needs of the family following a fatal road traffic accident. *Public Health*. **95**, 353–5.

Sanders, C. M. (1980). A comparison of adult bereavement in the death of a spouse, child and parent. *Omega* (*Journal of Death and Dying*), **10**, 303–22.

Sanders, C. M. (1983). Effects of sudden versus chronic illness death on bereavement outcome. *Omega* (*Journal of Death & Dying*), **13**, 227–41.

Schilling, R. J. (1994). Should relatives watch resuscitation? *British Medical Journal*, **309**, 406.

Whitlock, M., Baskett, P. J. F. & Bloomfield, P. (1994). Should relatives be allowed to watch resuscitation? *British Medical Journal*, **308**, 1687–92.

Wright, B. (1991). *Sudden Death: Intervention Skills for the Caring Professions*. Edinburgh: Churchill Livingstone.

Wright, B. (1992). *Skills for Caring: Loss and Grief*, p. 10. Edinburgh: Churchill Livingstone.

Wright, B. (1993). *Caring in Crisis*, 2nd edn. Edinburgh: Churchill Livingstone.

4

Immediate life support

G. S. SAMRA and R. M. BINGHAM

Introduction

Trauma has surpassed infectious disease as the leading cause of childhood death and disability in the developed world (Rivara, 1982). In the UK, three children die each day and 10 000 are permanently disabled as a result of trauma each year. Between the age of 5 and 14 years injury causes seven times as many deaths as leucaemia in this country (Teanby et al., 1994).

An analysis of paediatric trauma deaths over 3 years in Canada identified three major categories of preventable trauma deaths: respiratory failure, intracranial haemorrhage and inadequately treated haemorrhage. Respiratory failure was the major cause of pre-hospital deaths resulting in 19 of 42 (45%) pre-hospital deaths, with haemorrhage resulting in a further 17 of 42 (40%). In contrast, 17 of 33 (51%) of inhospital deaths resulted from potentially survivable central nervous system injury where intervention was delayed owing to failure to recognise clinical deterioration. Abdominal haemorrhage from liver or splenic injury was the cause of 15 of 33 (45%) inhospital deaths. In total, haemorrhage (predominately abdominal) accounted for 43% of all preventable deaths (Dykes et al., 1989).

The unique anatomical and physiological differences between small children and adults may lead to errors in management. The immediate care of the paediatric patient must therefore take account of these differences. Although the types of injury may vary, they often lead to common pathophysiological changes that may become life-threatening if untreated. Rational management of multitrauma patients must therefore include immediate restoration and maintenance of physiological functions to maintain tissue integrity and prevent further damage as well as the surgical treatment of traumatised tissues.

One of the fundamental principles in the immediate resuscitation of the injured child is the maintenance of oxygen delivery to the tissues especially the vital organs while definite therapy is instituted. In addition to this the resuscitation should be performed without causing further injury or exacerbating existing injuries.

Oxygen delivery is dependent on a physiological chain, which starts with the oxygen molecule in the inspired gas and ends with the uptake and utilisation of oxygen by the various cells of the body. Between these two points the movement of the oxygen molecule is dependent on its passage through the airway, the lungs, uptake by the haemoglobin molecule and movement through the circulatory system by the heart and finally on the unloading from the haemoglobin moiety to the tissues. This whole process depends on the movement of oxygen down a concentration gradient and is facilitated by high inspired concentrations of oxygen which should consequently be administered as early as possible.

Physical differences

Clearly size is one of the fundamental differences between the child and adult. There are however considerable variations, both within the paediatric age group and depending on whether body weight, height or body surface area (BSA) are used as the basis for size comparison. A newborn infant weighing 3 kg is 1/3.3 the size of an adult in length but 1/9 adult size in body surface area and 1/21 adult size in weight (Harris, 1957). Of these body measurements, BSA is probably the most important because it most closely parallels variations in basal metabolic rate and for this reason a better criterion than age or weight for judging fluid and nutritional requirements. Although BSA can be calculated from the height and weight using the Du Bois formula or from tables (Table 4.1), this is cumbersome for routine clinical use and most drug dosages and fluid requirements are based on body weight.

$$\text{BSA (m}^2) = 0.007184 \times \text{Height}^{0.725} \times \text{Weight}^{0.425}$$
(DuBois D & DuBois, 1916)

The process is further compounded during resuscitation because weight has to be estimated, which is notoriously unreliable, particularly for health care providers dealing with children on an infrequent basis. Recently a means of estimating a child's weight based on measurement of length has been developed (Schuman, 1991). This allows reasonably accurate estimates of weight on which to base resuscitative efforts.

Less obvious than the difference in overall size is the difference in relative size of body structures in infants and children. This is particularly true of the head which is relatively large at birth, larger for example than the chest circumference. Also at term, infants have a short neck and the chin meets the chest at approximately the level of the second rib. This anatomy has clear implications in the maintenance of the airway.

Table 4.1. *Age and body surface area*

Age (years)	Height (cm)	Weight (kg)	BSA (m^2)
Newborn	50	3	0.2
1	75	10	0.47
2	87	12	0.57
3	96	14	0.63
5	109	18	0.74
10	138	32	1.10
13	157	46	1.42
16 (female)	163	50	1.59
16 (male)	173	62	1.74

Based on a standard growth chart and DuBois formula (DuBois & DuBois, 1916).
BSA: body surface area.

The paediatric airway

Failure to adequately open and maintain the airway has been identified as major causes of preventable early trauma deaths (Dykes *et al.*, 1989). There are a number of anatomical differences between the paediatric and adult airway and a knowledge of these differences is vital in the correct management of injured children.

Compared with the adult, the child up to the age of about 3 years has a relatively large occiput. This causes the head to roll to the side and this may need to be controlled by using a head ring or sand bags. Additionally, the prominent occiput raises the head relative to the patients body in the supine position and thereby eliminates the need for material under the head to achieve the classical 'sniffing the morning air' position which aligns the axes of the trachea, posterior pharynx and oral cavity for optimal airway patency and visualisation. In some infants it may even be advantageous to correct for a large occiput by placing a small roll under the shoulders; however it must be remembered that excessive extension of the neck causes anterior displacement of the larynx and may be counterproductive.

In the newborn and young infant, the larynx is relatively high in the neck, situated opposite C3–4 vertebrae in the neonate. It descends during the first 3 years of life and again at puberty to its final position opposite C6 (Westhorpe, 1987). This high position forces the tongue to lie almost entirely within the oral cavity. It therefore tends to lie against the soft palate and may easily obstruct the oral airway and also make laryngoscopy more difficult. This is compounded because the epiglottis in the infant is relatively larger and more U-shaped. It is also floppy and angled in a more posterior direction (about 45°) tending to lie across the view of the glottis. In view of these differences tracheal intubation is usually easier if a straight blade laryngoscope is used to lift the epiglottis out of the way rather than a curved laryngoscope blade positioned in the vallecula. The angle of the vocal cords is also altered in the child, the anterior attachment being more caudally located. This predisposes the endotracheal tube tip to become caught in the anterior commissure especially during nasal intubation.

With the exception of the anterior nasal passages, the larynx is the narrowest part of the upper airway. It is shaped like an inverted cone with its apex at the cricoid cartilage which forms a complete ring, protecting the upper airway from compression. The cricoid ring is vulnerable to narrowing as mucosal oedema can only expand inwards diminishing the lumen. The mucosa covering the cricoid ring is the frequent site of trauma and oedema from a number of causes, but particularly from intubation with an oversized endotracheal tube (Koka *et al.*, 1977). As the cricoid ring is narrower than the glottic opening a tube passing through the glottis may compress the mucosa and cause ischaemia (Eckenhoff, 1951). This is particularly important because the average diameter of the trachea in the newborn infant is 6 mm in comparison to 14 mm in the adult. As resistance to gas flow through a tube is inversely related to the fourth power of the radius any oedema from inflammation or trauma may cause significant airway obstruction.

The cricoid ring is circular in cross-section, so a plain uncuffed tracheal tube will allow an adequate seal at this level allowing positive pressure ventilation and affording protection against aspiration of gastric contents. Not only is a cuffed tracheal tube potentially damaging, it is also unnecessary.

The length of the trachea correlates better with weight than with age, but shows large variations in babies under 6 kg, ranging from 3.2 to 7 cm. Endobronchial intubation is consequently a significant risk. The correct diameter and length of tracheal tube must be used and a small leak should be present on inflation of the lungs with a pressure of 25–30 cm H_2O.

Cervical spine

Spinal injuries are rare in children and cervical spine injury is less common in paediatric than adult trauma (Kewalraamani *et al.*, 1980). The disability that may result from a missed cervical spine injury is catastrophic, so airway management must include adequate management of the cervical spine.

The child's spine is much more elastic and mobile than the adult and the softer vertebrae are less likely to fracture with minor stress. The child's head is proportionally large in relation to the body and major inertial movements such as rapid deceleration may result in greater forces so cervical spine injury should always be suspected following head trauma. The spinal cord damage is usually the result of subluxation, most often at the atlanto–occipital or atlanto–axial joint in infants and toddlers or the lower cervical spine in school age children (Hill *et al.*, 1984).

Increased elasticity and mobility of the paediatric spine also more readily permits functional injury without associated bony vertebral injury. This is known as spinal cord injury without radiographic abnormality (SCIWORA) (Pang & Wilberger, 1982). SCIWORA is now recognised as an important cause of paediatric spinal cord injury (Pang & Pollack, 1989) and accounts for a number of pre-hospital deaths that were previously attributed to head trauma (Bohn, *et al.*, 1990).

By definition this type of spinal cord injury cannot be excluded by the standard radiographic techniques and cervical cord injury must be assumed in all children with multiple injuries and care must be taken during all airway management procedures to avoid exacerbating any injury.

Cardiorespiratory physiology

As blood pressure, heart rate and respiratory rates can be measured non-invasively, data is available on large populations of normal children. There are significant changes in these physiological parameters with age which are illustrated in Table 4.2.

Respiratory system

At full-term birth, the lungs are still maturing and the formation of adult type alveoli is just beginning. It may take several years for functional and morphological development to be completed. Similarly, control of breathing during the first weeks of extrauterine life differs notably from control in older children and adults. Of particular importance, during the first 2–3 weeks of age, infants in a warm environment respond to hypoxaemia by a transient increase in ventilation followed by sustained ventilatory depression (Brady & Ceruit, 1966). Three weeks after birth hypoxaemia induces sustained hyperventilation as in older children and adults.

The full-term newborn infant has 20–50 million terminal airspaces, mostly primitive saccules from which alveoli later develop. During the early postnatal years, development and growth of the lungs continues at a rapid pace, particularly with respect to the development of new alveoli. By the age of 6 years the alveoli reaches the adult level of 300 million. Subsequent lung growth is associated with an increase in alveolar size (Dunnill, 1962).

Early workers believed that peripheral airways with small calibre were the major contributors to the total airway resistance. The studies of Weibel (1963), however, proved that the total cross-sectional area of each generation of airway increases toward the periphery. Indeed, about two-thirds of the total airway resistance exists

Table 4.2. *Normal cardiorespiratory parameters in infants and children*

Age (years)	Respiratory rate (per minute)	Heart rate (per minute)	Blood pressure (systolic, mmHg)
< 1	30–40	110–160	70–90
1–5	20–30	90–140	80–100
6–11	15–20	70–120	90–110
> 11	12–15	60–100	100–120

between the airway opening and the trachea, and most of the remaining resistance is in the larger central airways. The airways smaller than a few millimetres in diameter (peripheral) contribute only about 10% of total resistance (Macklem & Mead, 1967).

Airflow resistance (R) is expressed as a unit pressure (P) per unit flow (V) (cm H_2O/l per second) and assuming laminar flow, is related to the length (l) and radius (r) of a tube and the viscosity (h) as shown in the Poiseuille's law:

$$R = 8lh/\pi r^4$$

It is apparent that the most important factor influencing flow resistance is the change in the radius of the air passages. Flow resistance is related to $1/r^5$ when turbulence is present such as crying; therefore infants and small children have higher absolute resistances than larger children and adults. Furthermore, relatively small changes in radius following trauma caused by oedema, secretions or blood may lead to severe and life-threatening upper airways obstruction which is exacerbated further by turbulent flow characteristics during crying.

In adult the nasal airway is the primary pathway for normal breathing. During quiet breathing the resistance through the nasal passages accounts for more than 50% of the total respiratory resistance or approximately 65% of the total airway resistance (Ferris *et al.*, 1964). This is more than twice the resistance of mouth breathing, although for air warming, humidification, and particle filtration it is important that one instinctively breathes through the nose (Proctor, 1977).

The newborn is an obligate nasal breather (Polgar, 1961). Factors contributing to this include the immaturity of the oropharyngeal motor output and sensory input resulting in a lack of coordination of respiratory and swallowing efforts. In addition, the relatively large tongue obstructs the oral airflow resulting in the nasal passages being the route of least resistance. Resistance to airflow in the nasal passage is one-fourth the total respiratory flow resistance and approximately one-half that in the adult (Polgar & Kong, 1965). This relatively decreased resistance provides for less work in nasal breathing for the infant compared with the adult. Obstruction to the nasal airway such as the insertion of too large a nasogastric tube may significantly increase total airway resistance (by as much as 50%) and may further compromise breathing (Stocks, 1980).

A number of upper airway muscles are involved in regulating upper airway calibre. Dilatation of nasal alae during inspiration, especially during exercise and dyspnoea, is well recognised. In animals the genioglossus, geniohyoid and pharyngeal and laryngeal abductor muscles have phasic inspiratory activity synchronous with phrenic nerve contractions (Bartlett *et al.*, 1973). Similar phasic activities in humans have been reported in the genioglossus as well as the scalene and sternomastoid muscles (Onal *et al.*, 1981). The activities of the genioglossus muscle and probably other abductors are easily depressed by alcohol ingestion, sleep and general anaesthesia (Nishino *et al.*, 1984, 1985). With depression of the genioglossus muscle during unconsciousness the tongue will fall back against the posterior pharyngeal wall and obstruct the upper airway; because of the aforementioned anatomical differences this is even more likely in the child.

If there is airway obstruction active inspiration often results in paradoxical chest movement with sternal and intercostal retractions rather than chest and lung expansion. The high compliance of the paediatric airway also makes it very susceptible to dynamic collapse in the presence of airway obstruction (Wittenborg *et al.*, 1967). Upper airway obstruction such as epiglottitis or extrathoracic foreign body may cause airway collapse during inspiration whereas intrathoracic obstruction is worsened during expiration. The application of continuous positive airway pressure (CPAP) or positive end expiratory pressure (PEEP) often improves gas exchange by opposing the forces causing dynamic airway collapse.

The resting respiratory rate of a newborn infant is between 30 and 40 breaths per minute and this gradually falls to the adult level of 15–16 breaths per minute by late childhood. At rest, the child's minute ventilation depends on metabolic demands and the respiratory rate is set for minimum energy expenditure. When the work of breathing increases, as in airway obstruction, a much larger portion of the energy expenditure is needed to maintain adequate ventilation.

In the diaphragm and intercostal muscles of infants there are fewer Type I muscle fibres, which are the slow-contracting, high oxidative fibres adapted for sustained activity. This contributes to the early fatigue of these muscles when the work of breathing is increased. Type I fibres comprise 25% of the diaphragm muscle fibres in the newborn and reach mature proportion of 55% by 8–9 months of age.

Tidal volume (V_T), minute ventilation, and functional residual capacity have all been measured in babies. Dead space volume calculated from the Bohr equation averaged about 2.2 ml/kg. The ratio of dead space ventilation and tital ventilation V_D/V_T is about 0.3 in both infants and adults. The average minute ventilation in the first year of life is 220 ml/kg, and alveolar ventilation is 140 ml/kg. This about twice the adult figures of 100 ml/kg and 60 ml/kg, respectively, but if expressed in relation to surface area they are almost identical at about $2.3\,l/m^2$ per minute. The importance of the dead space (only 6–7 ml in a newborn) is that it can be increased considerably by apparatus dead space. Intubation reduces dead space and if ventilation is controlled, dead space is usually not a problem if purpose built paediatric equipment is used.

The shape of the chest wall in neonates and infants influences lung volume and the mechanics of breathing. With an intact pleura the ribs and sternum normally support the lungs and help them remain expanded. In adults contraction of the intercostal muscles make the downward sloping ribs become more horizontal, thus increasing the anteroposterior diameter of the thorax and increasing its volume. Contraction of the diaphragm also increases thoracic volume. The intercostal muscles and the diaphragm alter the intrathoracic volume and pressure causing air to move in and out of the lungs. In infants the ribs and intercostal cartilage are highly compliant and offer less support to the lungs. As a result the volume of air remaining in the lungs at the end of normal expiration (functional residual capacity; FRC) is reduced. The FRC is also reduced in the supine child. The closing volume, which is the volume at which airway collapse occurs during expiration, exceeds the functional residual capacity in infants and neonates and this leads to airway closure during normal tidal ventilation. The FRC serves as a buffer to minimise cyclic changes in pCO_2 and pO_2 during each breath and acts as a reservoir of oxygen.

In addition the lack of lung support and horizontal alignment of the ribs makes the tidal volume of infants or toddlers almost totally dependent on movement of the diaphragm. When this movement is impeded by high intra-abdominal pressure such as gastric distension or intra-abdominal haemorrhage respiration will be compromised and FRC further reduced.

Efficient exchange of gases between air and pulmonary blood requires that areas of the lung that are ventilated are perfused and vice versa. If airway closure occurs during tidal ventilation this relationship is disturbed and desaturated pulmonary arterial blood is shunted past unventilated alveoli leading to desaturation of pulmonary venous blood. This ventilation to perfusion relationship is also disturbed in the supine, hypovolaemic patient.

The child has an increased oxygen consumption (6–8 ml/kg per minute in the neonate compared with 3–4 ml/kg per minute in the adult) which is related to a higher basal metabolic rate. Together with the ventilation perfusion mismatch and decreased functional residual capacity this makes the child and infant far more likely to become hypoxaemic in hypoxic situations.

As the paediatric chest wall is so compliant severe blunt chest trauma may be sustained without associated rib fractures or overt evidence of trauma but may result in significant underlying lung contusion or myocardial injury. If a rib fracture is present then a greater transfer of energy will have occurred and there is a significantly increased likelihood of multisystem injury (Garcia *et al.*, 1990).

The cardiovascular system

Heart rate is the single most important factor in the control of cardiac output in the young child. The heart of the neonate is thick walled and non-compliant and its ability to increase stroke volume is limited: therefore the maintenance of heart rate is important in paediatric trauma resuscitation.

The average heart rate is highest at 3 months of age and gradually declines thereafter into adulthood. The influence of the autonomic nervous system and maturation have not been well defined. Doses of atropine that effectively decrease salivation and gastric motility, but that are too small to influence heart rate, are relatively constant on a mg/kg basis during the first 12 years of life (Unna *et al.*, 1950). This strongly suggests that heart rate is determined by the circulatory needs of the individual rather than by a background autonomic tone.

Between 6 months and adolescence there are two major types of changes in the cardiovascular system. The pulmonary circulation grows by branching and the heart increases in size. Heart size increases throughout childhood. After 3 months of age, both ventricles increase in weight; however the proportion of the ventricular weights remains constant, indicating that the ventricles have assumed their approximate adult proportions by this age. Some children with mild cardiovascular disease have been investigated by echocardiography and this data gives a further insight into cardiovascular development. The size of the left ventricular cavity increases linearly until the patient reaches 8–9 years of age (surface area $1.0\,\text{m}^2$) (Roge *et al.*, 1978). Thereafter, the left ventricular dimensions remain constant but the right ventricular cavity continues to enlarge throughout development.

With growth, there is a need for an increased cardiac output. As previously stated increases in cardiac output are primarily due to heart rate when the limits of diastolic stretch are approached, e.g. newborn. In these circumstances any decrease in heart rate will cause a fall in cardiac output. The fact that the heart rate decreases with increasing age indicates that growth of the cardiac ventricles is more than adequate to supply the required increase in cardiac output.

The arterial blood pressure changes with age. The systolic pressure gradually rises after the first day of life until adolescence. Diastolic pressure is relatively constant throughout development and is important for coronary perfusion especially to the subendocardial layer of the ventricular wall.

The combination of an increasing systolic pressure and decreasing cardiac index suggests that with growth there is a gradual increase in peripheral vascular resistance. This change in resistance might indicate a gradual reduction in the need for peripheral blood flow, i.e. the tissues may become more efficient in their utilisation of oxygen. Two sets of data suggest that this is the case (Hill & Rahimtulla, 1965; Cumming *et al.*, 1978).

Oxygen transport

For normal metabolism oxygen must be transported continuously to all body tissues, changes in demand are met by the integrated response of three major components of the oxygen transport system: pulmonary ventilation, cardiac output and blood haemoglobin concentration and characteristics.

The delivery of oxygen (DO_2) to the periphery can be calculated using the following formula.

$$Do_2 = CI \times 10 \times CaO_2 \text{ (ml/min per m}^2)$$

where CI = cardiac index (l/min per m^2); CaO$_2$ (arterial oxygen content) = (Hb × % saturation × K) + (0.0225 × PaO_2) (ml/dl); Hb = haemoglobin (g/dl); PaO_2 = partial pressure of arterial oxygen (Kpa); K = Hufner factor typically 1.39 (ml/g).

Haemoglobin

Peripheral oxygen delivery depends on haemoglobin concentration, cardiac output, and PaO_2. It also depends on the degree of oxygen unloading by haemoglobin, which is controlled in great part by 2,3 diphosphoglycerate (2,3 DPG). This substance competes with oxygen for binding sites on the haemoglobin molecule. The higher the 2,3 DPG level, the more oxygen is offloaded to the tissues. The newborn, despite adequate levels of 2,3 DPG, has reduced oxygen unloading at tissue level because 2,3 DPG binds weakly with fetal haemoglobin. As the infant gets older and produces adult haemoglobin, the 2,3 DPG binding increases. If the cardiac output and venous oxygen saturation remain constant the amount of oxygen unloaded at peripheral tissues increases constantly to 4–5 volumes percent by the age of 8–11 months, despite a fall in absolute haemoglobin level (physiological anaemia of infancy) (Oski, 1973).

Children usually tolerate anaemia well. Cropp (1969) studied patients between 7 months and 14 years who had severe iron deficiency or renal disease and found that their cardiac function was nearly double that of non-anaemic children. Their systemic vascular resistance decreased as their haemoglobin concentration decreased. Breathing 100% oxygen returned their cardiac index and systemic vascular resistance towards normal, indicating that the local regulation of blood flow and oxygenation by peripheral tissues is very important for overall circulatory control in anaemia.

Body water

At birth 75% of an infant's body weight is composed of water. By 1 year of age this has decreased to 65% and after 1 year it begins to approach adult values of 55–60%. Body water is compartmentalised into the extracellular fluid compartment (ECF) and the intracellular fluid compartment (ICF). The extracellular compartment is composed of the plasma volume and the interstitial fluid. It is the distribution of these that changes with maturation.

Numerous methods have been described over the years for maintenance fluids in paediatric patients. The calculations have been based on body surface area, body weight, metabolic rate and caloric expenditure.

Maintenance fluid replacement has been simplified into the familiar 4-2-1 formula for hourly fluid maintenance commonly used for intraoperative fluid maintenance shown in Table 4.3 (Halliday & Segar, 1957). These formulae are guidelines for the basic maintenance requirements and do not take into account other losses that may be important in the trauma situation. These losses can range in severity from third space losses secondary to tissue injury to frank haemorrhage from an open wound. Estimation of such losses can be quite difficult in trauma patients and can lead to significant fluid deficits, especially in clinical situations such as burns injuries or peritonitis. In a trauma patient requiring an operative procedure, third space losses are usually greatest and most problematic during the first 2–3 hours of surgery. Table 4.4 shows the approximate requirements for third space losses in surgery.

Shock

Shock may be defined as the inadequacy of oxygen supply or delivery to meet metabolic demand. The most common form of shock in both paediatric and adult trauma patients is hypovolaemic or haemorrhagic shock. In shock there are compensatory cardiac and peripheral vascular changes to maintain the circulating blood volume and perfusion of critical organs such as the brain heart.

Children in shock differ from their adult counterparts by their ability to maintain a near normal central blood pressure in the face of as much as a 25% decrease in circulating volume (Schwaitzberg *et al.*, 1988). This is accomplished by a strong sympathetic tone enabling peripheral vasoconstriction. Thus the blood pressure is a much less sensitive indicator of hypovolaemia in a child than in an adult. A more useful indicator of hypovolaemia is the heart rate and tachycardia is an early sign in shock.

As tachycardia is a non-specific sign of distress and hypotension is a late and ominous sign of impending cardiovascular collapse a number of other physiological indicators should be used in evaluating the haemodynamic status of the child. These include peripheral perfusion, capillary refill, central and distal pulses, level of consciousness and adequacy of urine output.

Decreased skin perfusion can be an early sign shock. In the presence of a warm ambient temperature when the cardiac output falls the cooling of skin begins from the

Table 4.3. *Maintenance fluid replacement in children*

Body weight (kg)	Fluid (ml/h)
< 10	4 ml/kg per hour
10–20	40 + 2 ml for each kg > 10
> 20	60 + 1 ml for each kg > 20

Source: Halliday & Segar (1957).

Table 4.4. *Approximate requirements for third space losses in surgery*

Operation	Volume (ml/kg per hour)
Intra-abdominal surgery	2
Peritonitis/perforation	4
Two cavity surgery	6

This replacement is in addition to maintenance fluid and may be as high as 10 ml/kg per hour (Shires *et al.*, 1961).

periphery and extends proximally towards the trunk. Delayed capillary refill (more than 2 seconds) after blanching is caused by shock or a cool ambient temperature.

Pulses readily palpable in healthy infants and children may show a discrepancy between central and peripheral pulses in situations of vasoconstriction caused by a cold ambient temperature or a decreased cardiac output. The pulse volume is related to the difference between the systolic and diastolic pressures. When the cardiac output decreases the pulse pressure narrows and the pulse becomes thready and progressively more difficult to feel.

The clinical signs of brain hypoperfusion are determined by the severity and duration of the ischaemia. When the ischaemic insult is sudden, few signs of neurological compromise precede the loss of consciousness. When the onset is more gradual the neurological symptoms are more insidious. Alteration of consciousness occurs with confusion, irritability and lethargy. In the absence of central nervous system injury these signs indicate a profound physiological insult.

Urine output is directly proportional to glomerular filtration rate and renal blood flow. Urine flow of less than 1 ml/kg in the absence of renal disease is a good indicator of renal hypoperfusion from hypovolaemia.

Shock from volume depletion is often underestimated in children. Blood volume is approximately 80 ml/kg for children 3–12 months and 70 ml/kg for children older than 1 year. Whereas a blood loss of 500 ml in an adult means a loss of 10% of total blood volume, the same amount in a 4-year-old indicates a loss of approximately 40% of total volume. Thus small children can die rapidly from blood loss. While external bleeding is very impressive and alarming, internal bleeding can be insidious and unrecognised. Intrathoracic or intra-abdominal bleeding and bleeding into soft tissues and retroperitoneal structures can be life-threatening. Even intracranial bleeding can lead to haemorrhagic shock in small children and infants can die from haemorrhagic shock as a result of intracranial bleeding.

Circulatory support of the paediatric trauma patient requires simultaneous control of external haemorrhage, assessment, restoration and maintenance of an adequate circulating volume. Blood transfusion is of paramount importance in the initial stabilisation of the child who has sustained significant blood loss in order to maintain oxygen delivery. Failure to recognise and control internal bleeding is thought to be a leading cause of preventable death in children with multiple injuries (Dykes *et al.*, 1989). Signs of shock may be observed immediately or evolve slowly; if acute haemorrhage totals more than 15% of the blood volume, signs of circulatory compromise such as tachycardia, decreased peripheral pulses, delayed capillary refill and cold extremities will be present. Hypotension will not be present until 25–30% of the child's volume is lost acutely (Schwaitzberg *et al.*, 1988).

Reliable vascular access is required preferably at two sites proximal to injuries, the intraosseous route is acceptable in children under 6 years of age. The efficacy of fluid resuscitation will be determined by the fluid volume, fluid type and speed of delivery.,

If systemic perfusion is inadequate but blood pressure is maintained, and mild to moderate hypovolaemia is present, then rapid replacement with a bolus of 20 ml/kg of isotonic solution such as Ringers lactate or normal saline should be given initially. The fluids used should be warmed if possible. Additional boluses should be given if peripheral perfusion does not improve. The debate over the superiority of colloid solutions versus crystalloid solutions for fluid resuscitation centres on which fluid optimises the circulatory status of the patient and hence tissue oxygenation. Several studies have compared colloids with crystalloids in resuscitation and the evidence remains inconclusive (Virgilio *et al.*, 1979; Tait & Larson, 1991).

Administration of blood must be considered after two crystalloid or colloid boluses. The presence of hypotension indicates a 25–30% volume loss and blood and volume infusion is required immediately. Blood should be administered in boluses of 10 ml/kg, warmed to maintain body temperature and also to facilitate infusion. Ideally blood should be type-specific and cross-matched, however, transfusion should not be delayed in shock unresponsive to crystalloid therapy and O-negative or group-specific blood may be administered. If shock persists in spite of control of external haemorrhage and volume resuscitation then an alternative hidden loss must be suspected. Internal bleeding is likely and this requires continued transfusion and surgical assessment with a view to urgent surgical exploration.

Central nervous system

Head injury results in significant mortality and morbidity in the paediatric trauma patient. The brain of the neonate is relatively large weighing about 1/10 of the body weight as compared with about 1/50 in the adult. The brain grows rapidly, its weight doubling by 6 months and triples by 1 year. The development of cells in the cortex and brain stem is nearly complete by 1 year of age. Children have different injury patterns than adults because of their smaller anatomies.

In infants and children the head to body ratio is greater and the cranial bones are thinner, offering less protection to the contents. Myelination of the brain cells is incomplete and the cells are therefore more vulnerable to hypoxic damage. Increased intracranial pressure occurs much more commonly (80% compared with 50%) in children with head injury than in adults. In addition diffuse swelling dominates (50% compared with 30%) over mass lesions in the paediatric head injury patient. Children, however, are more likely than adults to recover from serious head injury (Craft *et al.*, 1972). The outcome in both severe and moderate head injury depends on the prevention and control of secondary injury caused by hypoxia, hypercarbia, hypotension and raised intracranial pressure (Klauber *et al.*, 1985) (Chapters 10 and 14).

Temperature homeostasis

Following trauma the maintenance of body temperature is important to prevent the physiological consequences of hypothermia. The body loses heat by evaporation, radiation, convection and conduction. Evaporative loss from the skin is related to the amount of sweating and also the relative humidity. It is greater when the humidity is decreased. Respiratory heat loss is increased if the nasal rewarming mechanism is bypassed as it is when the patient is intubated. The cooling due to breathing cold dry gases can be reduced by warming and humidifying the inspired gases.

As the environmental temperature decreases, radiant heat loss increases absolutely and in proportion to other heat losing mechanisms (Hey & Katz, 1970). Radiant heat is lost to nearby objects and is independent of the intervening air temperature. Significant heat loss by radiation may occur when it is cold outside, if a naked or only slightly clothed infant is placed near a closed window. Clothing reduces radiant heat loss.

Convective heat loss is the transfer of heat by the movement of surrounding air. Draughts should be avoided to prevent lowering of temperature by convection.

Conduction is heat transfer between molecules and heat loss can occur from the body to the surface with which it is in contact. The use of warming mattresses can help reduce conductive heat loss.

Infants have a greater problem in maintaining body temperature than older children or adults because their surface area to body weight ratio is 2–2.5 times greater, their skin and subcutaneous fat are thinner and their total mass is smaller. Every effort must be made in the management of the paediatric trauma patient to prevent heat loss from occurring.

Although it is not within the scope of this chapter the traumatologist should always consider the child's emotional as well as physical needs and create an environment that will minimise or abolish fear and distress. The most intense fear of an infant or a young child (less than 2 years) is created by separation from its parents. Older children may be more concerned about painful procedures and loss of self-control.

The physical, physiological, pathological and psychological differences between children and adults make the immediate management of the injured child a difficult clinical challenge. Their tremendous powers of recovery ensure that it is also an extremely rewarding and worthwhile exercise.

References

Bartlett, D. Jr, Remmers, J. E. & Gautier, H. (1973). Laryngeal regulation of respiratory air flow. *Respiration Physiology*, **18**, 194–204.

Bohn, D., Armstrond, D., Becker, L. & Humphrey, R. (1990). Cervical spine injuries in children. *Journal of Trauma*, **30**, 463–9.

Brady, J. P. & Ceruit, E. (1966). Chemoreceptor reflexes in the newborn infant. Effects of varying degrees of hypoxia on heart rate and ventilation in a warm environment. *Journal of Physiology*, **184**, 631–5.

Craft, A. W., Shaw, D. A. & Cartlidge, N. E. F. (1972). Head injuries in children. *British Medical Journal*, **4**, 200–3.

Cropp, G. J. A. (1969). Cardiovascular function in children with severe anaemia. *Circulation*, **39**, 775–84.

Cumming, G. R., Everatt, D. & Hastman, L. (1978). Bruce treadmill test in children: normal values in clinic population. *American Journal of Cardiology*, **41**, 69–75.

DuBois, D. & DuBois, E. F. (1916). A height-weight formula to estimate the surface area of man. *Proceedings of the Society of Experimental Biology and Medicine*, **13**, 77.

Dunnill, M. S. (1962). Postnatal growth of the lung. *Thorax*, **17**, 329–33.

Dykes, E. H., Spence, L. J., Bohn, D. J. & Wesson, D. E. (1989). Evaluation of pediatric trauma care in Ontario. *Journal of Trauma*, **29**, 724–9.

Eckenhoff, J. E. (1951). Some anatomical considerations of the infant larynx influencing endotracheal anaesthesia. *Anesthesiology*, **12**, 401–10.

Ferris, B. G., Mead, J. & Opie, L. H. (1964). Partitioning of respiratory flow resistance in man. *Journal of Applied Physiology*, **19**, 653–8.

Garcia, V. F., Gotschall, C. S., Eichelberger, M. R. & Bowan, L. M. (1990). Rib fractures in children: a marker of severe trauma. *Journal of Trauma*, **30**, 695–700.

Halliday, M. A. & Segar, W. E. (1957). Maintenance need for water in parenteral fluid therapy. *Paediatrics*, **19**, 823–32.

Harris, J. S. (1957). Special pediatric problems in fluid and electrolyte therapy in surgery. *Annals of the New York Academy of Science*, **66**, 966–9.

Hey, E. N. & Katz, G. (1970). The optimal thermal environment for naked babies. *Archives of Diseases of Children*, **45**, 328–32.

Hill, J. R. & Rahimtulla, K. A. (1965). Heart balance and the metabolic rate of newborn babies in relation to environmental temperature: and the effect of age and weight on basal metabolic rate. *Physiology*, **180**, 239–42.

Hill, S. A., Miller, C. A., Kosnik, E. J. & Hunt, W. E. (1984). Pediatric neck injury: a clinical study. *Journal of Neurosurgery*, **60**, 700–6.

Kewalraamani, L. S., Kraus, J. F. & Sterling, H. M. (1980). Acute spinal cord lesions in a paediatric population: epidemiology and clinical features. *Paraplegia*, **18**, 206–19.

Klauber, M. R., Marshall, L. F., Toole, B. M. *et al.* (1985). Cause of decline in head injury mortality in San Diego County California. *Journal of Neurosurgery*, **65**, 528–31.

Koka, B. V., Jeon, S., Andre, J. M., MacKay, I. & Smith, R. M. (1977). Postintubation croup in children. *Anesthesia and Analgesia*, **56**, 501–5.

Macklem, P. T. & Mead, J. (1967). Resistance of central and peripheral airways measured by a retrograde catheter. *Journal of Applied Physiology*, **22**, 395–401.

Nishino, T., Kohchi, T., Yonezawa, T. & Honda, Y. (1985). Response of recurrent laryngeal, hypoglossal, and phrenic nerves to increasing depth of anesthesia with Halothane or Enflurane in vagotomised cats. *Anesthesiology*, **63**, 404–9.

Nishino, T., Shirahata, M., Yonezawa, T. & Honda, Y. (1984). Comparison of changes in the hypoglossal and the phrenic nerve activity in response to increasing depth of anesthesia in cats. *Anethesiology*, **60**, 19–24.

Onal, E., Lopata, M. & O'Conner, T. D. (1981). Diaphragmatic and genioglossal electromyogram responses to CO_2 rebreathing in humans. *Journal of Applied Physiology*, **50**, 1052–5.

Oski, F. A. (1973). Designation of anaemia on a functional basis. *Journal of Paediatrics*, **83**, 353–5.

Pang, D. & Pollack, I. F. (1989). Spinal cord injury without radiographic abnormality in children: the SCIWORA syndrome. *Journal of Trauma*, **29**, 654–64.

Pang, D. & Wilberger, J. E. Jr. (1982). Spinal cord injury without radiographic abnormality in children. *Journal of Neurosurgery*, **57**, 114–29.

Polgar, G. (1961). Airway resistance in the newborn infant. *Journal of Pediatrics*, **59**, 915–21.

Polgar, G. & Kong, G. P. (1965). The nasal resistance of newborn infants. *Journal of Pediatrics*, **67**, 556–67.

Proctor, D. F. (1977). The upper airways. I. Nasal physiology and defence of the lungs. *American Review of Respiratory Diseases*, **115**, 97–129.

Roge, C. L. L., Silverman, N. H., Hart, P. A. & Ray, R. M. (1978). Cardiac structure growth pattern determined by echocardiography. *Circulation*, **57**, 285–90.

Rivara, F. P. (1982). Epidemiology of childhood injuries. I. Review of current research and presentation of conceptual framework. *American Journal of Diseases of Children*, **136**, 399–408.

Schuman, A. J. (1991). The Broselow tape: taking the guesswork out of resuscitation. *Contemporary Pediatrics*, **8**, 101–3.

Schwaitzberg, S. D., Bergman, K. S. & Harris, B. H. (1988). A pediatric model of continuous haemorrhage. *Journal of Pediatric Surgery*, **23**, 605–9.

Shires, T., Williams, J. & Brown, F. (1961). Acute changes in extracellular fluids associated with major surgical procedures. *Annals of Surgery*, **154**, 803–10.

Stocks, J. (1980). Effect of nasogastric tubes on nasal resistance during infancy. *Archives of Diseases of Children*, **55**, 17–21.

Tait, A. R. & Larson, L. O. (1991). Resuscitation fluids for the treatment of haemorrhagic shock in dogs: effects on myocardial blood flow and oxygen transport. *Critical Care Medicine*, **19**, 1561–5.

Teanby, D. N., Lloyd, D. A., Gorman, D. F. & Bolot, D. A. (1994). Regional review of blunt trauma in children. *British Journal of Surgery*, **81**, 53–5.

Tepas, J. J., Di Scala, C., Ramenofsky, M. L. & Barlow, B. (1990). Mortality and head injury: the pediatric perspective. *Journal of Pediatric Surgery*, **25**, 92–6.

Unna, K. R., Glaser, K., Lipton, E. & Patterson, P. R. (1950). Dosage of drugs in infants and children. I. Atropine. *Pediatrics*, **6**, 197–207.

Virgilio, R. W., Rice, C. L. & Smith, D. E. (1979). Crystalloid vs colloid resuscitation: is one better? *Surgery*, **85**, 129–39.

Weibel, E. R. (1963). *Morphometry of the Human Lung*. New York: Academic Press.

Westhorpe, R. N. (1987). The position of the larynx in children and its relationship to the ease of intubation. *Anaesthesia and Intensive Care*, **15**, 384–7.

Wittenborg, M. H., Gyepes, M. T. & Crocker, D. (1967). Tracheal dynamics in infants with respiratory distress, stridor and collapsing trachea. *Radiology*, **88**, 653–62.

5

Evaluation of injury in children

B. M. PHILLIPS

The evaluation of an injured child is a process which has two distinct themes. These are:

1. The effect of the injury on the whole child.
2. The identification of the individual components of the injury.

The process of evaluation starts at the injury incident and may be initiated by the child itself. More often lay people, the attending parent or bystander, will evaluate the child's injury and its effect leading to a decision on whether to seek professional help. This process may then be repeated by an increasing series of professionals with differing skills, from the paramedic in the Ambulance Service to the staff in the Emergency department, the Trauma Surgeon and later the Rehabilitation Therapist.

Within this process of evaluation, both historical and physical information are necessary. The history of the incident itself is vital to an understanding of the forces involved and therefore the potential tissue damage caused by the incident. The child's own medical and trauma history reveals the baseline to which the new injury is added. Physical examination then completes the evaluation process. Evaluation leads to a choice of management and is also predictive, i.e. it suggests what further investigations may be needed, what level of hospital care will be required and the likely final outcome.

Triage

Triage is an evaluation and prioritisation process which ranks patients in order of need. It is an evaluation of the patient's injury in the context of prioritising the resources available to patients. Triage was developed as a rapid evaluation tool for use in war time when the medical services were dealing with large numbers of severely injured trauma victims. The scheme divided patients into three groups (hence the name 'triage'):

48

1. In need of immediate resuscitation.
2. In need of urgent treatment.
3. Stable patient.

Many triage systems now employ additional categories, particularly enlarging those of (2) and (3) in the list above. There are now usually at least two triaging events in civilian medical practice. The first is at the scene of an injury. Triaging here is conducted by paramedics from the ambulance service and especially in the USA the use of the trauma scoring system for triage in the field leads to the appropriate disposition of patients to level 1 or level 2 trauma centres. These are hospitals with differing capabilities in the management of trauma victims; level 1 trauma centre having the higher capability (Jubelirer *et al.*, 1990).

In the Emergency department triage is a process applied to all attendees, both those suffering from medical conditions and those presenting with trauma. The process aims to rank patients in order of need and also to identify needs that require immediate attention such as:

1. The physiological effect of the injury on the whole child; is there a risk to life?
2. The effect of the individual injury; is there a risk to limb, vascular compromise, etc?
3. Is there a need for immediate pain control?
4. Is there a need for immediate psychological support of the child or his carers?

During the triage process the patient's age is a relevant feature. Infants and young children have a lower physiological reserve than older children or fit adults and therefore the younger the child the higher the triage priority is likely to be. During this process also a recognition of the possibility of child abuse may be made. During the patient's stay in the Emergency department re-triaging will be carried out on several further occasions, e.g. to detect clinical change during waiting or to prioritise the use of investigative or treatment facilities.

Trauma scoring

A number of scoring systems have been developed for use with the injured patient to assist in both the initial assessment and triage of the patient and the later audit of the outcome of the injury episode and its treatment. In this next section I examine the Revised Trauma Score (RTS) and the Paediatric Trauma Score (PTS) which are both triage tools. I also examine the Injury Severity Score and its use together with the RTS in the Major Trauma Outcome Study, which is an audit system.

The Trauma Score

The Trauma Score was first described by Champion *et al.* in 1981. It is a system using four physiological parameters, namely systolic blood pressure, capillary refill, respiratory rate and respiratory effort combined with the Glasgow Coma Scale. The Trauma Score is shown in Table 5.1. The Trauma Score varies from 1 (worst prognosis) to 16 (best prognosis). Table 5.2 shows the Trauma Score and the probability of survival from an injury. As can be seen, this varies from virtually 100% with the top trauma score down to 0 at the lowest trauma score. A trauma score of 13 for example, corresponds to a mortality rate of approximately 10%. The trauma score has been used as a triage instrument in the field especially in the USA and was developed for adults. It has also been used as a mechanism for reviewing the appropriateness of pre-hospital care.

There are, however, significant deficiencies in the trauma score as in any other scoring system. In common with other physiological indices the trauma score has a sensitivity rate of about 80%. In other words, 20% of the patients with a significant injury will not be identified by this score. This is usually because they have compensated physiologically or because the score was applied so early after the injury that physiological decompensation had not occurred. Additionally, the trauma score has a specificity of 75%, e.g. it will overestimate the severity of injury when physiological changes are related to underlying medical factors.

A study of the Trauma Score in Table 5.1 shows that some physiological parameters are at levels inappropriate for children. Normal physiological parameters for children of different ages are shown in Table 5.3. For example, a respiratory rate of 10–24 is given a score of 4 (the top score for this index). In the infant and young child a respiratory rate in this range would be indicative of severe physiological disturbance as it is a slow rate for this age. A normal rate for the age group of infants and young children would in fact be scored at 3 on the trauma score. Similar problems obtain in the scoring of systolic blood pressure which could well be between 80 and 90 mm/Hg in a healthy infant.

Revised Trauma Score

More recently a revised trauma score has been developed (Champion *et al.*, 1989). This uses three physiological parameters: systolic blood pressure, respiratory rate and Glasgow Coma Scale. A coded value is assigned to a specific range of each parameter. This is shown in Table 5.4. The coded value for each variable is then multiplied by an assigned weight which has been derived from a regression analysis from over 25 000 patients in the US Major Trauma Outcome Study. The revised trauma score is the sum of these three products. A total score therefore ranges from 0 to 8 and is not usually a

Table 5.1. *Trauma score*

Respiratory rate		10–24	4
		25–35	3
		> 35	2
		0–9	1 - - - - - -
Respiratory effort	Normal		1
	Shallow, retractive		0 - - - - - -
Systolic blood pressure		> 90	4
		70–90	3
		50–69	2
		< 50	1
	No carotid pulse		0 - - - - - -
Capillary refill			
	Normal		2
	Delayed		1
	Absent		0 - - - - - -

Glasgow Coma Scale
Eye opening
   Spontaneous   4
   To voice   3
   To pain   2
   None   1
Verbal response
   Oriented   5
   Confused   4
   Inappropriate words 3
   Incomprehensible words 2
   None   1
Motor response
   Obeys commands   6
   Localises   5

		Total GCS points	
Withdraws	4	14–15	5
Abnormal flexion	3	11–13	4
Abnormal extension	2	8–10	3
None	1	5–7	2
		3–4	1 - - - - - -
Total GCS points	- - - - - -		
		Total trauma score	- - - - - -

GCS: Glasgow Coma Score
Source: From Champion *et al.* (1981).

Table 5.2. *Trauma score and probability of survival*

Trauma score	Probability of survival (%)
16	99
15	98
14	95
13	91
12	83
11	71
10	55
9	37
8	22
7	12
6	7
5	4
4	2
3	1
2	0
1	0

Source: From Boyd *et al.* (1987).

Table 5.3. *Physiological parameters in children*

Age (years)	Respiratory rate (breaths per minute)	Heart rate (beats per minute)	Systolic blood pressure (mmHg)
< 1	30–40	110–160	70–90
2–5	20–30	95–140	80–100
5–12	15–20	80–120	90–110
> 12	12–16	60–100	100–120

Source: Adapted from Mackway-Jones *et al.* (1993).

whole number. The same problems occur with the Revised Trauma Score as with the Trauma Score in its applicability to children. The physiological parameter ranges are not appropriate to young children and infants; however, despite this, there is evidence that the trauma score and the revised trauma score have a place in the triage assessment of children and in the audit of trauma outcome in children. There have been studies that have indicated that the 'adult' trauma scores have a significant ability to predict paediatric outcome. Proponents of the use of 'adult' trauma scores in children especially point out that in the field, paramedics who are not very experienced

Table 5.4. *The Revised Trauma Score*

Glasgow Coma Scale Score	Systolic blood (mmHg)	Respiratory rate (breaths/min)	Coded value
13–15	> 89	10–29	4
9–12	76–89	> 29	3
6–8	50–75	6–9	2
4–5	1–49	1–5	2
3	0	0	0

Source: Adapted from Champion *et al.* (1989).

with paediatric care may have more skill in applying a familiar score to children even though it may not be physiologically entirely adapted for this age group (Nayduch *et al.*, 1991).

The Paediatric Trauma Score

As there was no trauma scoring system specifically developed for use in the triage of the injured child, a Paediatric Trauma Score was developed by Tepas *et al.* in 1987. This system includes six determinants of the clinical condition in an injured child. The score includes both a degree of physiological assessment and a degree of anatomical assessment together with a weighting for age. This latter is to recognise the lower respiratory reserve in the young infant and its greater predisposition for loss of fluid and heat relative to size. The Paediatric Trauma Score is shown in Table 5.5.

Each of the six determinants is assigned a grade consisting of either + 2 (minimal or no injury), + 1 (minor or potentially major injury), or − 1 (major or immediate life-threatening injury). The system is arranged in a manner reminiscent of the Advanced Trauma Life Support protocols and thereby also provides a quick assessment scheme. The ability of the Paediatric Trauma Score to predict the Injury Severity Score (see later) showed a significant predictive capacity (Tepas *et al.*, 1987).

The first parameter of the Paediatric Trauma Score, size, stresses the importance of size and age, and the impact trauma has on the patient. The limited physiological reserves of infants and small children was mentioned above but, in addition, multisystem injury is more likely in small children because the energy of traumatic impact tends to be dispersed throughout the smaller body of the child.

Airway obstruction is one of the most important causes of death in cases of paediatric trauma. The child has narrow airway structures, lymphoid tissue in the nasopharynx and a relatively large head which contributes to the difficulty in pro-

Table 5.5. *Pediatric Trauma Score*

Competent	Category		
	+ 2	+ 1	− 1
Size	≥ 20 kg	10–20 kg	< 10 kg
Airway	Normal	Maintainable	Unmaintainable
Systolic blood pressure	≤ 90 mmHg	90–50 mmHg	< 50 mmHg
Central nervous system	Awake	Obtunded/LOC	Coma/decerebrate
Open wound	None	Minor	Major/penetrating
Skeletal	None	Closed fracture	Major/penetrating fractures
Sum total points			

LOC: loss of consciousness.
Source: From Tepas *et al.* (1987).

cedures. The Paediatric Trauma Score accords the airway a high priority by grading it according to the type of airway manoeuvre necessary. Systolic blood pressure is a physiological measure of blood loss and vascular tone. It is a very crude indicator of shock in children. There is considerable evidence to show that blood pressure fall is late and hypotension is an extremely serious sign during trauma in a child.

The neurological state of the child can be best predicted by the level of consciousness and the Paediatric Trauma Score divides patients into three categories from awake (the highest category) to coma or decerebrate (the lowest).

Finally, there are two anatomical scores detailing skeletal or integument injury. The component scores are added together with a maximum of 12 and a minimum of − 6. Children with a paediatric trauma score of 8 or less have been shown to have a risk of mortality and this figure is therefore taken in the USA to indicate the requirement to transport the child to a level 1 trauma centre. The Pediatric Trauma Score has been found in multiple studies to be both valid and reliable and its documented specificity ranges from 73 to 98% with its sensitivity from 78 to 86% (Ramenofsky *et al.*, 1988; Nayduch *et al.*, 1991).

Controversy still exists as to the best trauma score for use in injured children. Currently the Paediatric Trauma Score is largely being used as a triage tool both in the field and within the hospital setting to determine the need to alert the 'trauma team'. The Revised Trauma Score currently has its main role in paediatrics as a component of the Major Trauma Outcome Study audit methodology. It is perhaps worth noting that there is evidence that the Paediatric Trauma Score (and indeed clinical examination) are unable to predict consistently isolated liver and/or spleen injuries in children (Saladino *et al.*, 1991).

Injury Severity Score

The abbreviated injury score (AIS) is a measure of the severity of anatomical injury. It was developed in the 1970s in the USA as a tool for quantitating injuries received in motor vehicle accidents. It scores from 1 (minor) to 6 (fatal) in each of five body systems. A total of over 1200 injuries are included. Although a breakthrough in concept for scoring injuries, this system was not efficient at describing multiple injuries. Baker *et al.* in 1974 designed a method which was able to express the accumulative effect of injury on several body systems. Each of six anatomical regions is scored with the highest AIS grade for any injury in that region. The AIS values of the three highest scoring body regions are squared and then summed. The resulting score is known as the Injury Severity Score (ISS) (Baker *et al.*, 1974). A score of 6 in any one body system incurs the maximum overall score of 75, indicating a fatal injury. The Injury Severity Score has been found to correlate well with mortality. For example an ISS of 16 is predictive of 10% mortality. The system works best in scoring the severity of injury due to blunt trauma and is less predictive when scoring penetrating injuries, although revisions are attempting to improve the correlation.

The Triss methodology

The Triss method is a standardised approach for evaluating the outcome of trauma care (Boyd *et al.*, 1987). Anatomical, physiological and age characteristics are combined to quantify the probability of survival related to the severity of injury. The age in question in the Triss methodology refers to adults over the age of 55 years for which weighting is assigned. There is no similar weighting for childhood trauma.

The Triss methodology uses the Trauma Score and the Injury Severity Score that have been described above, combining them in association with co-efficients derived from regression analysis which had been applied to data from many thousands of patients analysed in the US Major Trauma Outcome Study. Using the Triss methodology the probability of survival (Ps) for any particular patient can be estimated from the following formula.

$$Ps = 1/(1 + e - b)$$

where $b = bo + b (TS) + b_2 (ISS) + b_3 (A)$; bo ... 3 are coefficients derived from Walker–Duncan regression analysis applied to data from thousands of patients analysed in the Major Trauma Outcome Study.

The Major Trauma Outcome Study

The Major Trauma Outcome Study originated in the USA where, using Triss methodology, participating trauma units submit data to a central research centre (Champion *et al.,* 1990). From this data, statistics are derived which compare the distribution of the predicted survival probability in the sample population with that of the main database. This audit tool can be used to give an overall picture of the success of the trauma system being analysed. By examination of the individual pieces of data, specific shortfalls or examples of good practice can be identified.

Participation in the UK Major Trauma Outcome Study involves the collection of epidemiological, trauma score and management data for all patients who are admitted to hospital for more than 3 days, die from their injuries or are transferred to another hospital for further or intensive care. In addition to the data on the patient, data is also collected to audit the time to various aspects of management and the seniority of staff providing care. At hospital discharge, data on the final injury severity score is included in the analysis (Yates *et al.,* 1992).

The Major Trauma Outcome Study is a useful if yet flawed tool for the comparative study of trauma care outcome. The completeness and accuracy of data collection remain significant problems.

Evaluation of the injured child

Traumatic injury is a dynamic process that may produce rapid changes in the patient's status, especially in the first few hours after the incident. Frequent re-evaluations are therefore mandatory. An airway that was initially adequate may become obstructed by blood or secretions. Respiration that was initially satisfactory may deteriorate from lung contusion, a developing tension pneumothorax or respiratory drive lowered by raised intracranial pressure. Ongoing blood loss may cause haemodynamic instability. In addition, at initial evaluation it is not apparent how many or of what severity are the injuries. Superficial injuries which are obvious are likely to be the least important and the child's life is endangered more by the 'hidden' injuries in the trunk and cranium.

Trauma evaluation and care must therefore proceed in an organised systematic fashion. The system devised and taught for the Advanced Trauma Life Support and the Advanced Paediatric Life Support Courses (Mackway-Jones *et al.,* 1993) provides a framework in which these problems can be practically addressed. The form of the structured approach is shown below.

> *Primary Survey*
> Resuscitation
> *Secondary Survey*
> Definitive Care

The primary survey addresses what has become known as the ABCs. The vital functions of the body are assessed as follows:

1. Airway with cervical spine control.
2. Breathing.
3. Circulation and haemorrhage control.
4. Disability (conscious level and localising cerebral signs).

During the primary survey any shortfall of one of these areas is immediately dealt with so that in fact the primary survey and resuscitation occur hand in hand. It is only after the patient has been stabilised that the secondary survey is started. This is a part of the evaluation which looks at the individual details of each injury and goes on to definitive care where the injuries are treated. This latter phase may of course extend over several days to weeks.

Primary survey and resuscitation

The primary survey begins immediately and is directed at the identification of an immediate threat to life. The first priority is to ensure an adequate airway while preventing cervical spine movement in case of injury to this area. If there is spontaneous breathing, a chin lift or jaw thrust airway opening manoeuvre is carried out and secretions or debris can be cleared from the mouth and pharynx. Supplemental oxygen is administered at as high a concentration as possible. It is important to avoid tilting the head so as to prevent cervical spine movement. The neck should be immobilised with a hard collar, sand bags and tape. If the patient is apnoeic or the airway cannot be maintained, an artificial airway must be placed. Orotracheal intubation is the most reliable means of protecting the airway and ventilating children with airway compromise. The appropriate endotracheal tube size is given by the following formula: Internal diameter (mm) = (age over 4) + 4. An uncuffed tube is used for children under the age of 8 years. The correct positioning of the tube is confirmed by auscultation of the chest, noting appropriate chest movements and the identification of adequate oxygen saturation by the saturation monitor.

Endtidal CO_2 detectors are also useful. Rarely, intubation attempts fail, particularly when there has been injury, especially a burn injury, of the face and neck. In this situation a needle cricothyrotomy is performed. Oxygen can be insufflated through a 14 bore needle inserted through the cricothyroid membrane. This does not ventilate the patient but merely oxygenates them and therefore CO_2 will be retained. A definitive airway must be provided within the next 45–60 minutes.

Breathing

Once an airway is secured the adequacy of ventilation must be evaluated. Observation of the excursion of the chest wall (or of the abdomen in a young infant), auscultation of the chest for breath sounds and assessment of the patient's oxygenation status using the pulse oximeter monitor will indicate whether ventilation is adequate in the short term. The patient should be receiving as close to 100% oxygen as is possible and if ventilation is still inadequate, ventilatory support, initially with bag and mask, or once intubated, via the endotracheal tube should be provided.

These manoeuvres may still fail to ensure adequate ventilation and oxygenation and if this is the case, then life-threatening complications such as tension pneumothorax or a haemopneumothorax should be suspected. The former is diagnosed by the presence of hyper-resonance on the affected side with a possible tracheal shift away from the affected side. In the latter instance, the affected side is dull to percussion. The tension pneumothorax is treated by the emergency insertion of a cannula into the second intercostal space in the midclavicular line. The release of tension enables the patient to be ventilated adequately. Subsequently a chest drain is formally placed. The treatment of haemopneumothorax is more complex and hazardous. While the blood and air must be evacuated from the chest to allow for lung expansion there is, in addition to the ventilatory embarrassment, the potential for very significant blood loss. The chest should be evacuated and the loss of blood replaced by a transfusion of whole, fresh blood.

Circulation

Visible haemorrhage must be controlled with direct pressure and the patient evaluated for signs of shock. It is important to note that the early signs of shock in a child may be subtle. The heart rate should be evaluated. The rate initially increases in shock because of catecholamine release and as compensation for decreased stroke volume. Particularly in small infants the rate may be very high (up to 200 per minute). The pulse volume gives a useful indication of perfusion. Absent peripheral pulses and weak central pulses are serious signs of advanced shock. The capillary refill test is useful, although care must be taken in assessing this sign in a child who may have been exposed to cold before arrival at hospital. The sign is evaluated by pressing on a digit for 5 seconds. Capillary refill should occur within 2 seconds after release of the pressure. A slower refill time than this indicates poor skin perfusion. It is a useful early sign in the patient who has not been exposed to significant chilling.

Blood pressure is traditionally measured as a sign of shock. It must be remembered, particularly in children, that hypotension is a late and pre-terminal sign of circulatory failure. Children compensate well for fluid loss and once the blood pressure has started to fall there has been at least a 25% loss of circulating volume and the child is in significant shock.

Evaluation of other organ systems can yield useful information on circulatory adequacy. In the shocked child a rapid respiration rate may be present with increased tidal volume but without rib recession. This is produced by the acidosis resulting from circulatory failure. Mottled, cold, pale skin indicates poor perfusion. Urinary output, although a later sign, is related to total body fluid and renal perfusion. A particularly useful evaluation sign, however, is the patient's mental status. The mildly shocked or hypoxic patient will be agitated and often apparently uncooperative. It is very important not to ascribe 'lack of cooperation' to the patient's volition as it is very often a physiological problem. Once circulatory embarrassment and hypoxia become severe, then the patient's conscious level starts to deteriorate.

The management of shock is to replace fluid and so, in addition to controlling visible haemorrhage, vascular access must be gained. The recommendation is that two short, wide bore cannulae are inserted. If, because of severe shock, this cannot be achieved then an intraosseous infusion will be necessary. Once circulatory access is gained an initial bolus of 20 ml/kg of either crystalloid or colloid can be given. The patient is re-evaluated after every bolus of fluid. If further 20 ml boluses are required, then it is likely the patient will require a blood transfusion and preparations should be made for this by sending the patient's blood for group and cross-matching. It is sometimes the case that a child's circulation cannot be stabilised even with a blood transfusion. This implies significant, unchecked internal truncal bleeding. In the presence of respiratory embarrassment the cause is likely to be a haemopneumothorax as described above; however, most unstable bleeding patients will have a ruptured abdominal vessel or damaged liver, spleen or kidney. Urgent laparotomy to control bleeding is therefore the final stage of haemorrhage control in the 'primary survey'.

A common concern when evaluating the injured child is the range of normal physiological values for pulse, respirations and blood pressure which are relevant to children of different age groups. Table 5.3 shows the ranges of these parameters at different ages.

Disability

The next priority is a brief evaluation of the child's neurological status. In the primary survey this consists of assigning the patient to one of the following four categories with regard to conscious level.

    A. Alert
    V. Responds to voice
    P. Responds to pain
    U. Unresponsive.

In addition to the above the pupils are checked for size, symmetry and briskness of response to light.

60   B. M. Phillips

Clinical evaluation of the individual injuries

Head and spine injuries

Head injury is the commonest single reason for death following trauma in children (Tepas et al., 1990). Some children die very rapidly from brain injuries that are incompatible with life. Of those who survive to be resuscitated in hospital, the commonest cause of head injury death is raised intracranial pressure. Children may, like adults, have expanding extradural, subdural or intracerebral haematomas, but the characteristic cause of raised intracranial pressure in childhood head injury is that caused by cerebral oedema. The understanding and management of cerebral oedema in the head injured child is one of the major research challenges in childhood trauma today.

In evaluating the head injury, it is vital to remember that a primary survey and resuscitation must be undertaken first. 'Secondary' brain injury is just as damaging as the primary traumatic insult. The effect of hypoxia and especially hypotension on children with severe head injuries is well documented (Pigula et al., 1993).

During the secondary survey the head should be observed and palpated for bruises, lacerations and depressed skull fractures. Scalp lacerations should be examined carefully for evidence of underlying fractures. The signs of a basal skull fracture are indicated clinically by blood or cerebrospinal fluid in the nose or ear, haemotympanum, racoon eyes or Battle's sign (bruising behind the ear) (Kitchens et al., 1991). The pupils should be examined for size and reactivity. A dilated non-reactive pupil indicates nerve dysfunction for which the cause is an ipsilateral haematoma until proven otherwise. Papilloedema is not seen in acutely raised intracranial pressure but the presence of retinal haemorrhages may indicate abuse in a young infant with unexplained injuries. Motor and sensory function should be assessed. This includes examination of the cranial and peripheral nerves. Any lateralising signs may indicate an intracranial bleed. A level of dysfunction may indicate a spinal injury.

Coma Scale

The use of the Glasgow Coma Scale in the assessment of patients after traumatic brain injury has become universally accepted and forms the foundation of the communication between clinicians responsible for the care of these patients (Teasdale & Jennett, 1974). Observations of the patient's eye, speech and motor responses to stimuli gives the physician a reliable estimate of the level of neurological function at the time of examination. The scale is based on a score between 3 and 15 and is the numerical sum of these three determinants. Table 5.6 shows the Glasgow Coma Scale (GCS).

Infants and toddlers are unable to speak or follow commands, therefore the Glas-

Table 5.6. *Glasgow Coma Scale*

Response	Score
Eyes	
Open spontaneously	4
Verebal command	3
Pain	2
No response	1
Best motor response	
Verbal command	
Obeys	6
Painful stimulus	
Localises pain	5
Flexion with pain	4
Flexion abnormal	3
Extension	2
No response	1
Best verbal response	
Orientated and converses	5
Disorientated and converses	4
Inappropriate words	3
Incomprehensible sounds	2
No response	1

Source: From Teasdale & Jennett (1974).

gow Coma Scale motor and verbal response evaluations cannot be applied to them. For this reason, children's coma scales have been developed but have not yet been validated.

Probably familiarity with a particular coma scale is the most important prerequisite for success in its use. Clearly, in some instances, the coma scale may not accurately reflect the prognosis. Depression of the conscious level by sedative drugs or spinal cord damage can influence the prognostic value of the Glasgow Coma Scale downwards. In addition, patients who are intubated cannot be assessed verbally and this intervention may have been for a ventilatory rather than a neurological problem. When using the coma scales to evaluate and communicate that evaluation to other specialists, these confounding factors must be taken into consideration.

The coma scale is used to direct management. A coma score of below 15 would be an indication for computerised tomography (CT) scanning even in the absence of a skull fracture. A coma score of 8 or less indicates a very significant loss of consciousness and such patients should be intubated and ventilated to both protect the airway and to induce mild hypocapnia in an effort to decrease cerebral oedema by slightly reducing cerebral blood flow.

Spinal injuries

Spinal injuries are rare in children but a high index of suspicion, correct management and prompt referral are essential to prevent worsening of an underlying cord injury. Any severely injured child should be considered to have a spinal injury until adequate examination and investigations have excluded it. Cervical spine injuries are rare in children under the age of 12 years because of the mobility and elasticity of the cervical spine in this age group (Orenstein *et al.*, 1994). The symptoms of cervical spine injury are threefold. They include pain which, of course, cannot be evaluated in the unconscious patient, neurological abnormalities which require detailed neurological examination and signs relating to the loss of autonomic tone from the circulatory system resulting in spinal shock. Additionally, some cord reflexes may be released and shown as priapism. Radiological evaluation is also necessary, but a normal radiograph does not exclude cervical spine damage as the SCIWORA syndrome (cervical spine injury without radiological abnormality) is even commoner in children than in adults (Pang & Pollack, 1989).

Injuries to the thoracic and lumbar spine are even more rare in children and account for less than 1% of all spinal injuries. They are more common in sporting activities. The most common mechanism of injury is hyperflexion and the most common clinical sign is the sensory level.

Neurological assessment is difficult in children and such a level may only become apparent after repeated examinations. These difficulties mean that the child with multiple injuries should be assumed to have a spinal injury and immobilised on a long spinal board until evaluation is complete.

Chest injuries

The evaluation of life-threatening chest injuries has already been referred to in the section on the primary survey under Breathing. Inadequate ventilation and oxygenation must be relieved by emergency procedures such as thoracocentesis before an evaluation even of potentially major injuries can occur.

A tension pneumothorax is a life-threatening emergency. Air accumulates under pressure in the pleural space. This pushes the mediastinum across the chest and kinks the great vessels. Venous return to the heart is thereby compromised and cardiac output reduced, in addition to the hypoxia caused by compression of the affected lung. The evaluation is a clinical one. The child will by hypoxic and possibly shocked.

There will be decreased air entry and hyper-resonance to percussion on the side of the pneumothorax. Some children may show distended neck veins and later the trachea will be deviated away from the side of the pneumothorax. With a massive haemo-pneumothorax both blood and air accumulate in the pleural space. This adds blood loss to the physiological problems of a tension pneumothorax. On evaluation the child will be hypoxic and shocked. There will be decreased chest movement, decreased air entry and decreased resonance to percussion on the side of the haemo-pneumothorax.

An open pneumothorax is a penetrating wound in the chest wall with its associated pneumothorax. This type of wound is more common in adults and is usually obvious, but it may be on the patient's back and therefore must be actively sought, either during the primary survey in the event of unexplained hypoxia, or during the secondary survey as part of the routine examination of the patient's back. The elasticity of the child's thorax reduces the incidence of flail chest, but if this injury does occur it is an indication of very severe truncal trauma. In flail chest there are sufficient rib fractures for a portion of the chest wall to move paradoxically, impairing ventilation. With this injury there is always significant underlying lung contusion which will also impair ventilation and oxygenation. The child with flail chest will be hypoxic, and will have abnormal chest movements, sometimes associated with rib crepitus.

Cardiac tamponade caused by trauma is an accumulation of blood in the pericardial sac (Langer *et al.*, 1989; Ildstad *et al.*, 1990). This reduces the volume available for the heart to fill during diastole. Cardiac output is therefore progressively reduced. The child with a pericardial tamponade will be in shock from a poor cardiac output. There may be muffled heart sounds and distended neck veins, although this latter may be less apparent if significant hypovolaemia co-exists.

All of the injuries referred to in the preceding paragraph are life-threatening and therefore their evaluation and prompt, effective management are vital. In addition, there are serious injuries that may be discovered on the secondary survey which can lead to major complications and permanent morbidity. A high index of suspicion is therefore necessary. Indicators that a child may have significant intrathoracic trauma involving heart, lungs and mediastinum can come from the history of the injury and external examination of the child and radiological investigations. Evaluation of the trauma history may suggest a chest crushing mechanism. Any evidence of bruising to the chest wall as a result of a crushing injury indicates a high likelihood of serious organ damage.

Children have a high incidence of pulmonary contusion because of the mobility of their ribs which fail to protect their lungs to the same extent as occurs in adults. There is often no overlying fracture as the child's ribs have deformed and then sprung back to their normal shape. This injury ruptures the pulmonary capillaries allowing blood to fill the alveoli causing hypoxia. Apart from some chest wall bruising, initial evaluation may be negative and there is often no change on the chest radiograph for the first few hours, but clinically there is increasingly poor gas exchange.

Tracheal or bronchial rupture should be suspected in a patient who has a continued significant air leak after a chest drain has been used to treat a pneumothorax, especially with associated subcutaneous emphysema (Hancock & Wiseman 1991). Disruption of the great vessels is usually rapidly fatal at the scene of the accident. Occasionally, a child with this injury survives to reach hospital. In this case, the tear in the vessel has tamponaded itself. Evaluation shows a shocked patient with often poorly palpable peripheral pulses. The diagnosis should be suspected if a widened mediastinum is seen on the chest radiograph.

A ruptured diaphragm may occur following blunt abdominal trauma. The child may be hypoxic due to pulmonary compression and may have signs of hypovolaemia if there has been injury to the viscera. A chest radiograph may show abdominal contents in the thorax.

Abdominal injuries

Abdominal injuries are common in children for a number of reasons. The truncal proportions of the child are such that the abdomen is more prominent than in adults. The abdominal wall is thin, offering relatively little protection. The diaphragm is more horizontal than in adults so that the liver and spleen lie in a position less protected by the ribs. The ribs themselves, being elastic, offer less protection to these organs. Additionally, the bladder is intra-abdominal in young children rather than pelvic and therefore more exposed.

The management of the bleeding intra-abdominal or pelvic injury has been mentioned in the earlier section on primary survey and resuscitation. Again, the stabilisation of the circulation by whatever means necessary is more important than the management of any individual injury. Once the child is stable, however, there are several significant types of injury that must be sought. The commonest of these is blunt trauma to a solid organ, e.g. the liver, spleen or kidneys. Evaluation of these injuries starts, as usual, with a history to see if there is any suspicion that such an injury may have occurred. The abdomen should be evaluated for bruising, lacerations and penetrating wounds and, as in thoracic injury, any evidence of bruising makes the likelihood of significant intra-abdominal damage high. The abdomen should be gently palpated to reveal any areas of tenderness or rigidity and the bowel sounds should be auscultated.

In adults, diagnostic peritoneal lavage is often carried out to ascertain whether there is any evidence of solid organ trauma or rupture of the bowel. In this investigation, saline is introduced into the peritoneum and then withdrawn and examined. The presence of a red cell count of over 100 000 per cubic millimetre, a white cell count of over 500 per cubic millimetre or the presence of enteric contents or bacteria are an indication that there is either blunt abdominal trauma or rupture of the bowel. In adults this would lead, certainly until recently, to immediate laparotomy.

In children there has over the last 10–15 years been a decreasing tendency towards operative management of blunt abdominal trauma (Pranikoff *et al.*, 1994). There are two main reasons for this. First, it has been recognised for many years that the removal of the spleen causes a life-long susceptibility to *Streptococcus pneumoniae* in the affected patients. Second, there is increasing evidence that in the well-managed case, the non-operative treatment of solid organ damage has a better outcome in terms of organ preservation and lowered morbidity than operative treatment (Pearl *et al.*, 1989; Velanovich & Tapper, 1993). This type of management, however, is only possible in a paediatric surgical centre where there is careful monitoring of the patient and the immediate availability of skilled surgeons and anaesthetists to undertake a laparotomy if life-threatening bleeding should supervene. Evaluation in these patients is clinical by means of monitoring of physiological parameters of pulse and blood pressure and also of repeated abdominal examinations, preferrably by the same surgeon. CT is an extremely useful tool in the evaluation of blunt abdominal trauma as the anatomy of the damaged organ can be readily visualised and monitored.

Pelvic injuries

Occult blood loss can occur during pelvic injury and this area requires careful evaluation. The pelvis forms a bony rim to protect the bladder and other pelvic organs but if the pelvis is fractured then there is a significant likelihood of the major iliac vessels being damaged. An indication of pelvic damage is the presence of blood at the external urethral meatus or bruising around the perineum. Pressure on the pelvic rim will be acutely painful in the conscious child with a pelvic fracture.

Radiological evaluation

There are three mandatory radiographs that must be taken at the end of the primary survey and resuscitation phase of trauma management. These are:

1. Lateral cervical spine radiograph.
2. Chest radiograph.
3. Pelvic radiograph.

As discussed above, the evaluation of the integrity of the cervical spine includes both the radiological and physical examination; neither is adequate without the other. To be useful, a cervical spine radiograph must show all the cervical spine from the base of the clivus to C7/T1. Widening of the anterior soft tissue space, loss of the lordotic lines, inequality of the disc spaces, process spaces or facet joints will suggest disruption to the integrity of the cervical spine (Bailey, 1952).

The chest radiograph must be taken so that the clavicles are well centred about the spine and appropriately exposed. In trauma one is looking especially at the width of the mediastinum to indicate any tamponaded great vessel damage, the integrity of the pleura to show any small pneumothorax and the lung fields for opacification indicating underlying contusion. There is a problem with assessment of the mediastinum in the infant. The normal thymus, a very variable structure, causes mediastinal 'widening' and interpretation can be difficult in this age group in trauma. The pelvic radiograph is assessed by following the integrity of the ring formed by the pelvic brim and the two obturator rings seen between the pubic bones and the ischium. A lack of symmetry in the pelvis suggests disruption, usually at a joint. The significance of this is not from the pelvic bony injury itself but the high likelihood of soft tissue, especially vascular injury, in the close vicinity. A minor disruption of the pelvic radiograph appearance may be the only indicator to show from where a severely shocked child is bleeding.

Secondary survey investigations

Once the patient is stable, any investigation may be appropriate depending on the injuries sustained and the urgency required to treat them. Investigations may range from plain radiographs through to ultrasonography and CT to arteriography and radioisotope scanning.

Ultrasonography has the advantage of portability, non-invasiveness and ease of use and is recommended by many as a preliminary investigation for the assessment of intra-abdominal injury in children (Akgur *et al.*, 1993). Its role really is to assess the presence of free fluid, which may be blood, in the abdomen and rectoperitoneal area. The most useful investigation for blunt abdominal trauma is almost certainly the contrast aided computer tomogram. Using this technique the integrity of solid organs, the function of the renal system, the possibility of bowel rupture and the presence of free fluid can all be ascertained.

In the chest, much useful information can be obtained from the primary survey chest radiography. It is unusual to require evaluation of the chest, but in a few instances of chest trauma, arteriography or CT is required (Palder *et al.*, 1991).

By far the most useful investigation in the head injured child is the computerised tomogram which will show the presence of extra or subdural blood collections requiring urgent drainage. CT is less effective at demonstrating raised intracranial pressure. Clinical examination is a better guide and the definitive test is direct measurement through an intracranial pressure monitoring device.

Evaluation of limb injuries

There are few life-threatening extremity injuries but these include:

1. Traumatic amputation of an extremity.
2. Massive open long bone fracture.

These should be dealt with immediately and take precedence over any other extremity injury.

Traumatic amputation of an extremity may be complete or partial. It is usually the latter that presents the greatest initial threat to life because completely transected vessels go into spasm, whereas partially transected vessels do not (Eren *et al.*, 1991). Once airway and breathing have been assessed and stabilised as discussed, exanguinating haemorrhage must be controlled by the application of local pressure and elevation. Occasionally a tourniquet is required. If so, it is best to use the orthopaedic pneumatic variety in which inflation pressure can be easily read and adjusted.

Some amputated limbs are suitable for reimplanatation. Great care needs to be taken to minimise the duration of ischaemia time and the amputated part should be cooled without being allowed to come into direct contact with ice.

More commonly, a serious extremity injury in childhood is not life-threatening but without appropriate treatment is limb threatening. Survival of the limb is particularly at risk where there is serious vascular injury or where there is such severe bone and soft tissue trauma as to make surgical reconstruction unlikely to be successful. Early evaluation of arterial insufficiency is vital. The signs of such are usually referred to as the six Ps.

> Pain
> Paraesthesiae
> Pallor
> Pulselessness
> Paralysis
> 'Perishing with cold'

Any of these signs should alert the surgeon to the possibility of significant arterial insufficiency. It is important to note that there can be a reasonably normal-feeling pulse in a threatened limb caused by collateral circulation which, however, is not sufficient to maintain the integrity of the limb. These children require urgent vascular reconstructive surgery to prevent further loss of tissue from ischaemia and the subsequent amputation.

The compartment syndrome is a more common cause of limb ischaemia in children than direct arterial injury. In some anatomical sites, especially the forearm and lower leg, the limbs are divided into discreet osteofascial compartments by tough fascia attached to the periosteum. Within the compartment, some tissue swelling can be accommodated, but after a certain point, additional swelling leads to increasing intracompartmental pressure and resultant occlusion of the arterioles which supply the muscles. Muscular ischaemia leads to further reactive swelling and a vicious circle develops. This clinical situation is recognised first, by being aware of its possibility, especially in severe injuries and particularly those associated with soft tissue crushing, and second, by the symptoms listed above which indicate muscle and soft tissue ischaemia. The emergency treatment of this condition is fasciotomy.

Evaluation of the child with a fracture

The majority of children attending the emergency department with a fracture will have had only a single injury caused often at play or at sport and frequently the result of a fall. The evaluation aims to obtain the maximum amount of information with the minimum of distress to the child. Examination should be carried out in an environment which makes children feel comfortable. This is often with the patient sitting on the parent's knee and distracted with toys. The child's confidence can be gained by starting the examination on the uninjured side. The examination consists of observation, palpation and, in some instances, movement of the affected extremity.

First, the limb posture should be observed. The child will refrain from movement in an injured limb. In the toddler, who although able to injure himself, is often unable to give an account of the event, the first sign of injury and that which precipitates hospital attendance may be the child's refusal to move the arm or walk upon the leg affected. Of course, other causes may produce pain in a limb, including septic arthritis, osteomyelitis or generalised bone infiltration. Deformity should be easily recognised at this stage.

Having gained all the information available from an observation of the limb both in its posture and shape, the next stage is gentle palpation. The greenstick or buckle fracture is often quite difficult to diagnose. The child is often still using the limb to some extent and there is no visible deformity. The classical feature of these fractures is localised bone tenderness. Although the radiograph will show the injury in most cases, the presence of bone tenderness identifies the area of radiograph to be closely examined and indeed in some instances the diagnosis may rest solely on this sign.

Another crucial part of the initial evaluation by palpation is the search for neurovascular compromise. Neurovascular injury most frequently complicates fractures around the elbow where the arterial blood supply into the forearm or the median or ulna nerves can be damaged. The limb should be evaluated by palpating the peripheral pulses, comparing injured with non-injured side; it is also useful to compare the skin temperature proximal to the site of the injury and more distally. It is often difficult to ascertain sensory loss in the hand in an injured child as approaching him/her with a sharp object to test reaction to pain usually produces distress. An alternative is to look for the absence of sweating on the hand. Increased sympathetic outflow is likely to cause marked sweating on the uninjured side, but fingers whose nerve supply is impaired will feel distinctly dry. Moving the affected limb needs to be done with care. Obviously if there is a displaced fracture with gross deformity, moving the limb is inappropriate; however, in more subtle injuries, moving the injured part and neighbouring joints can help to distinguish a fracture from septic arthritis.

Radiography of fractures

The standard projections for examining a limb radiographically are two views at 90° to one another. These are an anteroposterior and a lateral view. If a patient is thought to have a long bone fracture it is important to include the joints proximal and distal to the injury in the radiograph. This is in order to exclude the presence of a dislocation which may have been caused along with the fracture.

The interpretation of radiographs of injured limbs in children depends on an understanding of the type and position of the fracture. First one must ascertain if the fracture is complete or incomplete. The greenstick or buckle fracture is incomplete and therefore unlikely to become further displaced, but the complete fracture has the potential to move into displacement before bony union occurs. Thus, immobilisation must be effective. Complete fractures may break the bone into only two fragments or into several comprising a comminuted fracture, and the fracture line itself may be transvere, oblique or spiral.

Small bone fragments seen on a radiograph lying near to a joint surface and known as 'chip fractures' are in fact the child's equivalent of the adult 'sprain'. In childhood, because of the strength of the tendons and the limited calcification of bone an injury such as eversion of the ankle may result in a small piece of bone being torn from the main shaft at its attachment to the tendon.

Growth plate injuries

Growth plate injuries are unique to childhood. It is crucial that they are recognised early and managed correctly. There are a number of different types of growth plate injury and the widely accepted classification is that developed by Harrison and Salter in 1963 which has grouped these injuries into five broad categories.

Type 1 injury

The line of separation runs through the growth plate without involving the metaphysis or epiphysis. This injury is seen in younger children and the prognosis is usually good.

Type 2 injury

This is the commonest type of growth plate injury. The line of separation begins within the physis and exits through the metaphysis creating a triangular fragment of bone.

Type 3 injury

This injury starts in the growth plate and leaves through the joint via the epiphysis. It is not common.

Type 4 injury

The fracture line runs through the metaphysis, thence through the physis and exits via the epiphysis into the joint. This is a complex injury which may lead to growth problems.

Type 5 injury

This is a difficult injury to recognise radiologically. It is a lesion in which the growth plate is crushed between the metaphysis and the epiphysis. It may lead to limb shortening if the germinal layer of the growth plate is permanently damaged. Children who have had growth plate injuries therefore should be followed up until it is clear that no risk of impaired growth remains.

Initial recognition of child abuse

The diagnosis of child abuse is generally a complex one to which several agencies may contribute including physicians, radiologists, social workers, police, etc. The initial suspicion of child abuse is usually based on a combination of historical and physical features.

There are a number of different types of abuse:

1. Physical abuse (non-accidental injury).
   a. Bruises, abrasions and lacerations.
   b. Fractures.
   c. Internal injuries (truncal or intracranial).
   d. Thermal injuries.
2. Sexual abuse (acute or chronic).
3. Psychosocial deprivation (neglect).
4. Munchhausen's syndrome by proxy.

An individual child may and often does suffer from more than one type of abuse.

Historical features suggestive of physical abuse

1. The history of the injury is inconsistent with the findings made on a physical examination.
2. Inappropriate delay in seeking advice after the occurrence of a significant injury.
3. Significantly different explanations produced for the same injuries to different professionals.
4. The child or another child is said to have caused the injury in a manner inconsistent with that child's development (e.g. a non-mobile infant who is said to have injured himself spontaneously).

Physical findings in child abuse

In addition to the finding of an injury which is inconsistent with the history of the alleged incident, there are a number of characteristic physical findings in injured children which are suggestive (although in general not diagnostic) of child abuse. All such injuries must be evaluated in the light of the history given.

Fingertip bruising and slap marks, especially around the face, suggest inflicted injury. Injuries to the ear occur rather infrequently accidentally, so bruising on both sides of or inside the pinna is suggestive. Bruises caused by a stick or other artefact show as a line of bruising on either side of the object's impression and bruising of various ages as shown by a colour change from red to yellowish brown suggests injuries caused at different times.

Any bruising occurring in an infant who is not mobile should be regarded with caution as should a torn frenulum which may be caused accidentally but can be caused by the forceful thrusting of a bottle into a baby's mouth.

Fractures are more difficult to interpret as being clearly accidental or non-accidental; however, there are some characteristic fractures which are generally associated with child abuse. These include rib fractures which rarely occur accidentally except in a very significant major trauma incident. Multiple 'chip' fractures at the growing ends of bones can be caused when a child is shaken, pulled or twisted aggressively. Multiple fractures in different stages of healing in the absence of an underlying bone disease are highly suggestive of child abuse (Carty, 1993).

Again, in a non-mobile baby, any fracture must be considered very carefully in the light of the history given. The characteristics of non-accidental skull fracture in infants are that there is more likely to be underlying brain damage, more than one skull bone is involved and fracture of the occiput is especially characteristic, together with multiple wide branching fractures. Non-accidental burns and scalds are characterised by the 'glove' or 'stocking' scalds which are caused by forcing a limb into too hot water.

This type of injury may also be present on the buttock or perineum. Cigarette burns are characterised by being circular and deep with a raised indurated edge.

Occasionally, young infants are shaken violently causing both the 'chip' fractures mentioned above and also significant intracranial injury. The deceleration, acceleration and rotational forces which are acting on the brain within the cranium during the act of violent shaking causes tearing of blood vessels, disruption of axons and subsequent brain swelling and bleeding. These infants present to hospital in a coma or with convulsions and will usually not have an accompanying history of trauma. The child may at first be considered to have meningitis or septicaemia, but an examination of the retinae may show the characteristic retinal haemorrhage which occurs frequently in this injury (Carty & Ratcliffe, 1995).

References

Akgur, S. M., Tanyel, F. C., Akhan, O. *et al.* (1993). The place of ultrasonographic examination in the initial evaluation of children sustaining blunt abdominal trauma. *Journal of Pediatric Surgery*, **28**, 78–81.

Bailey, D. K. (1952). The normal cervical spine in infants and children. *Radiology*, **59**, 712–19.

Baker, F. P., O'Neill, B., Haddon, W. & Long, W. B. (1974). The Injury Severity Score: a method for describing patients with multiple injuries and evaluating emergency care. *Journal of Trauma*, **14**, 187–96.

Boyd, C. R., Tolson, M. A. & Copes, W. S. (1987). Evaluating trauma care: the Triss method. *Journal of Trauma*, **27**, 370–8.

Carty, H. (1993). Fractures caused by child abuse. *Journal of Bone and Joint Surgery*, **75**, 849–57.

Carty, H. & Ratcliffe, J. (1995). The shaken infant syndrome. *British Medical Journal*, **310**, 344–5.

Champion, H. R., Copes, W. S., Sacco, W. J., Lawnwick, M. M., *et al.* (1990). The Major Trauma Outcome Study: establishing national norms for trauma care. *Journal of Trauma*, **30**, 1356–65.

Champion, H. R., Sacco, W. I., Carazzo, A. J. *et al.* (1981). The Trauma Score. *Critical Care Medicine*, **9**, 672–6.

Champion, H. R., Sacco, W. I., Copes, W. S., Gann, D. S., Gennarelli, P. A. & Flanagan, M. E. (1989). A revision of the Trauma Score. *Journal of Trauma*, **29**, 623–9.

Eren, N., Ozgen, G., Ener, B. K., *et al.* (1991). Peripheral vascular injuries in children. *Journal of Pediatric Surgery*, **26**, 1164–8.

Hancock B. J. & Wiseman, N. E. (1991). Tracheobronchial injuries in children. *Journal of Pediatric Surgery*, **26**, 1316–19.

Ildstaf, F. T., Tollerud, D. J., Weiss, R. G., *et al.* 1990). Cardiac contusion in pediatric patients with blunt thoracic trauma. *Journal of Pediatric Surgery*, **25**, 287–9.

Jubelirer, R. A., Agarwal, N. N., Beyer, F. C. III, Ferraro, P. J., *et al.* (1990). Pediatric trauma triage: review of 1,307 cases. *Journal of Trauma*, **30**, 1544–7.

Kitchens, J. L., Groff, D. B., Nagaraj, H. S. & Fallat, M. E. (1991). Basilar skull fractures in childhood with cranial nerve involvement. *Journal of Pediatric Surgery*, **26**, 992–4.

Langer, J. C., Winthrop, A. L., Wesson, D. E., *et al.* (1989). Diagnosis and incidence of cardiac injury in children with blunt thoracic trauma. *Journal of Pediatric Surgery*, 4, 1091–4.

Mackway-Jones, K., Molyneux, E., Phillips, B. & Wieteska, S. (1993). *Advanced Paediatric Life Support*. London, England: British Medical Journal Press.

Nayduch, D. A., Moyland, J., Rutledge, R., Baker, C. C., *et al.* (1991). Comparison of the ability of Adult and Pediatric Trauma Scores to predict pediatric outcome following major trauma. *Journal of Trauma*, 31, 452–7.

Orenstein, J. B., Klein, B. L., Gotsdhall, C., Ochsenschlager, D. W., *et al.* (1994). Age and outcome in paediatric cervical spine injury: eleven year experience. *Paediatric Emergency Care*, 10, 132–7.

Palder, S. B., Shandling, B. & Manson, D. (1991). Rupture of thoracic trachea following blunt trauma: diagnosis by CAT scan. *Journal of Pediatric Surgery*, 26, 1320–2.

Pang, D. & Pollack, I. F. (1989). Spinal cord injury without radiographic abnormality in children: the SCIWORA syndrome. *Journal of Trauma*, 69, 654–64.

Pearl, R. H., Wesson, D. E., Spence, L. J., Filler, R. M., Ein, S. H., Shandling, B. & Superina, R. A. (1989). Splenic injury: a five year update with improved results and changing criteria for conservative management. *Journal of Pediatric Surgery*, 24, 121–5.

Pigula, S. A., Wald, S. L., Shackford, F. R. & Vane, D. W. (1993). The effects of hypotension and hypoxia on children with severe head injuries. *Journal of Pediatric Surgery*, 28, 310–15.

Pranikoff, T., Hirschl, R. B., Schlesinger, A. E., Polley, T. Z. & Curan, A. G. (1994). Resolution of splenic injury after non-operative management *Journal of Pediatric Surgery*, 29, 1366–9.

Ramenofsky, N. L., Ramenofsky, M. B. & Jurkovic, G. I. (1988). The predictive validity of the Pediatric Trauma Score. *Journal of Trauma*, 28, 1038–42.

Saladino, R., Lund, D. & Fleisher, G. (1991). The spectrum of liver and spleen injuries in children: failure of the Pediatric Trauma Score and clinical signs to predict isolated injuries. *Annals of Emergency Medicine*, 20, 636–40.

Teasdale, G. & Jennett, B. (1974). Assessment of coma and impaired consciousness: a practical scale. *Lancet*, 11, 81.

Tepas, J. J. III, Di Scala, C., Ramenossky, M. L. & Barlow, B. (1990). Mortality in head injury: the pediatric perspective. *Journal of Paediatric Surgery*, 25, 92–6.

Tepas, J. J. III, Mollitt, B. L., Talbert, J. L. & Bryant, N. (1987). The Pediatric Trauma Score as a predictor of injury severity in the injured child. *Journal of Pediatric Surgery*, 22, 14–18.

Velanovich, V. & Tapper, D. (1993). Decision analysis in children with blunt splenic trauma: the effects of observation, splenorrhaphy or splenectomy on Quality Adjusted Life Expectancy. *Journal of Pediatric Surgery*, 28, 179–85.

Yates, D. W., Woodford, M. & Hollis, S. (1992). Preliminary analysis of the care of injured patients in thirty-three British hospitals: first report on the United Kingdom Major Trauma Outcome Study. *British Medical Journal*, 305, 737–40.

6
Injuries of the developing brain

C. M. BANNISTER

Introduction

'Brain injury' is a term commonly used and accepted to mean that the cerebrum has been damaged by being exposed to severe mechanical forces which are sufficiently powerful to fracture the skull and/or harm the brain by subjecting it to violent, disruptive movements. The immediate or primary effects of such an injury can be to tear the surface of the brain, disrupt the white fibre tracts within the substance of the brain, rupture blood vessels or cause them to go into spasm together with other less easily identifiable consequences, such as interruption of normal transmission across synapses. The immediate effects of a head injury are often followed by delayed or secondary ones which are potentially as damaging. Blood vessels running through channels in the skull and on the outer surface of the dura may be torn and bleed to give rise, several hours later, to an extradural haematoma. Rupture of vessels running on the surface of the brain, both arteries and veins, can produce subdural haematomas which take time to develop. Tearing of vessels within the brain parenchyma can give rise some time later to intracerebral haematomas which can vary in size from tiny petechial haemorrhages to large blood clots. Haemorrhages close to the ventricles may burst into their cavities causing an intraventricular haemorrhage which can later lead to hydrocephalus if an obstruction of the ventricular system or subarachnoid spaces supervenes. Disruption or spasm of the larger cerebral arteries can lead to infarction of the territories they supply. Intracranial haematomas, whether extradural, subdural or intracerebral, and infarction accompanied by cerebral oedema may cause the intracranial pressure to rise, and this in turn will lead to further brain damage if it causes a critical fall in the cerebral perfusion pressure. Fractures of the skull can result in a separated segment of bone being pushed into the underlying brain and, if in addition the scalp is torn and infection supervenes, several days later a brain abscess can develop in the injured parenchyma.

During birth, the neonatal period and throughout infancy the developing brain is at risk of being injured in a conventional manner, but prenatally the foetus is protected from mechanical injury by the mother's abdominal wall, the uterus and the cushioning effect of the amniotic fluid. There are only a few reports in the literature of foetuses who have had mechanical head injuries, and those that have survived have had very severe brain damage (Fowler *et al.*, 1971; Cohen & Roessmann, 1994). In practical terms, therefore, human foetuses are not at great risk of being subjected to a primary head injury, but they are most certainly not immune from the many events which follow a primary head injury, namely cerebral infarction, cerebral oedema, intracerebral and intraventricular haematomas, secondary obstructive hydrocephalus and possibly raised intracranial pressure.

In this chapter the foetus will be judged to be 'head injured' if it has sustained any of the conditions included in the list of secondary head injuries. As the greater part of brain development has been completed by the end of infancy, the developmental period chosen to be considered extends from the onset of foetal life to the end of infancy.

Relevant aspects of brain development

As the stage of development reached by the brain at the time of injury profoundly influences the outcome, in the following section aspects of brain development of particular relevance are emphasised.

The embryonic period is the first 8 weeks of gestation. During the first 4 weeks the neural groove is formed by the rapid division of the cells in the neural plate. With further division of the cells the edges of the neural groove roll towards one another and fuse to form the neural tube. During the latter part of the embryonic period evagination of two vesicles from the lateral aspects of the rostal end of the neural tube and other changes in the geometry of the tube results in the adult configuration of the ventricular system being reached. Throughout the embryonic period cells lining the lumen of the neural tube are dividing rapidly and even before the start of the foetal period, some have begun to migrate toward the periphery.

By the eighth week of gestation, the beginning of the foetal period, the germinal matrix is well defined and lines the walls of the ventricular system. At this stage the germinal matrix is mainly producing neuroblasts but not exclusively as some glial cells are known to be present, the best known of these being the radial glial cells. Their cell processes extend from the lumen of the ventricles to the pial surface of the developing brain. The processes form a scaffolding up which the neuroblasts climb to reach their destinations in the developing cortical plate (Rakic, 1972). These processes, first described in animals (Rakic, 1972), have subsequently been seen in human foetuses (Choi & Lapham, 1978; Larroche & Houcine, 1982; Gadisseux & Eurard, 1985). In the cerebral hemispheres the innermost layers of the cortical plate are laid down first, neuroblasts produced later migrate through the already formed deeper layers to reach their more peripheral final destinations (Angevine & Sidman, 1961; Sidman & Angevine, 1962; Altman, 1966). In this way the laminar structure of the cortex is gradually built up and by the 24th week of gestation all six layers of the cortex are present (Larroche, 1962). While younger neuroblasts are being produced, those that have already migrated into position are producing cell processes which gather together to form fibre tracts. At this stage of development the cortical mantle of many mammals, as demonstrated by the brain of the 17-day-old rat foetus (Figure 6.1), is divided into four zones. The deepest is the ventricular zone or germinal matrix lying adjacent to the ventricular lumen. The cells in the ventricular zone about to migrate are densely packed together and lined up in columns (Figure 6.2). The intermediate zone contains tracts of unmyelinated cell processes lying parallel to the cortical surface. The cortical plate is formed by the neuroblasts which have already migrated. The marginal zone is a thin acellular layer lying between the cortical plate and the pial surface of the brain. In the human foetus a transient layer of granular cells is laid down beneath the pia between the 12th and 22nd weeks of gestation. Later the layer is gradually removed and the last traces of it disappear from the frontal and occipital cortices during the 39th week of gestation. Synapses between axons and dendrites have been seen as early as the seventh week of gestation (Larroche, 1981) which is before the cortical plate is formed at 10 weeks. By 15 or 16 weeks of gestation axons can be seen running vertically in the deeper layers of the cortical plate (Molliver et al., 1973).

Large-scale production of neurons is over by the 16th week of gestation and from then on the volume of the germinal matrix steadily decreases so that by the 32nd or 33rd week of gestation it is represented only by relatively discrete masses of cells covering the head of the caudate nucleus, and lying in the thalamostriate groove close to the foramen of Monro, in the roof of the temporal horn and in the external wall of the occipital horn. Most neurons originate in the germinal matrix, but a few are produced elswhere within the developing parenchyma. Although the majority of neurons are produced in the early part of gestation, some production continues in selected parts of the brain throughout the foetal period, in particular the cerebellum, where it continues to a limited extent up to the end of the first postnatal year.

During the second half of foetal life, when the bulk of neuron production is over, there is a progressive increase in the volume of the cell bodies of individual neurons and a rapid multiplication of their cell processes. There is also a proliferation of glial cells, although in the white matter glial cells do not appear in large numbers until just before myelination begins. At the same time as these changes are taking place there is a vast multiplication of the capillaries. The combined effect of the growth of all these structures not only leads to a dramatic increase in the size of the brain but also to an increase in the surface area of the cortex. To accommodate the increase in brain bulk

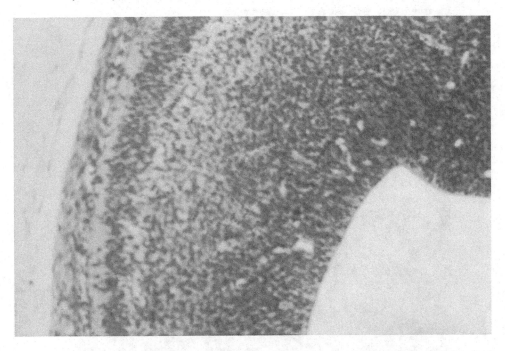

Figure 6.1. Developing cortical mantle of a foetal rat showing the germinal matrix and the intermediate zone through which neuroblasts are migrating to reach the cortical plate. Haematoxylin and eosin. × 60.

within the limited space available in the calvarium, the cortical surface becomes convoluted. At about 20 weeks of gestation the Sylvian fissure can be identified ultrasonographically in the human foetus (Figure 6.3). It is followed by the development of other sulci so that by the end of gestation two-thirds of the cortical surface is buried within their folds. The size of the lateral ventricles, as measured at the confluence of the body with the occipital and temporal horns, the atrium, alter little throughout gestation although the proportion of brain they occupy progressively diminishes throughout foetal life (Johnson *et al.*, 1980; Leanty *et al.*, 1981; Pretorius *et al.*, 1986).

Myelination contributes little to the increasing size of the foetal brain. It commences in the spinal cord and brainstem and only reaches the basal parts of the brain by the end of gestation. After birth myelination and glial cell proliferation, together with increasing arborisation of the dendrites and the formation of synapses, account for the continuing rapid growth of the brain which occurs throughout the neonatal period and the whole of infancy. Myelination of the brain is not complete until the seventh postnatal year of life.

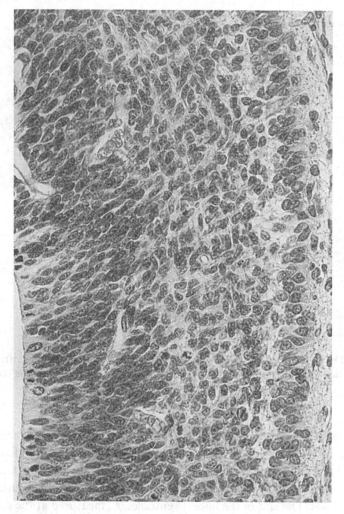

Figure 6.2. Germinal matrix of the developing cortical mantle of a foetal rat showing neuroblasts lined up in columns prior to migrating to the cortical plate. Haematoxylin and eosin. × 120.

The development of the brain takes place in a series of precisely defined steps, each step being rigorously controlled by sequentially triggered activity of numerous growth factors switched on and off by the appropriate genes. Discussion of the details of this exquisitely complex system is beyond the scope of this chapter. Once the requisite number of neurons has been produced, the genes ordering their multiplication are switched off permanently, and new neurons cannot be produced to make up for any losses. Neuronal loss starts in the foetal cortex due to overproduction of cells. Surviv-

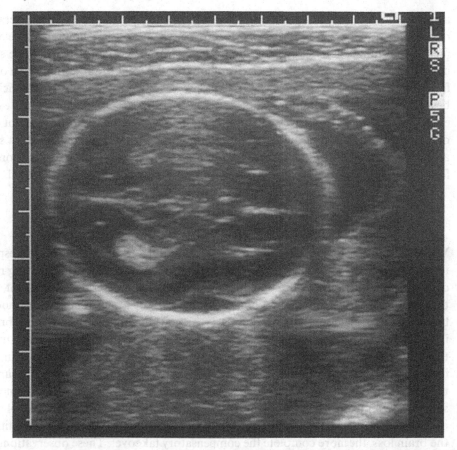

Figure 6.3. Ultrasound scan of a human foetus at 20 weeks of gestation showing early
development of the Sylvian fissure.

ing neurons are targeted by axons and make synaptic connections in an orderly,
programmed manner, while the fate of untargeted cells is destruction. This infinitely
complex process of linking up neurons with axons not only has to take place quickly, it
also has to be error-proof and it involves not only adjacent parts of the brain, but the
central nervous system as a whole.

Once brain development is underway, and neurons have started to move into their
definitive locations and have begun to make connections with nearby and distant cells,
it is understandable how it would be impossible and organisationally chaotic for
neurons produced later to be incorporated meaningfully into the system whether it be
to make up for neurons lost because of disease or any other mishap. The permanent
and irreversible switching off of the genes which direct the orderly and sequential
production of neurons protects the brain from this ever happening. As a consequence if

a part of the brain is destroyed, even at the beginning of the foetal period, regeneration of neurons cannot occur to replace the lost tissue. The brain does, however, have other methods of functionally compensating for lost tissue. There does appear to be some degree of functional overlap between most areas of adjacent brain so that some of the functions of the lost brain are taken over, a process known as plasticity. Plasticity is best expressed in the young foetal brain but it is still operational to a limited extent even in the mature brain. How well plasticity is able to compensate depends not only on the age of the brain at the time of injury, but also on the region affected. In some areas the compensatory processes are far more effective than others and occasionally, for example in the primary visual cortex, they do not appear to operate at all.

Pathological response of the developing brain to injury

While there are many similarities in the way that mature and immature brains respond to injury, there are also major differences. As the immature brain is undergoing rapid development, injuries have the potential to interfere, to a greater or lesser extent, with that process both locally and in more distant parts of the brain. While the methods of breaking down and removing dead tissue is the same in immature and mature brains, in the immature one it is much more rapid. Final healing in the immature brain, unlike the mature one, is accomplished with very little gliosis. The features which both injured immature and mature brains have in common is that in neither does neuronal regeneration play a part in the repair processes and in both loss of tissue is compensated for to a greater or lesser extent by plasticity, i.e. the functional take over of some of the lost activities by the remaining brain. The more immature the brain at the time of the brain loss, the more complete the compensatory takeover. These observations will be discussed in the following sections by reference to experimental studies of animal models and to findings in humans who have experienced brain injuries at different times during development.

Pathological changes following injury of the foetal brain in animal models

Most studies describing changes in the developing brain after injury have been carried out in the laboratory on animal models. Some years ago a colleague and I made a study of the effects of injury on the foetal rat brain (Bannister & Chapman, 1986). The rat pup is born on the 23rd day of gestation. At birth its brain is estimated to have reached the same stage of development as an 16 to 18-week-old human foetus. Lesions made in the rat foetal brain on the 18th day of gestation means that they were inflicted at a time when the germinal matrix was actively producing neurons and neuroblasts were still migrating out of the ventricular zone and into the cortical plate to form the cortex. We made lesions in the cerebral hemispheres of Sprague-Dawley rat foetuses on the 18th day of gestation by passing a 25 French gauge hypodermic needle bent at a right angle through the wall of the uterus and into one or other of the hemispheres. The needle was swept through 360° to create the lesion. Some foetuses were sacrificed immediately after the lesion had been made and their brains were examined histologically to determine the extent of the damage. They were found to have intracerebral haematomas of varying sizes as well as disruption of the adjacent cerebral substance. The remaining pups delivered spontaneously at term and were sacrificed at birth, 2 days, 2 weeks, and 4–16 weeks after birth. Histological examination of the brains of the pups sacrificed at birth or 2 days after birth showed that there were areas of necrosis in the cortex. Numerous macrophages were present in the necrotic areas and the surrounding tissues. Remnants of the haematoma were present in some of the brains but were actively being broken down as evidenced by the number of haemosiderin granules in the area. Stains for glial fibrillary acid protein (GFAP) were sometimes positive indicating that a few astrocytes in the area had undergone reactive change in response to the trauma (Figure 6.4). All of the brains of the pups sacrificed 2 weeks after birth had a cyst of considerable size in the traumatised hemisphere (Figure 6.5). In addition to the loss of cortical tissue, the ipsilateral hippocampus and the whole of the midbrain were smaller than normal. There was only a little gliosis in the tissues around the cyst. The findings in the brains of the pups sacrificed 4–16 weeks after birth were very similar to those of the 2-week-old pups. None of the pups examined before sacrifice exhibited any abnormal neurological signs.

These studies were pursued further by carrying out a unilateral excision of the occipital lobe in foetal lambs (Chapman & Bannister, 1989). At about the 70th day of gestation the same stage of development has been reached by the foetal lamb brain as the foetal rat brain at 18 days. The germinal matrix is present and actively producing neuroblasts. The intermediate zone contains tracts of fibres and neuroblasts are in the process of migrating to the cortical plate. The cortical plate is comprised of numerous cells which are stratified into laminae. The occipital lobe excision was carried out after a uterotomy had been carried out and the lamb's head delivered through it. An incision was made in either of the parieto-occipital regions and after a small bone flap had been raised the dura was opened and the occipital lobe was removed by a combination of suction and blunt dissection. After the bone flap had been replaced and the scalp sutured, the foetal head was returned to the uterus. The lambs were delivered spontaneously at term. All the lambs were allowed to survive for between 84 and 133 days after birth before being sacrificed. The brains were perfused fixed in situ prior to removal. In each of the brains the area of excision in the occipital lobe could be clearly identified (Figure 6.6). In all animals the excised area had a uniformly smooth surface which, in some of the brains, was in continuity with the cavity of the adjacent lateral ventricle. In some brains there were a few positive GFAP fibres and occasional

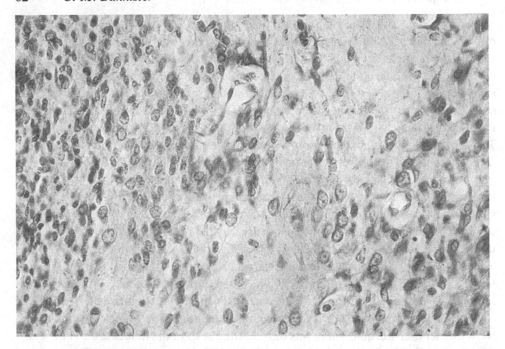

Figure 6.4. A few glial fibres in the traumatised parenchyma of the foetal rat brain stain positively with gial fibrillary acid protein indicating that some reactive glial cells are present. × 120.

astrocytes lying immediately beneath the smooth surface. No signs of regeneration or attempts to reform the excised cortex were seen in any of the brains. In more than half of the brains examined the dorsolateral geniculate nucleus in the operated hemisphere was reduced in size compared with the unoperated one (Figure 6.7). In addition, there were striking changes in the frontal lobes of the operated hemispheres. There was a consistent distortion of the sulcal pattern, the transverse sulcus, one of the principal convolutions in the sheep's brain, was displaced posteriorly (Figure 6.8), and in addition the white fibre tracts in the frontal lobes were reduced in size (Figure 6.9). These findings illustrate the profound and widespread changes which occur in at least the ipsilateral hemisphere after the foetal brain has been subjected to trauma at an early stage of foetal life. It is probable that the loss of projection fibres from the occipital lobe to the frontal region and other parts of the brain was responsible either directly or indirectly for the altered gyral pattern and the reduction in size of the dorsolateral geniculate nucleus.

These experimental findings confirm that loss of tissue at an early stage of brain development cannot be replaced and that dead tissue is removed rapidly by macrophages and is followed by repair processes in which remarkably little reactive gliosis

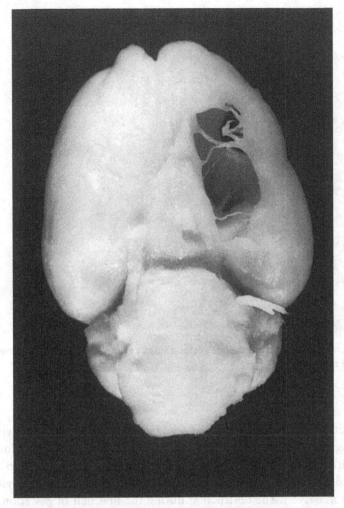

Figure 6.5. Rat pup with a cyst in the right cerebral hemisphere at the site where it was traumatised in utero.

occurs. The consequences of loss of the tissue have profound effects both locally and in distant parts of the brain.

Pathological changes in the human brain following injury

The findings of our experimental studies are in accord with those of Spatz who in 1921 reported that trauma-induced necrosis in human foetal brains was followed by excep-

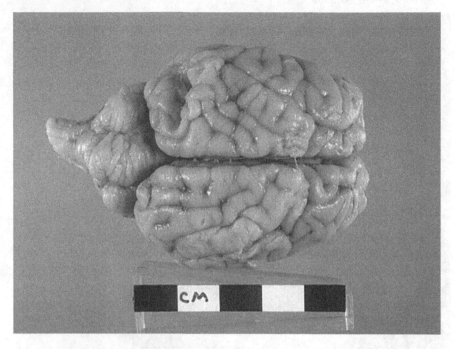

Figure 6.6. Lamb with a cyst in the left occipital lobe at the site where the excision had been carried out in utero.

tionally fast liquefaction and dissolution of the dead tissue as a result of the activity of rapidly disappearing macrophages. Spatz also noted that there was little or no forma- tion of glial scars around the residual lesion which was often a smooth-walled cyst. Friede (1989) found in human foetuses that while practically no residual gliosis occurred even after massive tissue destruction during the first half of gestation, the capacity of the astrocytes to react by proliferation does begin to develop during the last trimester of human gestation, and is well developed in the full-term newborn infant. On the other hand, as we found in our animal models, the macrophage–monocyte– microglial system is active at a much earlier stage. Monocytes have been found in the human foetal circulation as early as the fourth week of gestation, and numbers approximately the same as those in full-term infants are present from the 20th week of gestation (Playfair *et al.*, 1963). By the end of gestation the foetal brain deals with trauma by removing dead tissue and forming of a gliotic scar in a way which is progressing rapidly towards the adult method of healing.

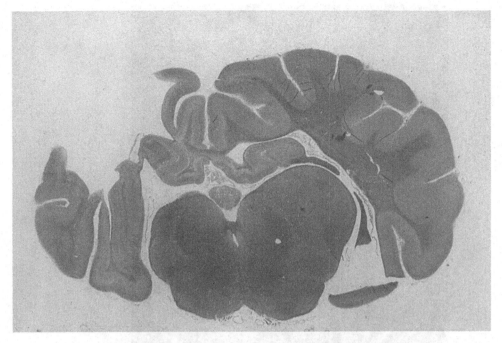

Figure 6.7. Dorsolateral geniculate nuclei of a lamb that had undergone excision of cortical material from the left occipital lobe at about the 70th day of gestation. The left dorsolateral geniculate nucleus is considerably smaller than the right one.

Traumatic events suffered by the developing brain at different ages

Whatever the cause of cell death and necrosis, whether it be mechanical injury, infarction from loss of the arterial blood supply, compression of the surrounding parenchyma by a haematoma within the brain following spontaneous or traumatic rupture of a blood vessel, or an extradural or subdural haematoma reducing the blood supply of the underlying brain to below the critical level, the healing processes and removal of the haematoma are the same. It is only the age of the subject at the time when the lesion occurred which causes differences in the healing processes. While the end points of different injuries are the same, however, age is also a major influence on how the injury is caused.

Injuries of the foetal brain

A wide diversity of conditions are now acknowledged to have adverse effects on the foetal cerebral circulation leading to intracranial haemorrhages, ischaemia and in-

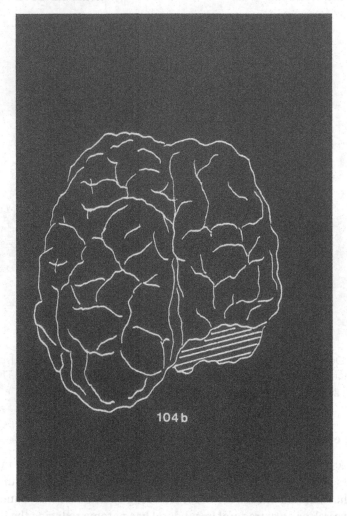

Figure 6.8. Drawing of the brain of a lamb which had undergone excision of material from the right occipital lobe at about the 70th day of gestation. The transverse sulcus of the left side is displaced posteriorly; the right sulcus is in the normal position.

farction. The fault may be in the mother, the foetus, the placenta and umbilical cord, or unknown. Maternal causes include systemic disorders, pre-eclampsia leading to a rise in the maternal blood pressure (Sibony *et al.*, 1993), carbon dioxide (Schweden- berg, 1959) and butane gas poisoning (Gosseye *et al.*, 1982), trauma (Fowler *et al.*, 1971; Cohen & Roesmann, 1994) and drug abuse, particularly cocaine (Levene, 1993). Among the foetal causes are immune (rhesus incompatibility) and non-immune hy- drops foetalis caused, among other things, by heart failure from severe congenital

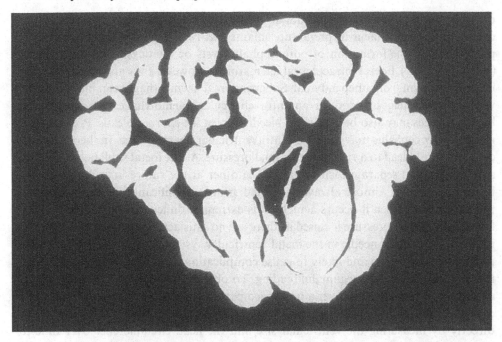

Figure 6.9. Drawing of a coronal section of the frontal lobes of a lamb which underwent excision of material from the left occipital lobe at about the 70th day of gestation. The left frontal lobe is generally smaller than the right one, and its white fibre tracts are considerably reduced in size compared with the normal.

heart anomalies such as Fallot's tetralogy and blood dyscrasia particularly thrombocytopenia, the foetal platelets being low because of destruction by maternal antibodies. Intrauterine infection by one of the TORCH organisms, or the mother having had a previous splenectomy (Carloss *et al.*, 1980; Aster, 1990) are also possible causes. Multiple pregnancies may lead to unequal sharing of placental resources resulting in the discordant growth of one of the foetuses or, if aberrant placental vessels are present, the twin–twin transfusion syndrome may develop allowing the recipient twin to grow at the expense of the donor. Infarction and calcification of the placenta increases the risk of the foetal cerebral circulation being impaired, as does a knot in the umbilical cord. In the greatest number of affected foetuses, however, the causes of intracranial haemorrhage or ischaemic lesions remain unknown. This may change in the future as ultrasound imaging becomes even more sophisticated than it is at present and nuclear magnetic resonance imaging (MRI) is adapted more successfully to examine the foetus.

Ischaemic infarcts resulting from occlusion of a major cerebral artery may occur in foetuses although the presence of an extremely good collateral circulation probably protects the brain unless an additional problem co-exists. Necrosis of white matter resembling leucomalacia in premature infants has been reported and described as proceeding to the formation of porencephalic cysts or multicystic encephalopathy (Larroche, 1993). Foetal intracerebral haematomas, however they are caused, may be intraparenchymal or subependymal. Subependymal haemorrhages can burst into the ventricular system to produce an intraventricular haemorrhage. Intraventricular haemorrhages may also be caused by bleeding from the choroid plexus. Posthaemorrhagic hydrocephalus may follow an intraventricular haemorrhage. In theory hydrocephalus could lead to a rise in intracranial pressure. As the foetal skull bones are thin and pliable and separate easily from one another at the suture lines, however, the brain is probably almost always protected from a significant rise in intracranial pressure except when it occurs acutely. It is extremely difficult to be certain that the foetal intracranial pressure is raised as there are no satisfactory methods of measuring it directly. Placing a needle in the foetal ventricular system is possible but is not only potentially dangerous and likely to cause complications, it is also painful and, therefore, unlikely to give a meaningful reading. To obtain useful information it would be necessary to take readings over a prolonged period and that at the present cannot be carried out non-invasively. Currently it is only possible to assess the pressure indirectly by measuring the ventricular size and the head circumference over time to decide whether they are increasing disproportionately quickly. If they are it is probable that the brain is being stretched, and if this becomes extreme the blood supply to the cortex and other areas of the brain may be reduced below the critical level even though the intracranial pressure is not particularly high.

Injuries of the postnatal brain

Premature infants

Premature infants are at risk of brain injury from ischaemia, hypoxia and intraparenchymal and intraventricular haemorrhages. Currently, premature infants born as early as the 24th or 25th week of gestation are kept alive by intubation and ventilation. Parts of the germinal matrix are present up to about the 36th week of gestation, and together with the choroid plexus, are a source of haemorrhage into the ventricular system and brain parenchyma. Liquefaction and removal of the haemorrhagic infarct leaves porencephalic cysts of varying size which almost invariably communicate with the adjacent lateral ventricle. Haemorrhages from the germinal matrix bursting into the ventricular system, as in the foetus, may give rise to posthaemorrhagic hydrocephalus due to structural blockage of part of the ventricular system or the subarachnoid space by the blood. The younger the premature infant at birth the greater the risk of it developing a brain injury because the more immature the lung the greater the difficulty of achieving adequate oxygenation. Hypoxia can cause white matter necrosis and leukomalacia which, if extensive enough, can lead to the formation of porencephalic cysts or multicystic encephalopathy.

Full-term infants at birth

From the onset of labour, there are many risk factors which place the infant in danger of sustaining brain damage. Anoxic brain damage can result from early separation of the placenta or if the placental circulation is compromised during uterine contractions. During passage of the head through the birth canal excessive mounding of the calvarium may also traumatise the brain. Babies born in the breech position are at risk because the head has little time to mould before it has to pass rapidly through the birth canal, or if the head cannot be delivered quickly enough the baby may become anoxic before breathing is established. A too short umbilical cord or a cord wrapped around the baby's neck can lead to anoxic brain damage. Cephalopelvic disproportion necessitating the use of forceps to assist the delivery of the infant's head may also result in brain damage. Depressed fractures may be caused by faulty application of forceps or by the infant's head being compressed against the wall of the mother's pelvis. In the majority of these so-called pond fractures, the overlying scalp is intact and there is, therefore, no risk of infection and cerebral abscess occurring.

Anoxia can lead to areas of necrosis scattered throughout the brain. Compression of the skull may cause subdural haematomas and intracerebral haemorrhages in both the cerebral hemispheres and the cerebellum. A tear of the tentorium accompanied by haemorrhaging over the surface of the cerebellum and an intracerebellar haematoma are characteristic of a birth injury caused by compression of the skull.

Neonates and young infants

In neonates and young infants accidental brain injuries are caused by them being dropped, and having their heads being hit against hard objects. Non-accidental injuries are caused by violent shaking, blows aimed at the head or the head being deliberately hit against hard objects. Rupture of blood vessels on the surface of the brain leads to the formation of subdural haematomas and subarachnoid haemorrhages. Infarction and intracerebral haematomas follow disruption of brain's arterial blood supply. The long, white fibre tracts may be torn by shearing forces which traverse the brain. Extradural haematomas are uncommon in this age group because the dura is still tightly bound to the inner aspect of the calvarium but they do occasionally occur. Road traffic accidents which are a common cause of head injuries in older subjects account for relatively few head injuries in infants of all ages.

Older infants

Older infants are at risk of the same traumatic events as younger ones; however, once they become mobile they face the additional hazards of falls in the home, either off furniture, down stairs or out of windows and they occasionally pull heavy objects onto themselves. The risk of depressed fractures with scalp wounds become more common, and the risk of infection with abscess formation is therefore present. In the older infant the incidence of extradural haemorrhages rises.

Diagnosis and management of head injuries of the developing brain

The diagnosis and management of brain injuries depends on the age of the subject at the time of the injury. It is inappropriate in this chapter to give more than a brief outline of how in the different age groups the diagnosis is established and the injuries are managed.

Foetuses

Developments in ultrasonography have made it possible to make a detailed examination of the human foetal brain from about the 20th week of gestation. Recently shed haemorrhages in the brains are imaged as bright echogenic areas. These become echolucent after the blood has liquefied and been removed to leave an intraparenchymal or porencephalic cyst (Figure 6.10). Haemorrhages into the ventricular system can also be clearly identified by ultrasound. Foetuses with this diagnosis are scanned at intervals to see if they are developing hydrocephalus. If they do and the hydrocephalus is progressive, provided their lungs are mature enough to allow spontaneous breathing after birth (generally at a gestational age of about 33 weeks), the foetus is delivered by caesarean section to allow an indwelling cerebrospinal fluid (CSF) diversion system to be inserted. Attempts to drain CSF from one of the ventricles into the amniotic cavity with an indwelling ventricular catheter (Clewell *et al.*, 1982; Frigoletto *et al.*, 1982; Glick *et al.*, 1984) have largely been abandoned because of poor results (Manning *et al.*, 1986). Fetuses at risk of developing thrombycytopenia have blood samples taken by puncturing one of the vessels in the umbilical cord. If necessary platelet infusions can be given into a cord vessel (Nicolini *et al.*, 1988). Foetuses in a multiple pregnancy have frequent ultrasound scans to detect any problems which might be developing. Using a uteroscope attempts have been made to divide with a laser beam aberrant vessels present in the placenta in the twin–twin transfusion syndrome.

Premature infants

All premature infants who are less than 36 weeks of age at birth are at risk of developing a germinal matrix haemorrhage; the younger the infant the greater the risk.

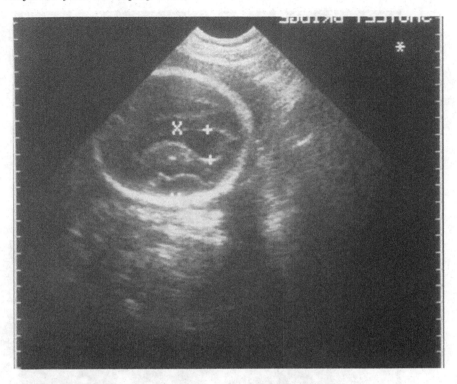

Figure 6.10. Ultrasound scan of a 25-week-old human foetus with a porencephalic cyst (+ +) in communication with the left lateral ventricle (×).

Any premature infant who collapses, has repeated episodes of bradycardia and/or has fits should be considered to have had a subependymal haemorrhage and an ultrasound scan of the brain should be obtained (Figure 6.11). Infants known to have had a haemorrhage into the ventricular system are examined regularly to test the tension of the anterior fontanelle. Repeated ultrasound scans are carried out to observe the resolution of the haematoma and at the same time the ventricular system is assessed to determine whether hydrocephalus is developing, and if it is whether it is progressing. If the infant develops hydrocephalus with raised intracranial pressure while it is still being ventilated or if its weight is very low, CSF is removed from the ventricular system either by repeated ventricular taps or by external drainage. If the infant still requires CSF after removal it becomes ventilator independent and its weight has risen above an agreed target value, generally 2 kg, then an indwelling CSF diversion system, usually a ventriculoperitoneal shunt, is inserted.

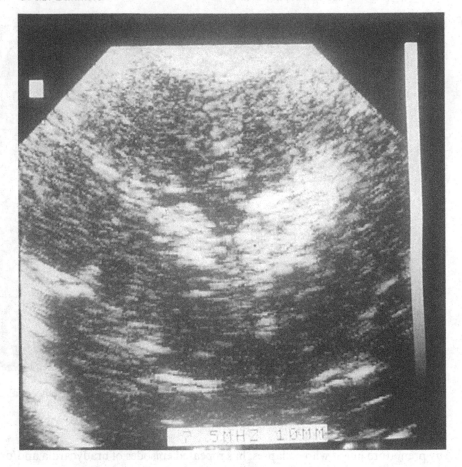

Figure 6.11. Ultrasound scan of a premature infant born at 27 weeks of gestation with bilateral intraventricular haemorrhages.

Full-term infants

With most infants who sustain a head injury during birth there is a history of a prolonged, difficult and complicated labour, and it has often been necessary to use forceps to assist the delivery, or an emergency caesarean section has had to be carried out. The baby may have required resuscitation after birth before breathing was established. As the baby's head is large in size relative to the rest of its body, enough blood can accumulate within the skull to cause hypovolemic shock. Every pale, newborn baby with a rapid pulse and a tense fontanelle should therefore be suspected of having sustained a head injury at birth. While many details of the intracranial damage can be diagnosed by an ultrasound scan, a more detailed picture can generally be obtained with a computed tomographic (CT) or MRI scan. If subdural haematomas are present they frequently need to be drained and this can generally be carried out by aspirating them with a needle passed through the lateral angles of the anterior fontanelle. Only rarely is it necessary to evacuate a haematoma from the parenchyma of the cerebral hemispheres or the cerebellum. Depressed pond fractures are visible through the thin neonatal scalp. If they are judged to need elevation, a burr hole is made close to the edge of the depression and an elevator is passed beneath the depressed bone and is used to lever it back into position.

Neonates, younger and older infants

Head injuries in neonates and infants of all ages can range in severity from concussion to deep coma. The first priority is to ensure that the infant has a clear airway and is breathing adequately, if not it should be intubated and ventilated. Bleeding into the calvarium and from the scalp can lead to hypovolemic shock and must be treated promptly by transfusion. Neurological assessment of the infant includes testing the tension of the anterior fontanelle. Retinal haemorrhages indicate that there has been a sudden increase in intracranial pressure. Ultrasound scans through the anterior fontanelle can generally only be carried out up the age of about 8 or 9 months; beyond that age the anterior fontanelle has become too small for a successful examination to be carried out. Ultrasound at any age in this group of infants does not provide as much information as a CT scan and this investigation should be carried out in all infants suspected of having had a traumatic intracranial haemorrhage. CT scan will generally allow extradural and subdural haematomas to be distinguished from one another. Subdural haematomas in the neonate and younger infants can often be drained by tapping them through the anterior fontanelle, older infants will require drainage to be carried out through burr holes. Extradural haematomas are best dealt with by evacuation after a craniotomy has been made. If an intracerebral haematoma causes raised intracranial pressure it should be removed through either a small craniotomy or a burr hole. Cerebral oedema causing life-threatening, raised intracranial pressure may have to be controlled by hyperventilation carried out after the infant has been intubated and paralysed.

Long-term outcome of traumatic events suffered at different ages

The long-term outcome of the lesions listed above depends on many factors. Age is a crucial factor as is the extent of the primary injury and the secondary events that follow it. The area of the brain affected is also of prime importance.

The primary injury often results in loss of tissue either by mechanical damage or the tearing apart of the tissues caused by the haemorrhaging which precedes the formation of a haematoma. As discussed above there is no evidence at any time from the onset of foetal life to old age that brain tissue once lost can be replaced. Yet it is a fact that substantial amounts of brain tissue can be missing and yet the patient may exhibit few abnormal neurological signs (Figure 6.12). The child illustrated in Figure 6.12 had a severe congenital heart lesion. It is likely that early in foetal life a catastrophic event occurred intracranially which may have resulted in the blood supply to the greater part of her left cerebral hemisphere being cut off. The only abnormal physical sign this girl has is a right homonomous hemianopia, her mentation is normal, as is the function of the right side of her face and right limbs. The function of the greater part of her left cerebral hemisphere appears to have been taken over, with the exception of the left visual cortex, by the remainder of the brain. This is a dramatic example of the brain's ability to exhibit plasticity. Similar sized porencephalic cysts occurring in premature infants between the ages of 25 and 33 weeks of gestation following haemorrhages from the germinal matrix do not generally have nearly such a good functional outcome. Many children so affected have demonstrable hemiparesis, although admittedly less severe than that seen after a similar lesion in a fully mature brain. It is apparent that the ability of the brain to compensate for loss of tissue is best seen in the very young foetus and from then on gradually diminishes. The mechanisms underlying plasticity are poorly understood. It can be hypothesised that plasticity employs either newly formed axon–dendritic connections, or takes over already formed connections which are not being used. Whatever the mechanism, it seems that as the brain matures and passes through its various stages of development, it gradually but never completely loses much of its flexibility.

The brain at any age withstands stretching and compression far better than loss of its blood supply; therefore, the secondary events that follow a primary head injury play an important role in the outcome. If a head injury results in an extradural or subdural haematoma which compresses the brain but has been removed successfully then the outcome is likely to be excellent. If, on the other hand, secondary events result in infarction of the brain or the intracranial pressure rises above the critical level so that the cerebral perfusion pressure of the brain fall below the critical level, then it is likely there will be extensive and permanent brain loss and the outcome will depend on the extent and site of the tissue lost. Management of the primary brain injury is prevention; management of the secondary head injury is aimed at maintaining the blood supply to the brain by every means available.

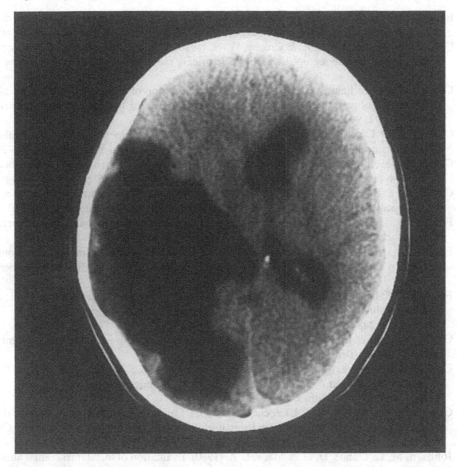

Figure 6.12. CT scan of 14-year-old girl with a congenital heart lesion and a huge porencephalic cyst in her left cerebral hemisphere.

References

Altman, J. (1966). Autoradiographic and histological studies of postnatal neurogensis. II. A longitudinal investigation of the kinetics, migration and transformation of cells incorporating tritiated thymidine in infant rats, with special reference to postnatal neurogenesis in some brain regions. *Journal of Comparative Neurology*, **128**, 431–74.

Angevine, J. B. & Sidman, R. L. (1961). Autoradiographic study of cell migration during histogenesis of the cerebral cortex in the mouse. *Nature*, **192**, 766–8.

Aster, R. H. (1990). 'Gestational' thrombocytopenia. A plea for conservative management. *New England Journal of Medicine*, **323**, 264–6.

Bannister, C. M. & Chapman, S. A. (1986). Response of the foetal rat brain to trauma during the 17th to 21st days of gestation. *Developmental Medicine and Child Neurology*, **28**, 600–9.

Carloss, H. W., McMillan, R. & Crosby, W. H. (1980). Management of pregnancy in women with immune thrombocytopenic purpura. *Journal of the American Medical Association*, **244**, 2756–8.

Chapman, S. A. & Bannister, C. M. (1989). Effect of excision of occipital lobe tissue on about the 70th day of gestation on the growth and development of the sheep's brain. *Surgical Neurology*, **32**, 98–104.

Choi, B. H. & Lapham, L. W. (1978). Radial glia in the human foetal cerebrum; a combined Golgi, immunofluorescent and electron microscopic study. *Brain Research*, **148**, 295–311.

Clewell, W. H., Johnson, M. L. & Meier, P. R. (1982). A surgical approach to the treatment of hydrocephalus. *New England and Journal of Medicine*, **306**, 1320–5.

Cohen, M. & Roessmann, U. (1994). In utero brain damage: relationship of gestational age to pathological consequences. *Developmental Medicine and Child Neurology*, **36**, 263–70.

Fowler, M., Brown, C. & Cbrera, K. F. (1971). Hydranencephaly in a baby after an aircraft accident to the mother: case report and autopsy. *Pathology*, **3**, 21–30.

Friede, R. L. (1989). Some features of basic reactions characteristic for immature nervous system. In *Developmental Neuropathology*, ed. R. L. Friede. Springer: Berlin, Heidelberg, p. 22.

Frigoletto, F. D., Birnholtz, J. C. & Greene, M. F. (1982). Antenatal treatment of hydrocephalus by ventriculoamniotic shunting. *Journal of the American Medical Association*, **248**, 2496–7.

Gadisseux, J. F. & Eurard, P. L. (1985). Glial–neural relationship in the developing central nervous system. *Developmental Neuroscience*, **7**, 12–37.

Glick, P. L., Harrison, M. R., Nakayama, D. K., Edwards, M. S. B., Filly, R. A., Chinn, D. N., Callen, P. W., Wilson, S. L. & Globus, M. S. (1984). Management of ventriculomegaly: the foetus. *Journal of Pediatrics*, **105**, 97–105.

Gosseye, S., Golaire, M. C. & Larroche, J. C. (1982). Cerebral, renal and splenic lesions due to foetal anoxia and their relationship to malformations. *Developmental Medixine and Child Neurology*, **24**, 510–18.

Johnson, M. L., Dunne, D. G. & Mack, L. A. (1980). Evaluation of foetal intracranial anatomy by static and realtime ultrasound. *Journal of Clinical Ultrasound*, **8**, 311–12.

Larroche, J. C. (1962). Quelques aspects anatomiques du développment cérébral. *Biologie de Neonatale*, **4**, 126–53.

Larroche, J. C. (1981). The marginal layer in the neocortex of a 7 week old human embryo. A light and electron microscopic study. *Anatomy and Embryology*, **162**, 301–12.

Larroche, J. C. (1993). Fetal cerebral pathology of circulatory origin. *Fetal Diagnosis Therapy*, **8** (Suppl. 2), 32–33.

Larroche, J. C. & Houcine, O. (1982). Le néocortex chez l'embryon et le foetus humain. Apport du microscope électronique et du Golgi. *Reproduction Nutritione et Developmente*, **22**, 163–70.

Leanty, P., Dramaix-Wilmet, M. & Delbeke, D. (1981). Ultrasonic evaluation of foetal ventricular growth. *Neuroradiology*, **21**, 127–30.

Levene, M. (1993). Late insults to the foetal brain: causes and protection. *Fetal Diagnoses Therapy*, **8** (Suppl. 2), 33–4.

Manning, F. A., Harrison, M. R. & Rodeck, C. (1986). Catheter shunts for foetal hydronephrosis and hydrocephalus. *New England Journal of Medicine*, **307**, 336–9.

Molliver, M. E., Kostavio, I. & Van Der Loos, H. (1973). The development of the synapses in cerebral cortex of human foetus. *Brain Research*, **50**, 403–7.

Nicolini, U., Rodeck, C. H. & Kochenour, N. K. (1988). In-utero platelet transfusion for alloimmune thrombocytopenia. *Lancet*, **ii**, 506–8.

Playfair, J. H. L., Wolfendale, M. R. & Kay, H. E. M. (1963). The leucocytes of peripheral blood in the human foetus. *British Journal of Haematology*, **9**, 336–44.

Pretorius, D. H., Drose, J. A. & Marco-Johnson, M. L. (1986). Fetal lateral ventricular ratio determination during the second trimester. *Journal of Ultrasound Medicine*, **5**, 121–5.

Rakic, P. (1972). Mode of cell migration to the superficial layers of foetal monkey cortex. *Journal of Comparative Neurology*, **145**, 61–84.

Schwendenberg, T. H. (1959). Leukoencephalopathy following carbon monoxide asphixia. *Journal of Neuropathology and Experimental Neurology*, **18**, 597–608.

Sibony, O., Fondacci, C., Oury, J.-C., Benard, C., Vuillard, E. & Blot, P. (1993). In utero foetal cerebral interparenchymal hemorrhage associated with an abnormal cerebral doppler. *Fetal Diagnosis Therapy*, **8**, 126–8.

Sidman, R. L. & Angevine, J. B. (1962). Autoradiographic analysis of time of origin of nuclear versus cortical components of mouse telencephalon. *Anatomical Record*, **142**, 326–7.

Spatz, H. (1921). Uber der Vorgange nach experimenteller Ruckenmarksdurchtrennung mit besonderer Beruckstigung der Underschlichen Pathologie (Porenzephalie und Syringomyelie). In: Nissel, F. and Alzheimer, A. eds, pp. 49–367, *Histologische und Histopathologische Arbeiten, Erganzungsband*. Jena: Fischer.

7

Wound healing in children

J. G. ANDREW

Wound healing in children is fundamentally the same as that seen, and classically described, in adults. Thus, while foetal wound healing is radically different from that seen after birth, that of children and adults differs only in detail. These details, however, result in clinically important features of wound healing in children.

The typical features of wound healing are illustrated in Figure 7.1. Wounds may be of various degrees of contamination and severity, but in an incised wound in which the edges are approximated healing occurs in predictable stages. First, a haematoma is formed in the wound. This acts as a source of growth factors (particularly from platelets) which act to 'kick start' the process of acute inflammation and wound repair. In addition, the blood clot contains a network of fibrinous material; this forms a substratum for migrating cells during the initial stages of wound repair. Both of these features are currently thought to be important in starting healing, although formal investigations of the effect of removal of the haematoma in some healing situations has revealed varying results.

The next stage of healing is the development of granulation tissue. The haematoma is invaded by granulocytes and macrophages. These cells (especially macrophages) are thought to play a vital coordinating role in wound healing. The evidence for granulocytes being important in preventing infection, both in wounds and elsewhere is clear (Weening *et al.*, 1992). The role of macrophages is currently less clear cut. They undoubtedly act as a prolific source of growth factors *in vitro*, but the relevance of this observation to wound healing *in vivo* is not completely clear. Endothelial cells grow into the haematoma and form capillaries. At the same time, undifferentiated mesenchymal cells proliferate and start to lay down connective tissue. The nature of this tissue changes during wound healing. At first, 'transitional' glycoproteins are most prominent (cellular fibronectin, tenascin and vitronectin). After this, collagen III is expressed as the major collagenous protein, and is then gradually replaced by collagen I. During the later stages of wound repair, the collagens initially laid down are remodelled to strongly cross-linked collagens with an ordered scar structure of high

Haematoma: infiltration of inflammatory cells
Capillary buds

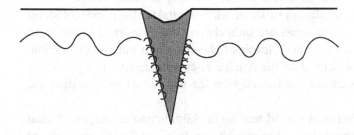

Granulation tissue: capillaries and fibroblasts

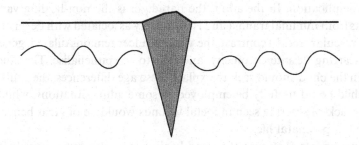

Scar formation: fibrosis and scar contracture
closes wound; re-epithelialisation

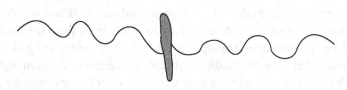

Figure 7.1. Wound healing.

tensile strength. Epidermal proliferation occurs at an early stage after wounding, and migration of keratinocytes results in healing of the superficial parts of the skin. There have been several useful reviews of adult wound healing (Janssen *et al.*, 1991; Gailit & Clark, 1994). It must be appreciated that such wound healing results in a replacement of the normal dermal structures by an organised scar. This consists of mature fibrous tissue which is at best thin and aligned with the scar but may be extensive and matted. It replaces the ordered dermal collagen structure which is vital for the normal function of the skin. In addition, scarred areas are unlikely to contain normal amounts of dermal appendages such as sweat glands, leading to further alteration in skin function. Restitution of the epidermal elements of the skin (i.e. re-epithelialisation) may also be a problem, and has been specifically addressed with the use of cultured keratinocyte grafts for burn patients.

Despite the similarities between wound healing in children and adults, the clinical problems associated with the process change with age. In the child, the paradigm of wound healing, and the commonest cause of wound healing problems, is the burn. This results from severe trauma. The common problems with burn healing in the child are excessive scarring, contracture and burn hypertrophy. Failure of re-epithelialisation is a relative rare complication. In the adult, the paradigm is the non-healing varicose ulcer. This results from minimal trauma and is intimately associated with degenerative problems in the vascular tree. In contrast, the varicose ulcer remains dilated, generally without severe scarring despite chronicity, and fails to re-epithelialise. The study of wound healing in the child should seek to explain these age differences; the exuberant healing of the child could usefully be employed in some adult situations, while it is believed that the lack of scarring seen in foetal wounds would be of great benefit if it could be induced in postnatal life.

There are many reports of studies of wound healing in adults, but relatively few in children. The effect of age on the rate of wound healing was recognised many years ago. Recently, studies in adult wound healing have concentrated on three areas: angiogenesis, the matrix elaborated at different stages of repair and the tensile strength of the wound, and the role of growth factors and cytokines in controlling wound repair. There are few reports of the biology of clinical wound healing in children or adults, but there are data of the effect of age from animal studies. These should be interpreted with caution, but most of the described effects of age from these studies do fit with clinically observed phenomena. Angiogenesis is vital in wound healing (Arnold & West, 1991); however, there are few studies of this phenomenon in children, with that of Raekallio and Viljanto (1983) being limited to observing inflammatory cell infiltrate and capillary formation in children's wounds using the Cellstic device. The initial matrix deposited in children's wounds appeared similar to that in adults, being rich in fibronectin (Viljanto *et al.*, 1981). This study did not address the presence of tenascin or other glycoproteins, but in a study of lip wounds in the neonatal mouse, Whitby and

Ferguson (1991a) found that fibronectin deposition in the wound was the same as for foetal and adult mice. The deposition of tenascin, however, was intermediate between foetal and adult wound healing, being first present at 12 hours in the neonate (1 hour in the foetus, 24 hours in the adult). This group has previously postulated that rapid deposition of tenascin is associated with rapid wound healing. This antiadhesive glycoprotein is thought to be important in cell migration in wound healing, permitting cells to modulate their degree of adhesion to the underlying matrix (one matrix protein for adhesion in this case being fibronectin). Various cells may be responsible for the production of these glycoproteins, including macrophages, endothelial cells and fibroblasts. Rapid recovery of the cellular population of wounds is a feature of foetal wound healing, and in this study the cellularity of neonatal wounds appeared intermediate between foetus and adult.

The deposition of collagen in the wound is the stage of definitive matrix formation. The two principal collagens of wounds are collagens I and III. The fully healed wound will have a scar consisting largely of collagen I which is heavily cross-linked and whose fibre orientation will resist the stresses on the wound. The first collagen to be laid down in the wound is probably collagen III. This is an embryonic form of collagen, which is only found transiently in processes such as wound healing in postnatal life. The ratio of collagen I to III increases as wound healing progresses, but in an elegant series of experiments Raekallio *et al.* demonstrated that the amount of collagen III in children's wounds is unusually high (Gay *et al.*, 1978). To do this, they employed a perforated silastic tube ('Cellstic') containing a removable wick which was left in the wound. The tube was removed from the wound between 1 and 5 days after operation, and its contents (cells or matrix) analysed. Whitby & Fersugon (1991a) reached similar conclusions in the lip wound model in the neonatal mouse. Collagen III was deposited earlier in the neonatal wound, but was associated with less alteration of the reticular structure of the dermis than in adult wounds. In the neonatal wound, the reticular structure had been restored at 5 days, while parallel bundles of scar tissue were still visible at 12 days in the adult wound. There is some evidence that collagen deposition varies because of intrinsic differences in wound fibroblasts with age, and not just due to the amount of growth factor 'drive' associated with the wound (Takeda *et al.*, 1992; Horiuchi & Ryan, 1993). These data tend to credit foetal fibroblasts with maximal collagen production, which is not in accordance with the demonstrated lack of scarring in foetal wounds. Thus Takeda *et al.* (1992) examined fibroblasts from foetuses and donors of varying age. They found that *in vitro* collagen III mRNA levels in the fibroblasts decreased predictably with age. More surprisingly, collagen I levels probably decreased with age but only in a rather haphazard fashion. They also examined the deposition of other collagens V and VI. These collagens were also examined in the neonatal mouse lip wound, the amounts found being intermediate between those of foetus and adult in a similar way to that for collagen III. It is of interest that the transition from foetal to adult type of wound healing may not be complete by birth. Hallock *et al.* (1993) examined the transition from foetal to adult collagen deposition in rat wounds. They found that the characteristics of foetal wound healing were maintained for approximately 15 days postpartum. While the persistence of a foetal pattern of healing after birth in humans is speculation at present, they note that several reports of cleft plate repair in the neonatal period have noted superior results. They speculate that the reason for this is the persistance of a low scar type of repair into the postnatal period. If this lack of scarring could be confirmed, it would support the development of several operations in the neonatal period, and might obviate the need for some projected developments in foetal surgery.

There is little information about the relative contributions of growth factors to paediatric and adult wound healing. One feature of foetal wound healing is the lack of inflammatory cells (Morykwas *et al.*, 1991), and it is thought that these may act as a source of growth factors in adult wounds. Thus, Whitby & Ferguson (1991b) demonstrated that one of the principal cells in the neonatal and adult lip wound containing TGFβ1 was the macrophage. It is thought that this growth factor is important in promoting both neovascularisation of the wound and connective tissue formation. Similarly, it has been demonstrated that one method of restoring wound healing in older animals to its youthful vigour is to transfer circulating macrophages (monocytes) to the wound area; macrophages from young animals were more effective than those from older ones (Danon *et al.*, 1989). The differences between inflammatory cell infiltrate in wounds between children and adults does not seem to have been examined, and would seem to be a possible candidate for future modulation of wound healing in children. There is a small amount of information on the presence of inflammatory cells in paediatric wounds (Raekallio & Viljanto, 1975), but this does not provide information about white cell function. Similarly, there are few data on the relative amounts of growth factors in child and adult wounds. Whitby and Ferguson were not able to demonstrate any significant differences between neonatal and adult lip wounds for the presence of TGFβ1 or 2, bFGF or PDGF. There is evidence that scar fibroblasts are more responsive to growth factor stimulation than control cells (Moriyama *et al.*, 1991). This emphasises that modulation of growth factor receptor expression is at least as important as the expression of growth factors. The idea that the differences between paediatric and adult wound healing are due to variations in growth factor expression remain, at present, largely supposition (albeit probably a correct supposition).

As noted earlier, the clinical problems associated with paediatric wounds are different from those in adults. Following burns in children, contractures and hypertrophy are more common than in adults (McDonald & Deitch, 1987; Kramer *et al.*, 1988). Burn contractures may be devastating in their effect on children, requiring recurrent surgical attention throughout growth. They cause persisting difficulty in the use of the associated joint. They are associated with burns which cross the flexor surfaces of joints; the scarred skin fails to grow in pace with the underlying joint structures, and gradually causes a relative shortening of the overlying skin. The contractures can involve considerable soft tissue tension, and distort the development of the underlying bone and joint structures. Results of surgical treatment are often poor. In addition to the scarred skin failing to grow, the scar may actively contract. The major cell type associated with contracture is the myofibroblast; this contractile fibroblast is thought to generate tension in wounds, promoting contracture (Baur *et al.*, 1978). The unique connection of the contractile intracellular actin bundles with the surrounding extracellular matrix ('the fibronexus') has been the subject of several investigations (Eyden, 1993). It is possible to modulate the presence of such cells by application of growth factors such as PDGF and TGFβ (Pierce *et al.*, 1991), although they noted that the reduction in the numbers of myofibroblasts present in experimental wounds was associated with increases in collagen content, so it is debatable whether more satisfactory scarring would have occurred. Recent evidence does support the concept that modulation of the amounts of growth factors in wounds can reduce undesirable scarring. Shah *et al.* (1992) initially demonstrated this by use of an anti TGFβ antibody (Shah *et al.*, 1992). Subsequently it has become apparent that the ratio of TGFβ3 to TGFβ1 and 2 is important in controlling scarring, with less scarring apparent in wounds with more TGFβ3 (Shah *et al.*, 1995).

Burns in children are also associated with hypertrophy, which is a particular feature of wound healing in black people (McDonald & Deitch, 1987). These are a particular problem in skin grafted wounds. Hypertrophic wounds are associated with enhanced fibronectin, collagen and TGFβ expression relative to non-hypertrophic wounds (Babu *et al.*, 1989; Peltonen *et al.*, 1991). They are also the site of rather obvious abnormalities of microvessels, including endothelial proliferation and occlusion (Kischer *et al.*, 1982). It is thought that hypoxia in wounds may be partially responsible for hypertrophy because of the known stimulatory effects of hypoxia and reactive oxygen species on fibroblasts (McDonald & Deitch, 1987). Similar appearances of microvessel occlusion have been noted in other conditions involving hypertrophic scarring such as Dupuytren's disease. The development of hypertrophy in burn wounds appears to be related to the absence of residual dermal elements in the graft recipient bed (McDonald & Deitch, 1987). The reconstitution of dermal elements after burns is variable, but adequate reconstitution of normal dermal elements is associated with minimal hypertrophy or scarring. In contrast, if the normal rete pattern of the dermis is replaced by a haphazard array of scar collagen, the cosmetic (and probably functional) results will be unsatisfactory. The relationship between the epidermis and underlying dermis is complex and outside the scope of this chapter, but has been particularly studied in relationship to the use of cultured epidermal allografts. Compton (1992) found that cultured keratinocyte allografts were more likely to develop a normal dermal pattern eventually than burns treated by split thickness skin graft. Others have also reported that cultured cells can give better cosmetic results than meshed split thickness grafts (Bettex-Galland *et al.*, 1988; Kumagai, *et al.*, 1988). The treatment of hypertrophic wounds has developed empirically, with pressure garments having become an important mode of treatment. The reason for the apparently satisfactory results of pressure garments, and the way in which this mechanical force modulates cellular behaviour, is not clear.

Fracture healing in children demonstrates significant differences from that seen in adults. The process of healing consists of the formation of a haematoma followed by the development of a granulation tissue mass. This includes blood vessels and mesenchymal progenitor cells. These progenitor cells give rise to chondrocytes and osteoblasts, generating bone by either endochondral or intramembranous ossification. The mass of new bone which is formed lies around the ends of the fractured bone rather than between them, and is known as the callus mass. Development of the callus is faster in children than in adults, and generally speaking fracture healing is faster and more reliable in children (Moseley, 1992). The rate of restoration of function to the bone has been found to hold a log normal relationship to the age of the patient (Skak & Jensen, 1988). It is, however, difficult to determine whether the restoration of function reflects genuinely faster healing or the lower mechanical demands placed on bones by smaller patients. The other striking feature of fracture healing in children, particularly those under the age of 10 years, is the rapid and extensive remodelling that occurs. Remodelling occurs by coupled osteoclasts and osteoblasts removing and laying down bone. This results in the callus mass being completely remodelled over a period of 1–2 years, and eventually becoming almost undiscernible on X-ray. The bone will remodel according to the functional demands placed upon it (Wolff's Law), and provided these are relatively normal (i.e. there is no gross degree of shortening or malunion), the fracture will eventually remodel completely. This satisfactory state is almost never attained in fractures of the cortex of adult long bones, although fractures through cancellous bone may eventually become completely remodelled. The excellent remodelling of children's fractures probably reflects their faster rate of bone turnover, associated with the normal processes of growth. The process of growth may actually be enhanced by long bone fractures in children; the complication of overgrowth is particularly recognised in femoral fractures. In general, fracture healing is a reliable process in children, giving relatively few complications. Recently, the reliability of fracture healing in both children and adults has been exploited in the technique of callotasis. In this technique, bone is induced to grow by stretching a callus mass at an early stage of its development, usually by means of an external fixation device. This has been used in both bone transport (filling a defect in a bone) and in limb lengthening. The process of callotasis has been found to be more reliable and more rapid in children than in adults.

The processes of wound and fracture healing in children have received relatively little specific research, despite many investigations of adult and foetal wound healing. This may reflect the general reliability of this process in the young. It may be noted that the results of extensive wounds in the young (e.g. burns) remain unsatisfactory, being particularly liable to contracture and hypertrophy. Both of these processes may prove amenable to manipulation in the near future by alteration of the growth factor content of the wound. The process of wound healing in the young, and its differences from adult healing, require further study.

References

Arnold, F. & West, D. C. (1991). Angiogenesis in wound healing. *Pharmacology and Therapeutics*, **52**, 407–22.

Babu, M., Diegelmann, R. & Oliver, N. (1989). Fibronectin is overproduced by keloid fibroblasts during abnormal wound healing. *Molecular and Cellular Biology*, **9**, 1642–50.

Baur, P. S., Barratt, G., Linares, H. A., Dobrkovsky, M., de la Houssaye, A. J. & Larson, D. L. (1978). Wound contractions, scar contractures and myofibroblasts: a classical case study. *Journal of Trauma*, **18**, 8–22.

Bettex-Calland, M., Slongo, T., Hunziker, T., Wiesmann, U. & Bettex, M. (1988). Use of cultured keratinocytes in the treatment of severe burns. *Zeitschrift Kinderchirurgie*, **43**, 224–8.

Compton, C. C. (1992). Current concepts in pediatric burn care: the biology of cultured epithelial autografts: an eight-year study in pediatric burn patients. *European Journal of Pediatric Surgery*, **2**, 216–22.

Danon, D., Kowatch, M. A. & Roth, G. S. (1989). Promotion of wound repair in old mice by local injection of macrophages. *Proceedings of the National Academy of Sciences of the United States of America*, **86**, 2018–20.

Eyden, B. P. (1993). Brief review of the fibronexus and its significance for myofibroblastic differentiation and tumour diagnosis. *Ultrastructural Pathology*, **17**, 611–22.

Gailit, J. & Clark, R. A. F. (1994). Wound repair in the context of extracellular matrix. *Current Opinion in Cell Biology*, **6**, 717–25.

Gay, S., Vijanto, J., Raekallio, J. & Penttinen, R. (1978). Collagen types in early phases of wound healing in children. *Acta Chirurgica Scandinavica*, **144**, 205–11.

Hallock, G. G., Merkel, J. R., Rice, D. C. & DiPaolo, B. R. (1993). The ontogenetic transition of collagen deposition in rat skin. *Annals of Plastic Surgery*, **301**, 239–43.

Horiuchi, Y. & Ryan, T. J. (1993). A comparison of newborn versus old skin fibroblasts, their potential for tissue repair. *British Journal of Plastic Surgery*, **46**, 132–5.

Janssen, H., Rooman, R., Robertson, J. I. H. (ed.) (1991). *Wound Healing*. Wrightson Biomedical Petersfield, England.

Kischer, C. W., Shetlar, M. R. & Chvapil, M. (1982). Hypertrophic scars and keloids: a review and new concept concerning their origin. *Scanning Electron Microscopy*, 4, 1699–713.

Kraemer, M. D., Jones, T. & Deitch, E. A. (1988). Burn contractures: incidence, predisposing factors, and results of surgical therapy. *Journal of Burn Care and Rehabilitation*, **9**, 261–5.

Kumagai, N., Nishina, H., Tanabe, H., Hosaka, T., Ishida, H. & Ogino, Y. (1988). Clinical application of autologous cultured epithelia for the treatment of burn wounds and burn scars. *Plastic and Reconstructive Surgery*, **82**, 99–110.

McDonald, W. S. & Deitch, E. A. (1987). Hypertrophic skin grafts in burned patients: a prospective analysis of variables. *Journal of Trauma*, **27**, 147–50.

Moriyama, K., Shimokawa, H., Susami, T., Sasaki, S. & Kuroda, T. (1991). Effects of growth factors on mucosal scar fibroblasts in culture – a possible role of growth factors in scar formation. *Matrix*, **11**, 190–6.

Morykwas, M. J., Ledbetter, M. S., Ditesheim, J. A., White, W. L., Vander Ark, A. D. & Argenta, L. C. (1991). Cellular inflammation of fetal excisional wounds: effects of amniotic fluid exclusion. *Inflammation*, **15**, 173–80.

Moseley, C. F. (1992). General features of fractures in children. *Instructional Course Lectures*, **41**, 337–46.

Peltonen, J., Hsiao, L., Jaakkola, S., Sollberg, S., Aumailley, M., Timpl, R., Chu, M. L. & Uitto, J. (1991). Activation of collagen gene expression in keloids: co localization of type I and VI collagen and transforming growth factor betal mRNA. *Journal of Investigative Dermatology*, **97**, 240–8.

Pierce, G. F., Vande Berg, J., Rudolph, R., Tarpley, J. & Mustoe, T. A. (1991). Platelet-derived growth factor-BB and transforming growth factor beta 1 selectively modulate glycosaminoglycans, collagen, and myofibroblasts in excisional wounds. *American Journal of Pathology*, **138**, 629–46.

Raekallio, J. & Viljanto, J. (1975). Regeneration of subcutaneous connective tissue in children. A histological study with application of the Cellstic device. *Journal of Cutaneous Pathology*, **75**, 191–7.

Raekallio, J. & Viljanto, J. (1983). Signs of capillary formation in the early phase of wound healing in children. *Experimental Pathology*, **23**, 67–72.

Shah, M., Foreman, D. M. & Ferguson, M. W. (1992). Control of scarring in adult wounds by neutralising antibody to transforming growth factor beta. *Lancet*, **339**, 213–14.

Shah, M., Foreman, D. M. & Ferguson, M. W. (1995). Neutralisation of TGF-beta 1 and TGF-beta 2 or exogenous addition of TGF- beta 3 to cutaneous rat wounds reduces scarring. *Journal of Cell Science*, **108**, 985–1002.

Skak, S. V. & Jensen, T. T. (1988). Femoral shaft fracture in 265 children. Log-normal correlation with age of speed of healing. *Acta Orthopaedica Scandinavica*, **59**, 704–7.

Takeda, K., Gosiewska, A. & Peterkofsky, B. (1992). Similar, but not identical, modulation of expression of extracellular matrix components during in vitro and in vivo aging of human skin fibroblasts. *Journal of Cellular Physiology*, **153**, 450–9.

Viljanto, J., Penttinen, R. & Raekallio, J. (1981). Fibronectin in early phases of wound healing in children. *Acta Chirurgica Scandinavica*, **147**, 7–13.

Weening, R. S., Bredius, R. G., Vomberg, P. P., van der Schoot, C. E., Hoogerwerf, M. & Roos, D. (1992). Recombinant human interferon-gamma treatment in severe leucocyte adhesion deficiency. *European Journal of Pediatrics*, **151**, 103–7.

Whitby, D. J. & Ferguson, M. W. (1991a). The extracellular matrix of lip wounds in fetal, neonatal and adult mice. *Development*, **112**, 651–68.

Whitby, D. J. & Ferguson, M. W. (1991b). Immunohistochemical localization of growth factors in fetal wound healing. *Developmental Biology*, **147**, 207–15.

8

The lung after injury in children

J. GRIGG

Introduction

The paediatric lung is not a fully developed organ. From birth to the age of 8 years the number of alveoli in the lungs increase from 20 to 300 million. Lung growth after 8 years of age is due to an increase in alveolar size alone (Phelan *et al.*, 1994). Structural immaturity of the lung in early childhood could result in an increased vulnerability to injury. Alternatively, an increased capacity for repair and regeneration may limit the degree of damage. Given the same insult, however, the mechanisms of lung tissue damage are often identical in the adult and child. In this chapter I describe how oxidants, inflammatory cells and oedema injure the lung. The role of these mechanisms in paediatric neurogenic pulmonary oedema, adult respiratory distress syndrome in children and neonatal chronic lung disease are reviewed.

Mechanisms of pulmonary injury

Oxidant injury

Pulmonary oxidant injury occurs when the rate of production of oxygen-derived reactive species (free radicals) overwhelms pulmonary antioxidant defences. If not removed immediately, free radicals oxidatively damage all components of cells. The key oxidants are the superoxide ($O_2{}^-$) and hydroxyl (OH.) radicals and the main pulmonary antioxidants are superoxide dismutase, catalase and glutathione. During normal cellular respiration some degree of intracellular free radical production occurs. The pulmonary production of intracellular and extracellular free radicals is substantially increased by high concentrations of oxygen, reperfusion injury (Jenkinson *et al.*, 1988) and activated neutrophils (Farber *et al.*, 1990). During an oxidant stress, the first radical to be produced is superoxide. It is formed when a free electron is transferred onto oxygen. The antioxidant enzyme superoxide dismutase specifically deals with this

107

reactive species, converting superoxide to hydrogen peroxide. Hydrogen peroxide per se is relatively harmless, but if superoxide radicals are not removed completely, they react with hydrogen peroxide to form the hydroxyl radical, the most destructive of the oxygen-derived species. The formation of the hydroxyl radical via hydrogen peroxide requires iron as a catalyst (Farber *et al.*, 1990). The enzyme catalase and the tripeptide glutathione (glutamyl-cysteinyl glycine) do not remove oxidants directly but limit the availability of hydrogen peroxide. Catalase has less affinity for hydrogen peroxide than glutathione, but is explosively fast. It is not present in the mitochondria, a major site of oxygen-derived free radical generation. Glutathione, on the other hand, plays a pivotal role in both cytosolic and mitochondrial antioxidant defence. The reduced form of glutathione (GSH), in conjunction with the enzyme glutathione peroxidase, converts hydrogen peroxide to water. In animal models, pulmonary glutathione depletion enhances hyperoxia-induced free radical damage (Denke & Fanburgh, 1989). Glutathione has a high affinity for its substrate, but is relatively slow in removing hydrogen peroxide (Farber *et al.*, 1990). The resulting oxidised glutathione (GSSG) is regenerated by the enzyme glutathione reductase. The alveolar surface is an important site for the generation of extracellular free radicals. Not surprisingly, the alveolar epithelial lining fluid (ELF) is rich in antioxidants. The reduced form of glutathione accumulates in the ELF in concentrations up to one hundred times those of the plasma (Cantin *et al.*, 1987) and the extracellular form of superoxide dismutase is present in the ELF of normal children (J. Grigg, unpublished results). ELF also contains a range of nonspecific antioxidants including surfactant (Ghio *et al.*, 1994).

Although it is very difficult to measure free radical production directly, it is possible to detect pulmonary free radical damage *in vivo*. Free radical damage to unsaturated fatty acids releases conjugated dienes, malondialdehyde, lipid hydroperoxides and the gases ethane and pentane. These compounds can be measured in lung tissue, bronchoalveolar lavage fluid and in the exhaled breath. Accumulation of oxidised glutathione within the lung is also a marker of oxidant stress (White *et al.*, 1986); however, these indirect markers of free radical production do not necessarily reflect pulmonary damage. For example, an increase in breath ethane is associated with free radical damage to the lipids in parenteral infusions (Wispe *et al.*, 1985) and accumulation of oxidised glutathione may only reflect efficient activation of the glutathione system rather than pulmonary injury.

Inflammatory injury

Mediators released from leucocytes have significant tissue-destructive potential. The histotoxic mediators of neutrophils have been well described and include the chlorinated oxidant, hypochlorous acid, and proteolytic enzymes (serine proteinase, elastase and the two metalloproteinases, collagenase and gelatinase) (Weiss, 1989). Anti-proteinases such as α_1-proteinase inhibitory leucoproteinase inhibitor and α_2-macro-globulin limit the degree of proteinase-mediated tissue injury. Like antioxidants, proteinase inhibitors accumulate in human alveolar ELF (Watterberg *et al.*, 1994).

Recruitment of intravascular cells is critical to neutrophil-mediated pulmonary injury. Leucocytes cannot enter the pulmonary interstitium without the expression of specific adhesion molecules on the pulmonary endothelium. Vascular leucocytes (mainly neutrophils) constantly make random contact to the pulmonary endothelium. In health, permanent sticking does not occur; however, if the endothelium is activated by an extravascular stimulus, leucocytes randomly touching endothelial cells will initially roll along the endothelial surface. This form of adhesion is delicate and can be overcome by increased blood flow. 'Shear-stress sensitive' rolling is mediated via increased expression of the endothelial proteins P- and E-selectins interacting with normal levels of sialyl Lewis X carbohydrate on the neutrophil surface (Carlos & Harlan, 1994). Additional adhesion during rolling is provided by normal levels of neutrophil L-selectin interacting with an unknown structure on the endothelial surface. Firm 'shear-stress resistant' sticking (activation-firm adherence) is then mediated by a different set of adhesion molecules. To stop the neutrophil requires the combination of increased levels and affinity of neutrophil β_2 integrins (the transmembrane proteins, CD11a/CD18, CD11b/CD18, CD11c/CD18) interacting with increased expression of endothelial 'immunoglobulin-like' adhesion proteins. These endothelial molecules include intercellular adhesion molecule-1 and -2 (ICAM) and vascular cell adhesion molecule-1 (VCAM-1). The β_2 leucocyte integrin classification describes a common β chain (CD18), noncovalently associated with one of three different α chains (CD11 a, b or c). Finally, if a chemotactic gradient exists, leucocytes will transmigrate. For neutrophils, the leucocyte β_2 integrins, the endothelial immunoglobulins platelet/ endothelial cell adhesion molecule-1 (PECAM-1) and ICAM-1, are important determinants of transmigration (Carlos & Harlan, 1994). PECAM-1 (CD31) is normally expressed on the intercellular junctions of endothelial cells and controls diapedesis between cells (Muller *et al.*, 1993). In animals, pulmonary injury can be significantly attenuated by intravenous monoclonal antibodies blocking adhesion molecule function (Lo *et al.*, 1994). This form of therapy is ineffective if the targeted adhesion molecule plays only a minor part in the leucocyte influx (Keeney *et al.*, 1994). In humans, blocking leucocyte-endothelial adhesion will probably be best suited to conditions where leucocyte influx can be anticipated. Caution will be required in manipulating adhesion mechanisms in humans as in certain circumstances inflammation may be essential. For example, blocking CD18 worsens endotoxaemia and cardiovascular injury in the dog model of septic shock (Eichacker *et al.*, 1993).

The degree of inflammatory injury is dependent on not only the balance of pulmonary histotoxic/antihistotoxic compounds, but also on the efficiency of resolution response. After fulfilling their function, neutrophil disintegration within the lung would be counterproductive. The release of stored mediators can cleave matrix components into fragments chemotactic for intravascular neutrophils thereby maintaining inflammation (Vartio et al., 1981). Two processes that limit the proinflammatory effect of neutrophil breakup are neutrophil apoptosis and removal of neutrophils by macrophages.

Aged neutrophils can undergo apoptosis, or programmed cell death. During apoptosis cells retain their membrane integrity and do not release stored histotoxic mediators (Savill et al., 1989). Apoptic neutrophils are then rapidly recognised and engulfed by macrophages. Once within the macrophage phagosome, neutrophil mediators are inactivated without causing activation of the macrophage itself (Meagher et al., 1989). Removal of 'normal' neutrophils in vivo has not been observed and it has been thought that apoptosis is important in triggering the surface changes required for macrophage recognition and removal (Savill et al., 1989). Recent research into the bcl-2 proto-oncogene in transgenic mice has called this concept into question. Apoptosis is blocked in aged neutrophils expressing bcl-2. Despite the absence of apoptosis in these cells, macrophages engulf the aged, bcl-2 neutrophils (Lagasse & Weissman, 1994). Thus, while apoptosis may prevent neutrophil disintegration and limit inflammation, macrophage removal of neutrophils may, in certain circumstances, be dependent on cell surface changes associated with aging per se. Irrespective of the precise mechanisms governing neutrophil removal, inflammatory mediators such as granulocyte colony-stimulating factor inhibit neutrophil apoptosis and prolong its ability to cause tissue damage (Lee et al., 1993). Furthermore in leukaemic cell lines in vitro, low intracellular levels of GSH push cells to disintegrate rather than undergo apoptosis in response to a toxic stimulus (Fernandes & Cotter, 1994). Substances that stimulate leucocytes to undergo apoptosis rather than disintegrate may be important during the resolution phase, but to date they have not been demonstrated in the lung. Turning off the 'stickiness' of the pulmonary endothelium for neutrophils is another important phase of the resolution process. It remains unclear which endogenous factors downregulate pulmonary endothelial 'immunoglobulin-like' adhesion molecules.

Pulmonary oedema

The mechanisms underlying the formation and the resolution of pulmonary oedema have recently been re-evaluated. Pulmonary oedema has been divided into either 'hydrostatic' or 'permeability' forms. In hydrostatic oedema, elevations in the pulmonary microvascular pressure (e.g. from increased left atrial pressure) increase transvascular fluid flow into the interstitium. At high microvascular pressures, the most important protection mechanism for oedema is the ability of the lung to increase pulmonary lymph flow (Parker *et al.*, 1981). In the traditional view of hydrostatic oedema, the pulmonary endothelium does not increase its permeability to protein. As the intact alveolar epithelium is virtually impermeable to protein (Berthiaume *et al.*, 1988), alveolar oedema formed hydrostatically should be protein-depleted (Staub, 1974). In contrast, permeability oedema is characterised by damage to the pulmonary endothelium and alveolar epithelium. This allows leakage of both serum proteins and fluid into the pulmonary interstitium and alveolar space. The alveolar epithelium is very sensitive to direct mechanical injury. Even short periods of lung overinflation damage the air–blood barrier and lead to the formation of high protein permeability oedema (Dreyfuss *et al.*, 1992).

There has previously been no evidence to suggest that hydrostatic pressure per se increases the protein permeability of the air–blood barrier; however, bronchoalveolar lavage of rabbits has recently demonstrated an increase in both ELF volume and protein concentration during elevations in pulmonary microvascular pressure (Tsukimoto *et al.*, 1994). The concept that hydrostatic oedema may transform into permeability oedema is supported by histological studies. In rabbits, moderate elevations of microvascular pressure produce inequalities in the protein density of interstitial and alveolar fluid pools, which suggest local differences in protein sieving (Bachofen *et al.*, 1993a). In the same model, frank disruptions can be seen in the type I alveolar epithelial cells in the regions of alveolar oedema (Bachofen *et al.*, 1993b). In other experimental protocols, hydrostatic forces also injure the alveolar epithelium/ pulmonary endothelium (Tsukimoto *et al.*, 1991). Whether tissue disruption occurs in human forms of hydrostatic oedema is unclear, although vascular/epithelial injury could explain high protein concentrations in some patients with 'pure' cardiogenic oedema (Carlson *et al.*, 1979). The amount of tissue injury/protein leak associated with hydrostatic pulmonary oedema is important clinically. The accumulation of protein-depleted fluid has less potential to initiate other forms of tissue injury. High concentrations of protein in the alveolar space inactivate surfactant proteins and stimulate the formation of fibrin strands (Hallman *et al.*, 1991). Furthermore, an intact alveolar epithelium is required for oedema resolution (Matthay & Wiener-Kronish, 1990).

Paediatric neurogenic pulmonary oedema

The association between pulmonary oedema and acute intracranial injury has been well described (Demling & Riessen, 1990). Neurogenic pulmonary oedema (NPE) usually has an immediate onset and is clinically significant 2–12 hours after head injury. Dyspnoea is a predominant symptom and is accompanied by the clinical signs of tachypnoea, hypoxaemia, decreased pulmonary compliance and 'fluffy' infiltrates on chest radiographs. Oedema resolution takes hours to days, if the patient does not succumb from the other complications of trauma (Kaufman *et al.*, 1993). Many cases may be subclinical (Pender & Pollack, 1992) and the true incidence is unknown, although up to 50% of comatose adults after intracranial injury have significant elevations in pulmonary extracellular water (Mackersie *et al.*, 1983). Fulminant NPE with pink frothy oedema welling up from the trachea is rare. The pattern of NPE in children appears to be similar to adults. In children, clinical onset of oedema ranges from 1 to 12 hours after head injury and the fulminant form occurs (Milley *et al.*, 1979; Mulroy *et al.*, 1985; Pender & Pollack, 1992; Jourdan *et al.*, 1993). A more delayed onset form of NPE has been reported in adults (Kaufman *et al.*, 1993), and paediatric NPE occurring 3 days after neurological recovery from a subarachnoid haemorrhage has been described (Lear, 1990). Treatment of clinical NPE is supportive with positive pressure mechanical ventilation.

The prevailing view on the formation of NPE is that it is caused by a massive, transient central nervous system neural discharge which activates the sympathetic nervous system resulting in pulmonary hypertension and hydrostatic pulmonary oedema. Studies in small mammals have confirmed that extravascular lung water (EVLW) can increase after activation of the sympathetic nervous system (Minnear & Connel, 1981). In the dog model of NPE, intracisternal injection of the compound veratrine causes massive sympathetic activation, translocation of blood from the systemic circulation to the pulmonary circulation and a transient degree of pulmonary hypertension. Pulmonary oedema occurs within minutes, but only in those animals with extreme elevations in the pulmonary arterial pressure (> 60 Torr) (Maron *et al.*, 1994). The recent evidence suggesting a continuum of endothelial/epithelial injury with 'hydrostatic' oedema would predict that in some of these dogs with NPE, 'permeability' oedema should occur. The significant variability in the increase in EVLW in the canine NPE model with extreme elevations in microvascular pressure may indeed reflect individual differences in the susceptibility of the vascular endothelium to pressure-induced damage. Furthermore, the airway fluid-to-plasma protein concentration ratios in canine NPE form a continuum lying between pure 'hydrostatic' oedema caused by moderate volume overload (ratio 0.54) and pure 'permeability' oedema caused by alloxan (ratio 0.98) (Maron, 1987).

How pulmonary hypertension is initiated in NPE is far from clear, but pulmonary venous constriction may be an important factor. In the rat model of NPE, alveolar flooding with pink proteinaceous material occurs after head trauma. Resin casts of the rat lung after head injury show narrow focal constriction in the pulmonary veins. This venous contraction increases with maturation (Schraufnagel *et al.*, 1994). Contraction is not present in the pulmonary arteries or arterioles (Schraufnagel & Patel, 1990) and although the innervation of these venous 'sphincters' has not been completely defined, contraction can be blocked by α-adrenergic blockade (Schraufnagel & Thakkar, 1993).

The sympathetically-driven model of NPE is not universally accepted. Capsaicin is an extract of red peppers and selectively depletes the sensory neuropeptide, substance P. Rats systemically treated with capsaicin have destruction of primary sensory neurones (unmyelinated C-fibres) and depletion of sensory neuropeptide substance P in the spinal cord, vagus nerve and lung tissue (Levasseur *et al.*, 1993). Substance P depleted rats do not develop pulmonary oedema following severe head injury; however, the increase in pulmonary artery pressure remains essentially unchanged (Levasseur *et al.*, 1993). This result implies that (1) NPE is not necessarily a direct consequence of pulmonary hypertension, and (2) there is a link between neurogenic oedema (oedema subsequent to head injury) and neurogenic inflammation (neuropeptide driven inflammation). The mechanisms underlying sensory fibre activation and the anatomical site of activation are unknown. If the initial sensory stimulus is due to direct chemical stimulation of peripheral receptors within the lung, local release of substance P could secondarily initiate pulmonary vasoconstriction.

How relevant these models are to the head injured child remains to be determined. Changes in lung function in combination with bronchoalveolar lavage may help to resolve some of the apparent contradictions seen in the animal experiments.

Adult respiratory distress syndrome in children

Adult respiratory distress syndrome (ARDS) describes a clinical pattern seen in patients requiring endotracheal intubation and mechanical ventilation for life support and has both similarities and differences to neonatal respiratory distress syndrome. Its hallmarks are respiratory distress, need for mechanical support with positive end-expiratory pressure, diffuse alveolar infiltration on chest radiographs, impaired pulmonary compliance, decreased lung volumes and capacities and increased alveolar–arterial oxygen gradient (Pfenninger *et al.*, 1991). For the definition of ARDS, patients should have previously normal lungs and an acute triggering injury. In trauma patients developing ARDS, radiological infiltrates develop simultaneously with the abnormalities in pulmonary function, with the earliest changes most visible in the upper and middle lung fields (Johnson *et al.*, 1994). ARDS has been described in children (Effmann *et al.*, 1985) and neonates (Faix *et al.*, 1989; Pfenninger, 1993) although the initiating factors differ (Table 8.1). In the paediatric population, ARDS behaves as a single disease regardless of the underlying cause with four clinical stages: acute lung injury, latent period, acute respiratory failure and a phase of severe physiological derangement (Sarnaik & Lieh-Lai, 1994). During a 24-month surveillance period in a paediatric intensive care unit in the USA, 2.4% of admissions developed ARDS with a mortality rate of 62%. The highest incidence (12%) was in the group admitted for sepsis, viral pneumonia, smoke inhalation and near drowning. The

Table 8.1. *Causes of the adult respiratory distress syndrome in neonates and children*

Neonates	Children
Group B *Streptococcus* septicaemia	Systemic sepsis
Birth asphyxia	Infectious pneumonia
	Aspiration of gastric contents
	Smoke inhalation
	Near drowning
	Circulatory arrest
	Multiple trauma
	Haemorrhagic shock

lowest incidence (< 3%) was in children admitted with pulmonary contusion or multiple trauma (Davis *et al.*, 1993).

Initiation of ARDS

ARDS behaves as a single entity because the final common pathway is breakdown of the alveolar–capillary barrier and the formation of 'permeability' oedema. The initial clinical course is dependent on the degree of alveolar injury (Davis *et al.*, 1993). Within 12–48 hours of the insult, there is accumulation of debris and inflammatory cells within the alveolar space and interstitium with epithelial sloughing. Increased vascular permeability may not just be limited to the lung (Gosling *et al.*, 1994). The mediator of endothelial injury depends on the initial trigger factor. Both oxidants and inflammatory cells have been implicated in the pathogenesis of the catastrophic failure of the endothelial/epithelial barrier. In smoke inhalation, oxidant histotoxicity appears to predominate. Adult sheep exposed to smoke develop severe respiratory failure associated with airway damage, moderate pulmonary oedema, doubling in soft tissue lymph flow, an increase in bronchoalveolar lavage lipid peroxides and carboxyhaemoglobin levels between 40 and 50% (LaLonde *et al.*, 1994). Remarkably, aerosolised desferrioxamine-pentastarch given 30 minutes after smoke inhalation and continued for 24 hours, completely attenuates the physiological, histological and lipid peroxide responses. In this model, desferrioxamine chelates pulmonary iron thereby attenuating the formation of the hydroxyl radical from hydrogen peroxide.

The relative contribution of oxidants and inflammatory mediators in the development of ARDS after trauma is far more complex. Immediately after severe trauma in humans, plasma lipid peroxidation products (conjugated dienes) increase rapidly with a secondary increase during the second week (Marzi *et al.*, 1993). In a small prospective, randomised trial, intravenous recombinant superoxide dismutase significantly attenuated both diene peaks and attenuated cardiovascular and pulmonary indices of organ failure (Marzi *et al.*, 1993); however, it still remains possible that in trauma-associated ARDS, inflammatory mediators other than oxidants initiate pulmonary endothelial damage. Indeed, after severe trauma increases in plasma neutrophil elastase levels parallel conjugated dienes (Marzi *et al.*, 1993). The role of intravascular neutrophils in the latent phase of ARDS is controversial. ARDS patients do exhibit a significant neutrophil chemotactic gradient between the pulmonary vascular and alveolar space before the onset of clinical pulmonary injury (Donnelly *et al.*, 1993). This gradient results from increased concentrations of interleukin 8 (IL-8) in the alveolar space. Alveolar IL-8 levels are not increased in patients with similar predisposing factors who do not develop ARDS. There is also evidence of alterations in adhesion molecule expression on intravascular neutrophils before the development of ARDS. As previously discussed, L-selectin on neutrophils interacts with an unknown adhesion molecule on the pulmonary endothelium. When neutrophils become activated during shear-sensitive rolling, L-selectin is shed from the neutrophil surface as the soluble form (Carlos & Harlan, 1994). Proteolytic cleavage of selectins on the neutrophil surface also increases soluble levels. In patients at risk from developing ARDS, there is a significant correlation between low levels of plasma soluble L-selectin and the subsequent development of ARDS (Donnelly *et al.*, 1994). The pathological significance of low levels of L-selectin remains unknown but could reflect increased binding of the soluble selectin to activated endothelial cells. Clearly something is happening to adhesion molecule expression on circulating neutrophils during the latent phase of ARDS, but the changes in intravascular leucocytes could all be secondary to endothelial damage/activation from another cause.

An alternative pathogenic mechanism not dependent on adhesion of circulating leucocytes, is activation of cells resident within the lung interstitium and on the surface of the alveolar epithelium. This mode of injury could explain why ARDS occurs in severely neutropenic children (Sivan *et al.*, 1990). High levels of mediators released into the alveolar space could damage both the alveolar epithelium and pulmonary endothelium. The alveolar macrophage is both a pro- and anti-inflammatory cell and is therefore a candidate for the key resident leucocyte. Alveolar macrophages are exquisitely sensitive to minute concentrations of lipopolysaccharide (Grigg *et al.*, 1994) and are activated by oxidants (Grundfest *et al.*, 1982). Alveolar fluid IL-8 in the latent period of ARDS is probably released by alveolar macrophages (Donnelly *et al.*, 1993). IL-8 is not known to initiate severe endothelial damage in its own right, but other locally generated mediators such as leukotrienes can directly injure cells. For example, in the septic cat model of ARDS, pretreatment with the new potent cysteinyl-leukotriene antagonist ICI 198,615, prevents the pulmonary microvascular protein leakage and significantly attenuates the fall in blood oxygenation (Schützer *et al.*, 1994).

Resolution of ARDS

Once ARDS is established, cells, mediators and oxidants all increase, making an assessment of their relative importance in the initial injury virtually impossible. There is a massive influx of neutrophils into the alveoli with a 10 to 40-fold increase in the protein content of the alveolar fluid (Fowler *et al.*, 1987). Resting peripheral neutrophils show upregulation of the integrin CD11b/CD18 (Laurent *et al.*, 1994) and the levels of reduced glutathione in the alveolar fluid are lower than normal controls (Bunnell & Pacht, 1993). Changes in cells, mediators and antioxidants after the first 48 hours of ARDS are less important to the short-term outcome than the initial endothelial injury. Clinical outcome can be identified as early as the second day of ARDS using a measure of oxygenation efficiency (Davis *et al.*, 1993). Furthermore, children dying within the first 5 days of ARDS show heavy, partly collapsed lungs, extensive hyaline membrane formation, marked capillary congestion and interstitial oedema (Effman *et al.*, 1985). Although inflammatory cells within the alveoli do not appear to be of primary importance within the first 48 hours of ARDS, they may be of significance during the resolution phase.

In adults and children, mortality from ARDS after the first week is related to a progressive fibroproliferative response within the lung (Effman *et al.*, 1985; Meduri *et al.*, 1994). A lack of improvement in ventilator settings and worsening alveolar infiltrates on chest radiographs after 7 days is suggestive of an abnormal fibroproliferative response (Heffner & Zamora, 1990). Fibroproliferation is characterised by accumulation of mesenchymal cells and their connective tissue products in the airspaces and the repair of damaged epithelial cells. Why do some children with ARDS develop this complication? Very high levels of the fibrogenic peptide platelet-derived growth factor are present in the alveolar lining fluid of patients with ARDS (Snyder *et al.*, 1991); however, these high levels occur irrespective of whether fibroproliferation progresses to fatal pulmonary fibrosis. Indeed some degree of fibroproliferation may be important in establishing an intact alveolar epithelial barrier and only those children capable of controlling this essential fibrosis will survive. In the initial stages of ARDS, containing the degree of fibrosis depends on re-establishing the correct balance between procoagulant and fibrinolytic systems (Andrew & Berry, 1994). Later stages of successful resolution may depend on the induction of neutrophil and fibroblast apoptosis. It is encouraging that the resolution phase is responsive to appropriate pharmacological interventions. Intravenous steroid therapy during the fibroproliferative phase increases survival in adults, especially if started before the development of dense acellular fibrosis and derangement of intra-alveolar architecture (Meduri *et al.*, 1994).

There is little data on the outcome in paediatric survivors of ARDS. In a follow-up of nine children 4 years after ARDS, three had some degree of exertional dyspnoea (Fanconi *et al.*, 1985). Larger studies in adults demonstrate that during the first year after ARDS there is continued improvement in lung function abnormalities, although most have persistent mild reductions in carbon monoxide transfer factor (TLCO) at 12 months (Hert & Albert, 1994). Deficits persisting at 1 year are unlikely to improve in adults (Hert & Albert, 1994), but in children any persisting deficits would be expected to improve with additional lung growth.

Neonatal chronic lung disease

Neonatal chronic lung disease is a result of lung injury originating in the first weeks of life. Chronic lung disease was originally described in infants ventilated for hyaline membrane disease (HMD) who developed gross radiological evidence of fibrotic and cystic changes by the first month of life (Northway et al., 1967). This clinical picture is associated with histological evidence of 'bronchopulmonary dysplasia' (BPD) (Taghizadeh & Reynolds, 1976). The final expression of BPD is chronic fibroproliferation with patchy intra-alveolar fibrosis alternating with hyperinflated air sacs (Robertson, 1989). The lung of fatal BPD is histologically very similar to the adult with fatal fibroproliferation (Hert & Albert, 1994); however, there are important differences between the two age groups. One point of divergence is that the adult lung prior to ARDS is structurally normal, whereas the premature lung is not only structurally immature but is also potentially deficient in anti-inflammatory and antioxidant defenses. In the past 'BDP' has been used interchangeably to describe both the clinical syndrome and the pulmonary pathology after HMD (i.e. surfactant deficiency). Recently, the term chronic lung disease (CLD) has been introduced (Robertson, 1989). This represents an important conceptual change as it does not exclude infants who do not initially have hyaline membrane disease. CLD without any evidence of prior HMD (CLD-noHMD) has been recognised since the 1980s (Edwards et al., 1980; Fitzgerald et al., 1990). Neonatal CLD may therefore be at least two separate conditions; CLD-HMD and CLD-noHMD.

Vulnerability for CLD at birth

By definition, surfactant deficiency is important in the aetiology of CLD-HMD. Infants developing CLD-HMD could have less functional surfactant at birth compared with those with an uncomplicated outcome. Alternatively, surfactant deficiency may just provide the setting for the extrauterine insults of barotrauma and oxidants to act on other areas of pulmonary vulnerability (e.g. antioxidant levels, structural immaturity). The clinical evidence points more to this second possibility. Ventilator settings in the first day of life are a surrogate for the degree of surfactant deficiency and do predict survival or death in the acute stages of HMD (Gray et al., 1993); however, ventilator settings at 24 hours do not predict which infants will develop CLD (Cooke, 1991). In addition, severe pulmonary damage still occurs with pulmonary surfactant replacement therapy. For example, in infants dying from HMD the extent of intraalveolar hyaline membranes, epithelial necrosis and interstitial oedema is unaffected by prophylactic surfactant therapy (Thornton et al., 1994). The degree of surfactant deficiency may therefore not be the primary mechanism leading to CLD-HMD.

There is little evidence to suggest a role for foetal inflammation in the development CLD-HMD. In complicated and uncomplicated HMD, the alveoli at birth are devoid of neutrophils (Ogden et al., 1984; Grigg et al., 1993a) which only appear in the lung after the first 24 hours of ventilation (Ogden et al., 1984). In comparison to CLD-HMD, there are data to suggest that foetal inflammation is critical to the development of CLD-noHMD. Neonatal pulmonary inflammation, acquired in utero, occurs frequently in premature infants (Grigg et al., 1993a), but why inflammation is rarely seen at birth in HMD is unclear. One explanation is that inflammatory products stimulate surfactant secretion (Oda et al., 1991). In babies without HMD, there is clear evidence of a link between inflammation in the newborn airway and amniotic inflammation. Increased numbers of neutrophils and concentrations of interleukin 6 (IL-6) in the airways of newborn premature infants are associated with clinical indicators of maternal chorioamnionitis (e.g. maternal fever) (Grigg et al., 1992a, 1993a). In situ hybridisation has conclusively demonstrated that the airway neutrophilia at birth represents a primary foetal response (Grigg et al., 1993a; Scott et al., 1994). The evidence that foetal pulmonary inflammation is detrimental is still incomplete; however, in intubated premature infants without the hyaline membrane disease, there is an association between elevated tracheal aspirate neutrophil elastase-α_1-proteinase inhibitor complex at birth and the development of CLD-noHMD (Fujimura et al., 1993). Furthermore, this form of CLD-noHMD is associated with a high incidence of maternal chorioamnionitis (Fujimura et al., 1993). One hypothesis incorporating all these findings is that that foetal pulmonary inflammation matures ('stresses') the surfactant system, but the price in some babies is neutrophil-mediated tissue injury. Although airway neutrophils at birth are not a risk factor for CLD-HMD (Watterberg et al., 1994), an association between high levels of airway IL-6 at birth and the development of CLD-HMD has been recently reported (Bagchi et al., 1994). It is unclear how this observation fits with the absence of inflammation in the airway of infants with HMD; however, the rare combination of neonatal lung inflammation and surfactant deficiency could be devastating.

There is some indirect evidence to suggest that CLD-HMD is associated with increased oxidant damage. In the first 24 hours of HMD, levels of expired pentane and ethane are low, but increase rapidly on the third day of life (Pitkänen et al., 1990). The highest levels are associated with either death or the development of CLD-HMD; however, the levels of inspired oxygen in the first 3 days of life do not predict the development of CLD-HMD (Cooke, 1991). Pulmonary antioxidant levels at birth and the ability to rapidly induce pulmonary antioxidant production may therefore be more important than differences in the amount of free radicals generated in the lung. In a small study, the total amount of glutathione in bronchoalveolar lavage fluid on the first day of life was significantly lower in those infants who subsequently developed CLD (both HMD and no HMD) (Grigg *et al.*, 1993b). Certainly, the concentrations of reduced glutathione in the plasma of premature babies are an order of magnitude less than those seen in adults (Smith *et al.*, 1993). Antioxidant deficiency as a cause of CLD is an attractive hypothesis. Aerosol therapy is feasible in intubated premature infants (Grigg *et al.*, 1992b) and antioxidants could be delivered by direct supplementation (Borok *et al.*, 1991). Differences in lung structure as the major risk for CLD would be far less amenable to therapy. Immaturity in the lung matrix leads to disruption of the epithelial lining and ripping open of alveoli during mechanical ventilation. For ethical reasons, the lung histology on the first day of life in survivors of HMD is unknown and any differences in structure remain undefined. Early measurement of respiratory mechanics may indirectly indicate structural differences. The lower dynamic compliance of the respiratory system of the first day of life in infants who subsequently develop CLD-HMD could reflect differences in lung matrix (Freezer & Sly, 1993); however, other studies have reported that lung compliance and resistance obtained during the first 3 days of life do not differentiate between CLD-HMD and uncomplicated HMD (Farstad & Bratlid, 1994). The effect of surfactant therapy has not clarified CLD aetiology. The reduction in mortality from CLD-HMD with surfactant therapy (Schwartz *et al.*, 1994) could indicate attenuation of barotrauma, but could equally reflect a reduction in the pulmonary oxidant burden.

Resolution of inflammation and CLD

It is very difficult to interpret the differences seen in pulmonary inflammation in uncomplicated HMD and CLD-HMD infants after the fifth day of life. The persistent neutrophilia (Ogden *et al.*, 1984; Groneck *et al.*, 1994), the increased concentrations of free elastase (Groneck *et al.*, 1994) and leukotrienes (Mirro *et al.*, 1990) in CLD-HMD could reflect important differences in the resolution process; however, these differences could be secondary to a more important oxidant/barotrauma injury. Unfortunately, our understanding of neonatal CLD parallels that of ARDS in that very little is known about the resolution phase of pulmonary inflammation. Neutrophil apoptosis and removal by macrophages has been seen in the premature lung (Figure 8.1), but its clinical significance is unknown (Grigg *et al.*, 1991). Furthermore, steroid therapy is clinically useful when given on the second week of CLD, but its mode of action is unclear (Silverman, 1994). Few researchers have applied the same insult to both

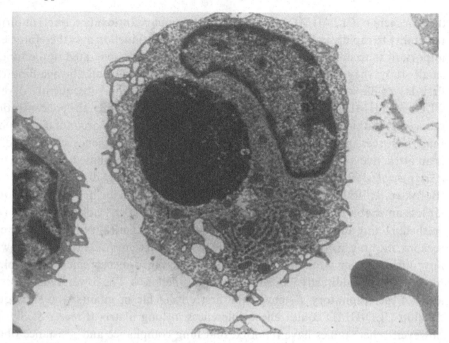

Figure 8.1. Electron micrograph of alveolar macrophage lavaged from the airway of a premature infant during the resolution of hyaline membrane disease. An intact apoptotic neutrophil is contained within the macrophage phagosome.

neonatal and adult animals and directly compared evolution/resolution phases. In the hyperoxic baboon model of 'adult' ARDS and neonatal CLD, intra-alveolar fibrinolysis is more deficient in the premature animal (Andrew & Berry, 1994). Deficient clearance of fibrin strands could increase the vulnerability of the newborn to intraalveolar fibrosis. On the other hand, in studies of adhesion molecule function, neonatal rabbits have significantly reduced CD18 and L-selectin-dependent neutrophil migration into inflammatory sites (Fortenberry et al., 1994). This relative deficiency in neutrophil/endothelial adhesion may increase vulnerability to infection, but it may also increase resistance to neutrophil-mediated lung injury.

In humans, the medium to long-term outcome of CLD survivors is good. Some infants will die with refractory failure, secondary to either pulmonary hypertension or the combination of alveolar disruption and bronchomalacia (Azizkhan et al., 1992). Children surviving to 10 years of age have, in general, a normal mean lung total capacity and functional residual capacity, although the majority have bronchial reactivity to methacholine (Blayney et al., 1991). The very long-term effects of CLD and ARDS are unknown. There is concern that after diffuse lung damage children will have less pulmonary reserve during the normal decline in lung function of adulthood, especially if this decline is accelerated by smoking.

Interpretation of future studies

The application of bronchoalveolar lavage and similar techniques to children has transformed our capacity to understand the nature of paediatric pulmonary injury; however, rather than simplifying the picture, analysis of alveolar fluid has demonstrated a complex and often confusing inter-relationship between mediators of injury and defence. In assessing this type of data there are two important questions to be asked. First, does the difference in mediator/cell/etc. reflect the initial mechanism of tissue damage, or is it a secondary event? Second, does the change predict a clinically important measure of outcome? Samples obtained from the intubated child after serious trauma and from the premature infant are most likely to provide an insight into aetiology if taken before the clinical appearance of pulmonary injury.

Conclusion

Clinical classifications of pulmonary disease have been useful in guiding supportive therapies and determining epidemiology. Over the next decade an understanding of the mechanisms underlying paediatric lung injury will be essential in establishing appropriate prophylactic therapies. It may also lead to a reclassification of pulmonary diseases in children based on underlying pathology and not just on clinical presentation.

References

Andrew, M. & Berry, L. (1994). Influence of lung maturity on bronchoalveolar fibrin deposition and clearance in lung injury syndromes. *American Journal of Respiratory and Critical Care Medicine*, **149**, 572–4.

Azizkhan, R. G., Grimmer, D. L., Askin, F. B., Lacy, S. R., Mesten, D. F. & Wood, R. F. (1992). Acquired lobar emphysema (overinflation): clinical and pathological evaluation of infants requiring lobectomy. *Journal of Pediatric Surgery*, **27**, 1145–52.

Bachofen, H., Schürch, S., Michel, R. P. & Weibel, E. R. (1993a). Experimental hydrostatic pulmonary edema in rabbit lungs: morphology. *American Review of Respiratory Disease*, **147**, 989–96.

Bachofen, H., Schürch, S., Michel, R. P. & Weibel, E. R. (1993b). Experimental hydrostatic pulmonary edema in rabbit lungs: barrier lesions. *American Review of Respiratory Disease*, **147**, 997–1004.

Bagchi, A., Viscardi, R. M., Taciak, V., Ensor J. E., McCrea, K. E. & Hasday, J. D. (1994). Increased activity of interleukin 6 but not tumor necrosis factor-α in lung lavage of premature infants is associated with the development of bronchopulmonary dysplasia. *Pediatric Research*, **36**, 244–52.

Berthiaume, Y., Broaddus, V. C., Gropper, M. A., Tanita, T. & Matthay, M. A. (1988). Alveolar liquid and protein clearance from normal dog lungs. *Journal of Applied Physiology*, **65**, 585–93.

Blayney, M., Kerem, E., Whyte, H. & O'Brodovich, H. (1991). Bronchopulmonary dysplasia: improvement in lung function between 7 and 10 years of age. *Journal of Pediatrics*, **118**, 201–6.

Borok, Z., Buhl, R., Grimes, G. J., Bokser, A. D., Hubbard, K. J., Roum, J. H., Czerske, B., Cantin, A. M. & Crystal, R. G. (1991). Effect of glutathione aerosol on oxidant-antioxidant balance in idiopathic pulmonary fibrosis. *Lancet*, **338**, 215–16.

Bunnell, E. & Pacht, E. R. (1993). Oxidized glutathione is increased in the alveolar fluid of patients with the adult respiratory distress syndrome. *American Review of Respiratory Disease*, **148**, 1174–8.

Cantin, A., North, S. L., Hubbard, R. C. & Crystal, R. G. (1987). Normal alveolar epithelial lining fluid contains high levels of glutathione. *Journal of Applied Physiology*, **63**, 152–7.

Carlson, R. W., Schaeffer, R. C., Michaels, S. G. & Weil, M. H. (1979). Pulmonary edema fluid: spectrum of features in 37 patients. *Circulation*, **5**, 1161–9.

Carlos, T. M. & Harlan, J. M. (1994). Leukocyte-endothelial adhesion molecules. *Blood*, **84**, 2068–101.

Cooke, R. W. I. (1991). Factors associated with chronic lung disease in preterm infants. *Archives of Disease in Childhood*, **66**, 776–9.

Davis, S. L., Furman, D. P. & Costarino, A. T. Jr. (1993). Adult respiratory distress syndrome in children: associated disease, clinical course, and predictors of death. *Journal of Pediatrics*, **123**, 35–45.

Demling, R. & Riessen, R. (1990). Pulmonary dysfunction after cerebral injury. *Critical Care Medicine*, **18**, 768–74.

Deneke, S. M. & Fanburg, B. L. (1989). Regulation of cellular glutathione. *American Journal of Physiology*, **257**, 163–73.

Donnelly, S. C., Strieter, R. M., Kunkel, S. L., Walz, A., Robertson, C. R., Carter, D. C., Graut, I. S., Pollock, A. J. & Haslett, C. (1993). Interleukin 8 and development of adult respiratory distress syndrome in at-risk patient groups. *Lancet*, **341**, 643–7.

Donnelly, S. C., Haslett, C., Dransfield, I., Robertson, C. E., Carter, D. C., Ross, J. A., Grant, I. S. & Tedder, T. F. (1994). Role of selectins in development of adult respiratory distress syndrome. *Lancet*, **344**, 215–9.

Dreyfuss, D., Soler, P. & Saumon, G. (1992). Spontaneous resolution of pulmonary edema caused by short periods of cyclic overinflation. *Journal of Applied Physiology*, **72**, 2081–9.

Edwards, D. K., Jacob, J. & Gluck, L. (1980). The immature lung: radiographic appearance, course and complications. *American Journal of Radiology*, **135**, 659–66.

Effmann, E. L., Merten, D. F., Kirks, D. R., Pratt, D. C. & Spock, A. (1985). Adult respiratory distress syndrome in children. *Radiology*, **157**, 69–74.

Eichacker, P. Q., Hoffman, W. D., Farese, A., Danner, R. L., Suffredini, A. F., Waisman, W., Banks, S. M. (1993). Leukocyte CD18 monoclonal antibody worsens endotoxemia and cardiovascular injury in canines with septic shock. *Journal of Applied Physiology*, **74**, 1885–92.

Faix, R. G., Viscardi, R. M., DiPietro, M. A. & Nicks, J. J. (1989). Adult respiratory distress syndrome in full-term newborns. *Pediatrics*, **83**, 971–6.

Fanconi, S., Kraemer, R., Weber, J., Tschaeppler, H. & Pfenninger, J. (1985). Long-term sequelae in children surviving adult respiratory distress syndrome. *Journal of Pediatrics*, **106**, 218–22.

Farber, J. L., Kyle, M. E. & Coleman, J. B. (1990). Biology of disease: mechanisms of cell injury by activated oxygen species. *Laboratory Investigation*, **62**, 670–9.

Farstad, T. & Bratlid, D. (1994). Incidence and prediction of bronchopulmonary dysplasia in a cohort of premature infants. *Acta Paediatrica*, **83**, 19–24.

Fernandes, R. S. & Cotter, T. G. (1994). Apoptosis or necrosis: intracellular levels of glutathione influence mode of cell death. *Biochemical Pharmacology*, **48**, 675–81.

Fitzgerald, P., Donoghue, V. & Gorman, W. (1990). Bronchopulmonary dysplasia: a radiographic and clinical review of 20 patients. *British Journal of Radiology*, **63**, 444–7.

Fortenberry, J. D., Marolda, J. R., Anderson, D. C., Smith, C. W. & Mariscalco, M. M. (1994). CD18-dependent and L-selectin-dependent neutrophil emigration is diminished in neonatal rabbits. *Blood*, **84**, 889–97.

Fowler, A. A., Hyers, T. M., Fisher, B. J., Bechard, D. E., Centor, R. M. & Webster, R. O. (1987). The adult respiratory distress syndrome: cell populations and soluble mediators in the air spaces of patients at high risk. *American Review of Respiratory Disease*, **136**, 1125–31.

Freezer, N. J. & Sly, P. D. (1993). Predictive value of measurements of respiratory mechanics in preterm infants with HMD. *Pediatric Pulmonology*, **16**, 116–23.

Fujimura, M., Kitajima, H. & Nakayama, M. (1993). Increased leukocyte elastase of the tracheal aspirate at birth and neonatal pulmonary emphysema. *Pediatrics*, **92**, 564–9.

Ghio, A. J., Fracica, P. J., Young, S. L. & Piantadosi, C. A. (1994). Synthetic surfactant scavenges oxidants and protects against hyperoxic lung injury. *Journal of Applied Physiology*, **77**, 1217–23.

Gosling, P., Sanghera, K. & Dickson, G. (1994). Generalized vascular permeability and pulmonary function in patients following serious trauma. *Journal of Trauma*, **36**, 477–81.

Gray, P. H., Grice, J. F., Lee, M. S., Richie, B. H. & Williams, G. (1993). Prediction of outcome of preterm infants with severe bronchopulmonary dysplasia. *Journal of Paediatrics and Child Health*, **29**, 107–12.

Grigg, J. M., Savill, J. S., Sarraf, C., Haslett, C. & Silverman, M. (1991). Neutrophil apoptosis and clearance from neonatal lungs. *Lancet*, **338**, 720–2.

Grigg, J. M., Barber, A. & Silverman, M. (1992a). Increased levels of bronchoalveolar lavage fluid interleukin 6 in preterm ventilated infants after prolonged rupture of membranes. *American Review of Respiratory Disease*, **145**, 782–6.

Grigg, J., Arnon, S., Jones, T., Clarke, A. & Silverman, M. (1992b). The delivery of therapeutic aerosols to intubated babies. *Archives of Disease in Childhood*, **67**, 25–30.

Grigg, J., Arnon, S., Chase, A. & Silverman, M. (1993a). Inflammatory cells in the lungs of premature infants on the first day of life: perinatal risk factors and origin of cells. *Archives of Disease in Childhood*, **69**, 40–3.

Grigg, J., Barber, A. & Silverman, M. (1993b). Bronchoalveolar lavage glutathione in intubated premature infants. *Archives of Disease in Childhood*, **69**, 49–51.

Grigg, J., Kukielka, G. L., Berens, K. L., Dryer, W. J., Entman, A. L. & Smith, C. W. (1994). Induction of intercellular adhesion molecule-1 by lipopolysaccharide in canine alveolar macrophages. *American Journal of Respiratory Cell and Molecular Biology*, **2**, 304–11.

Grundfest, C. G., Chang, J. & Newcombe, D. (1982). Acrolein: a potent modulator of lung macrophage arachidonic acid metabolism. *Biochemica et Biophysica Acta*, **713**, 149–59.

Groneck P., Götze-Speer, B., Oppermann, M., Eiffert, H. & Speer, C. P. (1994). Association of pulmonary inflammation and increased microvascular permeability during the development of bronchopulmonary dysplasia: a sequential analysis of inflammatory mediators in respiratory fluids of high-risk preterm neonates. *Pediatrics*, **93**, 712–18.

Hallman, M., Merritt, T. A., Akino, T. & Bry, K. (1991). Surfactant protein A, phosphatidylcholine, and surfactant inhibitors in epithelial lining fluid. Correlation with surface activity, severity of respiratory distress syndrome, and outcome in small premature infants. *American Review of Respiratory Disease*, **144**, 1376–84.

Heffner, J. E. & Zamora, C. A. (1990). Clinical predictors of prolonged translaryngeal intubation in patients with the adult respiratory distress syndrome. *Chest*, **97**, 447–52.

Hert, R. & Albert, R. K. (1994). Sequelae of the adult respiratory distress syndrome. *Thorax*, **49**, 8–13.

Jenkinson, S. G., Marcum, R. F., Pickard, J. S., Orzechowski, R. A., Lawrence, R. A. & Jordan, J. M. (1988). Glutathione disulphide formation occurring during hypoxia and reoxygenation of rat lung. *Journal of Laboratory and Clinical Medicine*, **112**, 471–80.

Johnson, K. S., Bishop, M. H., Stephen, C. M. II, Jorgens, J., Shoemaker, W. C., Shori, S. K. & Ordog, G. (1994). Temporal patterns of radiographic infiltration in severely traumatized patients with and without adult respiratory distress syndrome. *Journal of Trauma*, **36**, 644–50.

Jourdan, C., Convert, J., Rousselle, C., Wasylkiewicz, J., Mircevski, V., Mottolese, C. & Lapras, C. (1993). Étude hémodynamique de l'óedème pulmonaire aigu neurogène chez l'enfant. *Pédiatrie*, **48**, 805–12.

Kaufman, H. H., Timberlake, G., Voelker, J. & Pait, G. T. (1993). Medical complications of head injury. *Medical Clinics of North America*, **77**, 43–60.

Keeney, S. E., Mathews, M. J., Haque, A. K., Rudloft, E. & Schmalsteig, F. C. (1994). Oxygen-induced lung injury in the guinea pig proceeds through CD18-independent mechanisms. *American Journal of Respiratory and Critical Care Medicine*, **149**, 311–19.

Lagasse, E. & Weissman, I. L. (1994). bcl-2 inhibits apoptosis of neutrophils but not their engulfment by macrophages. *Journal of Experimental Medicine*, **179**, 1047–52.

LaLonde, C., Ikegami, K. & Demling, R. (1994). Aerosolized deferoxamine prevents lung and systemic injury caused by smoke inhalation. *Journal of Applied Physiology*, **77**, 2057–64.

Laurent, T., Markert, M., von Fliedner, V., Feihl, F., Schaller, M.-D., Tagan, M.-C., Chiolero, R. & Perret, C. (1994). CD11b/CD18 expression, adherence, and chemotaxis of granulocytes in adult respiratory distress syndrome. *American Journal of Respiratory and Critical Care Medicine*, **149**, 1534–8.

Lear, G. H. (1990). Neurogenic pulmonary oedema. *Acta Paediatrica Scandinavica*, **79**, 1131–3.

Lee, A., Whyte, M. K. & Haslett, C. (1993). Inhibition of apoptosis and prolongation of neutrophil functional longevity by inflammatory mediators. *Journal of Leukocyte Biology*, **54**, 283–8.

Levasseur, J. E., Patterson, J. L., Garcia, C. I., Moskovitz, M. A., Choi, S. C. & Kontos, H. A. (1993). Effect of neonatal capsaicin treatment on neurogenic pulmonary edema from fluid-percussion brain injury in the adult rat. *Journal of Neurosurgery*, **78**, 610–18.

Lo, S. K., Bevilacqua, M. B. & Malik, A. B. (1994). E-selectin ligands mediate tumor necrosis factor-induced neutrophil sequestration and pulmonary edema in guinea pig lungs. *Circulation Research*, **75**, 955–60.

Marzi, I., Bühren, V., Schüttler, A. & Trentz, O. (1993). Value of superoxide dismutase for the prevention of multiple organ failure after multiple trauma. *Journal of Trauma*, **35**, 110–19.

Mackersie, R. C., Christensen, J. M., Pitts, L. H. & Lewis, F. R. (1983). Pulmonary extravascular fluid accumulation following intracranial injury. *Journal of Trauma*, **23**, 968–75.

Maron, M. B. (1987). Analysis of airway fluid protein concentration in neurogenic pulmonary edema. *Journal of Applied Physiology*, **62**, 470–6.

Maron, M. B., Holcomb, P. H., Dawson, C. A., Rickaby, D. A., Clough, A. V. & Lineham, J. E. (1994). Edema development and recovery in neurogenic pulmonary edema. *Journal of Applied Physiology*, **77**, 1155–63.

Matthay, M. A. & Weiner-Kronish, J. P. (1990). Intact epithelial barrier function is critical for the resolution of alveolar edema in humans. *American Review of Respiratory Disease*, **142**, 1250–7.

Meagher, L. M., Savill, J. S., Baker, A., Fuller, R. & Haslett, C. (1989). Macrophage secretory responses to ingestion of aged neutrophils. *Biochemical Society Transactions*, **17**, 608–9.

Meduri, G. U., Chinn, A. J., Leeper, K. V., Wunderink, R. G., Tolley, E., Winer-Muram, H. T., Khare, V., & Eltorky, M. (1994). Corticosteroid rescue treatment of progressive fibroproliferation in late ARDS. *Chest*, **105**, 1516–27.

Milley, J. R., Nugent, S. K. & Rogers, M. C. (1979). Neurogenic pulmonary edema in childhood. *Journal of Pediatrics*, **94**, 706–9.

Minnear, F. L. & Connell, R. S. (1981). Increased permeability of the capillary-alveolar barrier in neurogenic pulmonary edema (NPE). *Microvascular Research*, **22**, 345–66.

Mirro, M., Armstead, W. & Leffler, C. (1990). Increased airway leukotriene levels in infants with severe bronchopulmonary dysplasia. *American Journal of Diseases in Children*, **144**, 160–1.

Muller, W. A., Weigl, S. A., Deng, X. & Phillips, D. M. (1993). PECAM-1 is required for transendothelial migration of leukocytes. *Journal of Experimental Medicine*, **178**, 449–60.

Mulroy, J. J., Mickell, J. J., Tong, T. K. & Pellock, J. M. (1985). Postictal pulmonary edema in children. *Neurology*, 403–5.

Northway, W. H. Jr, Rosan, R. C. & Porter, D. Y. (1967). Pulmonary disease following respirator therapy of hyaline membrane disease: bronchopulmonary dysplasia. *New England Journal of Medicine*, **276**, 257–68.

Oda, Y., Kai, H., Isohama, Y., Takahama, T. & Miyata, T. (1991). Stimulation of pulmonary surfactant secretion by activating neutrophils in rat type II pneumocytes culture. *Life Sciences*, **49**, 803–11.

Ogden, B. E., Murphy, S. A., Saunders, G. C., Pathak, D. & Johnson, J. D. (1984). Neonatal lung neutrophils and elastase/proteinase inhibitor imbalance. *American Review of Respiratory Disease*, **130**, 817–21.

Parker, R. E., Roselli, R. J., Harris, T. R. & Brigham, K. L. (1981). Effects of graded increases in pulmonary vascular pressures on lung fluid balance in unanesthetized sheep. *Circulation Research*, **49**, 1164–72.

Pender, E. S. & Pollack, C. V. Jr. (1992). Neurogenic pulmonary edema: case reports and review. *Journal of Emergency Medicine*, **10**, 45–51.

Pfenninger, J., Tschaeppeler, H., Wagner, B. P., Weber, J. & Zimmerman, A. (1991). The paradox of adult respiratory distress syndrome in neonates. *Pediatric Pulmonology*, **10**, 18–24.

Pfenninger, J. (1993). Adult respiratory distress syndrome in newborn infants. *Critical Care Medicine*, **21** (Suppl. 9), S362–S363.

Phelan, P. D., Olinsky, A. & Robertson, C. F. (1994). Lung growth and development. In

Respiratory Illness in Children, 4th edn, ed. P. D. Phelan, A. Olinsky & C. F. Robertson, pp. 1–7. London: Blackwell Scientific Publications.

Pitkänen, O. M., Hallman, M. & Andersson, S. M. (1990). Correlation of free oxygen radical-induced lipid peroxidation with outcome in very low birth weight infants. *Journal of Pediatrics*, **116**, 760–4.

Robertson, B. (1989). The evolution of neonatal respiratory distress syndrome into chronic lung disease. *European Respiratory Journal*, **2** (Suppl. 3), 33s–37s.

Sarnaik, A. P. & Lieh-Lai, M. (1994). Adult respiratory distress syndrome in children. *Pediatric Clinics of North America*, **41**, 337–63.

Savill, J. S., Wyllie, A. H., Henson, J. E., Walport, M. J., Henson, P. M. & Haslett, C. (1989). Macrophage phagocytosis of aging neutrophils in inflammation. *Journal of Clinical Investigation*, **83**, 865–75.

Schraufnagel, D. E., Kurtulus, M. M. & Patel, T. H. (1994). Effect of age on the contraction of pulmonary venous sphincters in rats. *American Journal of Respiratory and Critical Care Medicine*, **149**, 227–31.

Schraufnagel, D. E., & Patel, K. R. (1990). Sphincters in pulmonary veins: an anatomic study in rats. *American Review of Respiratory Disease*, **141**, 721–6.

Schraufnagel, D. E. & Thakkar, M. B. (1993). Pulmonary venous sphincter constriction is attenuated by α-adrenergic antagonism. *American Review of Respiratory Disease*, **148**, 477–82.

Schützer, K-M., Larsson, A., Risberg, B. & Falk, A. (1994). Leukotriene receptor antagonism prevents lung protein leakage and hypoxaemia in a septic cat model. *European Respiratory Journal*, **7**, 1131–7.

Schwartz, R. M., Luby, A. M., Scanlon, J. W. & Kellogg, R. J. (1994). Effect of surfactant on morbidity, mortality, and resource use in newborn infants weighing 500 to 1500 g. *New England Journal of Medicine*, **330**, 1476–80.

Scott, R. J., Peat, D. & Rhodes, C. A. (1994). Investigation of the fetal pulmonary inflammatory reaction in chorioamnionitis, using an in situ Y chromosome marker. *Pediatric Pathology*, **14**, 997–1003.

Silverman, M. (1994). Chronic lung disease of prematurity: are we too cautious with steroids? *European Journal of Pediatrics*, **153** (Suppl. 2), S30–S35.

Sivan, Y., Mor, C., Al-Jundi, S. & Newth, C. J. L. (1990). Adult respiratory distress syndrome in severely neutropenic children. *Pediatric Pulmonology*, **8**, 104–8.

Smith, C. V., Hansen, T. N., Martin, N. E., McMicken, H. W. & Elliott, S. J. (1993). Oxidant stress responses in premature infants during exposure to hyperoxia. *Pediatric Research*, **34**, 360–5.

Snyder, L. S., Hertz, M. I., Peterson, M. S., Harmon, K. R., Marinelli, W. A., Henke, C. A. & Greenbeck, J. R. (1991). Acute lung injury. Pathogenesis of intraalveolar fibrosis. *Journal of Clinical Investigation*, **88**, 663–73.

Staub, N. C. (1974). Pulmonary edema. *Physiological Reviews*, **54**, 678–811.

Taghizadeh, A. & Reynolds, E. O. R. (1976). Pathogenesis of bronchopulmonary dysplasia following hyaline membrane disease. *American Journal of Pathology*, **82**, 241–64.

Thornton, C. M., Halliday, H. L. & O'Hara, M. D. (1994). Surfactant replacement therapy in preterm neonates: a comparison of postmortem pulmonary histology in treated and untreated infants. *Pediatric Pathology*, **14**, 945–53.

Tsukimoto, K., Mathieu-Costello, O., Prediletto, R., Elliott, A. R. & West, J. B. (1991). Ultrastructural appearances of pulmonary capillaries at high transmural pressures. *Journal* of *Applied Physiology*, **71**, 573–82.

Tsukimoto, K., Yoshimura, N., Ichioka, M., Tojo, N., Miyazato, I., Marumo, F. & West, J. B. (1994). Protein, cell, and LTB_4 concentrations of lung edema fluid produced by high capillary pressures in rabbit. *Journal of Applied Physiology*, **76**, 321–7.

Vartio, T., Seppa, H. & Vaheri, A. (1981). Susceptibility of solute and matrix fibronectin to degradation by tissue proteinases, mast cell chymase and cathepsin. *Journal of Biological Chemistry*, **256**, 471–7.

Watterberg, K. L., Carmichael, D. F., Gerdes, J. S., Werner, S., Backstrom, C. & Murphy, S. (1994). Secretory leukocyte protease inhibitor and lung inflammation in developing bronchopulmonary dysplasia. *Journal of Pediatrics*, **125**, 264–9.

Weiss, S. J. (1989). Tissue destruction by neutrophils. *New England Journal of Medicine*, **320**, 356–76.

White, C. W., Mimmack, R. F. & Repine, J. E. (1986). Accumulation of lung tissue oxidized glutathione (GSSG) as a marker of oxidant induced lung injury. *Chest*, **89** (Suppl. 3), 111s–113s.

Wispe, J. R., Bell, E. F. & Roberts, R. J. (1985). Assessment of lipid peroxidation in new born infants and rabbits by measurements of expired ethane and pentane: influence of parenteral lipid infusion. *Pediatric Research*, **19**, 374–9.

9
Metabolic and endocrine stress responses to surgery

M. P. WARD PLATT

Introduction

The neuroendocrine stress response to surgical injury is well understood in adult humans. Although there remains a serious lack of published data on the stress response to accidental injury in children, the response to surgical injury is now much better understood. This chapter focuses on current knowledge in relation to the stress response to surgery in infants and children.

Most surgery in children and neonates is essentially safe. For 'general' surgery there is a low direct mortality and the morbidity is mostly that of the underlying disease process for which the surgery is being undertaken. In some areas of surgery, for instance cardiac surgery, opposing trends are evident. While some major procedures are now more common, because of technical advances (e.g. switch operations for transposition of the great arteries), the development of transluminal techniques for closure of patent arterial duct will reduce the exposure of children to open surgery for this condition. Laparoscopic techniques for general surgery will probably become more frequent in children as experience develops.

The importance of developing a scientific understanding of the processes involved in the response to elective surgery is threefold:

- it is a constant challenge to improve outcome among those children undergoing emergency surgery, including that for trauma
- surgery for conditions such as complex congenital heart disease carries much greater hazards than 'general' surgery: this challenges us to improve outcome further
- the 'model' of surgical injury may have relevance to our understanding of accidental injury, which remains a leading cause of death and disability in childhood.

128

Irrespective of age, neural impulses from the site of injury result in the release of neuroendocrine mediators, with the consequent mobilisation of metabolic fuels to optimise the healing process (Figure 9.1). The two solid afferent lines represent the somatic and visceral pathways, while the dotted line represents humoral mediators (now known to be cytokines) which both modulate the neuroendocrine response centrally and influence metabolism, particularly in the liver. This response is of fundamental biological importance, and from an understanding of its nature and purpose new therapeutic strategies have emerged for the management of patients recovering from injury and undergoing surgery.

The stress responses of neonates, children and adults to surgery are different from one another. The neonatal response occurs more rapidly and has a greater magnitude than that in the adult, but is also of a shorter duration. The different pattern of the stress response in the neonate may reflect a fundamentally different physiology, characteristic of the neonatal period, or it may represent a response unmodified by fear, the learned experience of pain, or other cultural factors which could potentially alter the endocrine and metabolic response in the adult. If the former hypothesis (a different physiology) were valid, children might be expected to mount a neuroendocrine response to surgery which was either similar to that of the adult or else had features unique to childhood and distinct from both the neonatal and the adult responses. If social and cultural influences were dominant, one might predict a gradual change in the pattern of the stress response through infancy and childhood as learned experiences of discomfort become more sophisticated. Until recently, there have been no data in the literature which give direct evidence for either hypothesis.

This chapter explores various aspects of the metabolic and endocrine response to surgical injury in infants and children which have been elucidated in recent years. The focus is on the neonate and the older child rather than the foetus, although the increasing use of invasive foetal investigation and surgery means that studies of the consequences of foetal injury will assume increasing importance in the future. An excellent recent review of stress in the foetus is that of Glover & Giannokoulopoulos (1995). Three other recent reviews which complement the approach of this chapter are that of Anand (1990), Schmeling & Coran (1991) and Stuart & Ward Platt (1995).

Cardiac surgery

Cardiac surgery has, quite appropriately, received special attention in view of its complex nature and its special anaesthetic requirements. The techniques employed, including cardiac bypass, various degrees of hypothermia and the transfusion of large volumes of donated blood and pump prime fluids (Ratcliffe *et al.*, 1986) potentially make endocrine and metabolic measurements difficult to interpret. The metabolic load

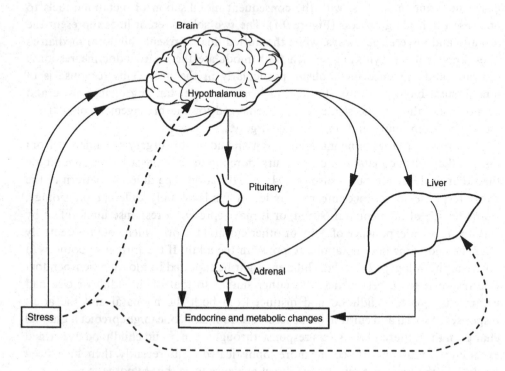

Figure 9.1. Afferent and efferent pathways of the neuroendocrine stress response.

of these fluids can be reduced, and this itself may reduce the metabolic impact of the anaesthesia and surgery (Ratcliffe *et al.*, 1988; Ridley *et al.*, 1990).

There is a very intense sympathoadrenal response to hypothermic circulatory arrest in neonates (Wood *et al.*, 1980), with large increases in glucose and insulin concentrations (Benzing *et al.*, 1983). Relative to other reasons for surgery, the morbidity and mortality of cardiac surgery was, and is, high. Yet efforts to manipulate the metabolic and endocrine response to improve this situation have only recently received attention, and remain controversial.

A detailed observational study by Anand *et al.* (1990) concluded that, as with non-cardiac surgery in the neonate, there was a very substantial metabolic and endocrine response; that sympathoadrenal hormone concentrations appeared to be well above those reported in the adult literature; and that non-survivors tended to have a more severe metabolic and endocrine response than survivors. These observations in turn led on to a randomised controlled trial (Anand & Hickey, 1992) which demonstrated the predicted reduction in the stress response, a reduced rate of complications, and a reduced mortality in the group treated with sufentanil compared with that receiving halothane-morphine. The inevitable controversy surrounding these results has centred on possible imbalances of high risk operations between the allocation groups, and it is to be hoped that other centres will soon publish data to support or refute the results of this trial.

Two complementary studies (Yamashita *et al.*, 1982, Milne *et al.*, 1986) described the sympathoadrenal response and the broader metabolic and endocrine responses, respectively, concentrating on infants and children outside the neonatal period. Yamashita *et al.* (1982) studied nine children between 2 and 8 years old, demonstrating increases in plasma adrenaline (> 30-fold) and noradrenaline (about two fold) in association with cardiopulmonary bypass; however, this study was neither comprehensive nor prolonged beyond an immediate postoperative sample. Milne *et al.* (1986) took a much more comprehensive approach in seven postneonatal infants of less than 10 kg. They measured concentrations of cortisol, insulin, glucagon, growth hormone, glucose and other intermediary metabolites. They demonstrated hyperglycaemia (to around 30 mmol/l) and hyperlactataemia (around 6 mmol/1) which were accompanied by large surges in concentrations of glucagon, cortisol, growth hormone and insulin. In both these studies the number of subjects was small, and it was not clear whether the findings could be extrapolated to general surgical conditions of less severity.

None of the above studies addressed concentrations of non-esterified ('free') fatty acids. These are released as a consequence of lipolysis which is in turn driven by the counter-regulatory actions of the catabolic stress hormones. The importance of free fatty acids lies in their ability to impair myocardial function, a property of obvious importance after cardiac surgery. It is therefore of concern that very high concentrations of free fatty acids should have been detected in infants undergoing cardiac surgery (Lopaschuk *et al.*, 1994), and these results reinforce the concept that anaesthetic strategies which can decrease lipolytic drive may well improve outcome.

There is relatively little literature on the metabolic effects of surface cooling alone. It is known that a metabolic acidaemia develops during cooling, and that this is associated with a small increase in blood lactate concentrations (Stayer *et al.*, 1994). It is unfortunate that more detailed studies have not been undertaken because the controlled conditions pertaining in the operating theatre would provide an ideal model of relevance to the understanding of drowning. Drowning remains an important cause of childhood death in several developed countries (Chapter 11), and its outcome may be modulated by hypothermia.

When energy expenditure has been studied in children after cardiac surgery, the expected increase, as seen in the adult (Tulla *et al.*, 1991), has either not been found (Gebara *et al.*, 1993) or found inconstantly (Puhakka *et al.*, 1994). Gebara *et al.* (1992) could only demonstrate that there was a shift towards fat utilization, consistent with the known pattern of the metabolic stress response. Their studies were performed relatively late (up to 3 days after surgery), and a short-lived increase in resting energy expenditure could therefore have been missed. Another possibility is that the children were actually hypermetabolic before the operation, and correction of their cardiac defect returned their metabolic rates towards normal (Puhakka *et al.*, 1993; Mitchell *et al.*, 1994).

Other surgical injury: the neonate

That the neonate was capable of mounting a metabolic and endocrine response to surgery at all was first shown definitely by Anand *et al.* (1985a,b). These papers demonstrated not only that there was indeed an endocrine and metabolic response, but that it was massive. This led the team on to two classic randomised controlled trials (Anand *et al.*, 1987, 1988) which compared the responses to surgery, under the then standard regimen of nitrous oxide and curare, with the additions of fentanyl and halothane, respectively. The control data from these trials potentially illuminates our understanding of the raw response to injury in neonates, because of the relatively homogeneous study groups, while the intervention group demonstrates the reduction in the stress response consequent on the use of potent analgesia and anaesthesia.

The randomised controlled trials of Anand *et al.* (1987, 1988) focused on changes in circulating concentrations of metabolites and hormones, and their published data do not include the absolute values of concentrations in either the treatment or intervention groups. This makes attempts at direct comparison with other situations of injury or surgery rather difficult, although some useful inferences can be made. Furthermore, two quite distinct populations of babies were studied. The first (fentanyl) trial examined preterm babies undergoing surgery for ligation of a patent arterial duct (Anand *et al.*, 1987), while the second (halothane), dealt with term babies undergoing a variety of operations (Anand *et al.*, 1988). Thus, even in the absence of absolute values for key metabolites and hormones, it is possible to form some tentative conclusions about the differences in the stress responses between preterm and term babies.

The conclusions of these studies of Anand *et al.* (1987, 1988) may be summarised as follows. Surgical injury in the neonate was accompanied by very large surges of noradrenaline and adrenaline, together with an adrenocortical response. Severe hyperglycaemia ensued, together with increases in the major gluconeogenic substrates, predominantly lactate; however by 24 hours from the end of surgery, most parameters returned to their baseline values. The magnitude and duration of these changes was greatly reduced by the administration of fentanyl (for duct ligation in preterm babies) or halothane (for surgery in the term babies). For the control groups, the adrenaline response was more prolonged, and the noradrenaline response of greater magnitude, in the preterm babies; but changes in cortisol concentrations were greater in the term babies. Insulin concentrations increased in a similar pattern in term and preterm babies, but hyperglycaemia was more prolonged in the preterm. Other metabolic parameters cannot be directly compared.

It is tempting to approach the measurement of stress hormones in the neonate as if the underlying physiology were the same as in the adult; however, adrenocortical steroid biosynthesis is quite different in term and preterm babies compared with older children and adults (Winter, 1985; Thomas *et al.*, 1986; Voutilainen & Miller, 1986; Hughes *et al.*, 1987), and has different patterns again in growth retarded babies (Doerr *et al.*, 1989). Anand took this into account by measuring cortisol precursors as well as cortisol itself. From the point of view of surgical injury, the key result is that as previous workers have recognised, the production of cortisol may be delayed in relation to the insult (Cathero *et al.*, 1969; Obara *et al.*, 1984; Hughes *et al.*, 1987), and increases in steroid precursors may dominate (Anand *et al.*, 1987).

The data of Anand *et al.* also have to be interpreted in the light of the metabolic capabilities of babies, about which relatively little was known at the time these surgical trails were carried out. More recent work has shown that the ability to undertake metabolic processes such as ketogenesis is strictly limited in both preterm and growth retarded term babies (Hawdon *et al.*, 1992; Hawdon & Ward Platt, 1993), which probably explains the very attenuated ketone body concentrations detected at the end of surgery by Anand *et al.* (1985a) in preterm babies. In the classical stress response, ketogenesis is seen as a consequence of the lipolysis which is driven by the catabolic neuroendocrine milieu; without an understanding of the metabolic immaturity of neonates, a blunted ketogenic response might be misinterpreted as evidence for 'less stress'.

The measurement of body composition and metabolic rate using indirect calorimetry has been used to understand the metabolic events following surgery in newborn infants (Winthrop *et al.*, 1987a). The high rates of postoperative accretion of carbohydrate, protein and fat shown by these workers suggests that the neonate has a high level of anabolic drive, and seems able to maintain protein balance even in the face of borderline calorie intake (Winthrop *et al.*, 1989; Jones *et al.*, 1995a).

In the adult the increased mobilisation of metabolic substrates at the time of surgery, including increased glucose utilisation, is reflected in a measurable increase in resting metabolic rate (Severino Brandi *et al.*, 1988; Tulla *et al.*, 1991), the magnitude of which is probably related to the severity of surgery (Lind, 1995). Not all attempts to demonstrate this in the neonate have been successful. Neither Groner *et al.* (1989), Shanbhogue *et al.* (1991) nor Shanbhogue & Lloyd (1992) were able to demonstrate the increase in resting energy expenditure predicted by the surges of stress hormones which had been described, and various ingenious explanations for this were proposed.

The suspicion lingered that these 'negative' results were a methodological artefact, and that changes in metabolic rate were simply passing undetected. Support for this suspicion was fuelled by subsequent reports (Jones et al., 1993, 1995b) that there was a definite but short-lived increase in energy expenditure and substrate utilization which was related to the severity of surgery as measured by the Oxford surgical stress score (Anand & Aynsley-Green, 1988). Resting energy expenditure increased by about 5% after minor, and 20% after major surgery. This demonstration of a 'dose–response' to surgical stress is powerful evidence that there is a true increase in postsurgical metabolic rate, rather than the results being an artefact. A further intriguing observation, which requires confirmation, was that infants undergoing surgery within the first 48 hours postnatally showed less increase in energy expenditure than those undergoing their surgery later. This may reflect once again the rapidly changing metabolic capabilities of the neonate during this time (Hawdon et al., 1992).

Other surgical injury: infants and children

Compared with the attention to metabolic and endocrine responses to surgery in the adult, there have been few studies in infants or children. As there was relatively high morbidity and mortality from cardiac surgery, most of the early work concentrated on open heart operations as described above.

There is a reasonable amount of information on cortisol concentrations after surgery in childhood. Boninsegni et al. (1983) demonstrated increases in circulating concentrations of cortisol during minor surgical procedures under halothane anesthesia in children aged between 5 and 12 years, but the values they found during surgery were highly variable, ranging from 130 to 2230 nmol/l, and no postoperative values were reported. In contrast, Sweed et al. (1992) found consistently high concentrations of cortisol during and after major surgery (abdominoperineal pull through for Hirschsprung's disease), with mean levels at the end of the procedure in excess of 1500 nmol/l.

More recently Khilnani et al. (1993), in a study of 98 subjects, found significantly elevated cortisol concentrations 3 hours after the end of surgery compared with baseline values. Unfortunately the interpretation of this study is made difficult by the heterogeneity of the population. A wide variety of premedications and anaesthetic techniques were used; some subjects received fentanyl during the operation, and some had local bupivacaine prior to skin incision. The age range was 2–20 years, no data on the nature of the operations were reported, and duration of surgery was used as a proxy for severity. Thus in spite of the large number of subjects, no useful inferences can be made.

Other authors have taken an interest in the neuroendocrine response to paediatric surgery as a way of evaluating the effects of anaesthetic agents. The effect on the cortisol response of adding halothane to a combination of nitrous oxide/oxygen/ pancuronium was assessed by Obara *et al.* (1984) who found that concentrations of cortisol in their group given halothane were considerably less than in controls. Although there was little difference between the groups by the end of surgery, halothane seemed to delay the rise in cortisol, suggesting that it can attenuate the hypothalamic–pituitary–adrenal response. Similar results were obtained by Sigurdsson *et al.* (1982) who evaluated the effect of adding morphine (150 μg/kg) to a premedication of diazepam in a randomised controlled trial. Both the rate of increase of cortisol concentrations, and the absolute values, were reduced in the group receiving morphine.

Epidural anaesthesia also appears to affect concentrations of cortisol in children. Murat *et al.* (1988) studied children undergoing relatively minor genital or lower limb surgery with and without the addition of epidural bupivacaine to a standard halothane anaesthetic, and measured plasma cortisol concentrations up to 24 hours after surgery. Cortisol concentrations in the control children were elevated at the end of surgery (mean 281 nmol/l), but reached a mean value of 367 nmol/l 3 hours later, falling thereafter. Children receiving an epidural anaesthetic had significantly reduced cortisol concentrations at the end of surgery, but their levels rose over the first postoperative day although never reaching those of the control children.

Sympathoadrenal responses to surgery have been used to evaluate the effects of halothane versus enflurane anaesthesia (Sigurdsson *et al.*, 1984), and halothane with and without caudal epidural anaesthesia (Dupont *et al.*, 1987). Sigurdsson *et al.* (1984) measured total catecholamines, rather than adrenaline and noradrenaline separately, which makes any comparisons with other studies impossible. Although they found a clear difference in total catecholamine concentrations by the end of surgery, this may simply have reflected a differential effect of the two agents on the release of adrenaline or noradrenaline secretory granules, as concentrations of neither cortisol nor adrenocorticotrophic hormone differed between the groups. Dupont *et al.* (1987) found that both adrenaline and noradrenaline concentrations during surgery were significantly higher in their halothane than epidural group, which suggests that caudal epidural anaesthesia could effectively abolish the sympathoadrenal response to surgery below the umbilicus.

The insulin response to a glucose load has been used in the assessment of the metabolic effects of inhalational anaesthesia with and without epidural anaesthesia (Gouyet *et al.*, 1993). Some authors have been concerned with blood glucose homeostasis, largely because of concern about hypoglycaemia in young children starved overnight for surgery, but initial studies paid no attention to other aspects of the counter-regulatory response, such as lipolysis and ketogenesis (Nilsson *et al.*, 1984; Redfern *et al.*, 1986; Welborn *et al.*, 1986). More recent investigations have shown that the provision of a small amount of glucose (2 mg/kg per minute) during minor surgery can abolish lipolysis without producing hyperglycaemia (Nishina *et al.*, 1995), as can 10 ml/kg of apple juice given 2 hours prior to surgery (Maekawa *et al.*, 1993). Whether lipolysis would be suppressed in the face of the catabolic drive associated with major surgery in children has not been investigated, but it is certainly not suppressed by glucose infusion in the neonate (Anand *et al.*, 1985a).

Not all the metabolic effects of tissue injury are the result the neuroendocrine response. There is now general awareness that the production of cytokines not only modulates the immune system, but has a variety of other effects on organs distant from the site of injury, including some profound effects on metabolism in general. The importance of this in relation to burn injury is dealt with in Chapters 12 and 13.

Surgical procedures have been shown to be associated with the production of interleukin 6 (IL-6) (Sweed *et al.*, 1992; Tsang & Tam 1994; Jones *et al.*, 1994), IL-1 receptor antagonist (IL-Ra) (ó Nualláin *et al.*, 1993), IL-8 (Tsang & Tam, 1994), and C-reactive protein (CRP) (Chwals *et al.*, 1993). Circulating concentrations of tumour necrosis factor, in contrast, do not appear to rise following major surgery (ó Nualláin *et al.*, 1993; Chwals *et al.*, 1993). There is some evidence that the degree of tissue damage may determine the amount of interleukin released, as both Tsang & Tam (1994) and Jones *et al.* (1994) were able to demonstrate a positive correlation between the Oxford Surgical Stress Score and peak concentrations of IL-6. Chwals *et al.* (1993) found a relation between concentrations of CRP and prealbumin, and mortality, with non-survivors having higher peak concentrations of CRP and lower peak concentrations of prealbumin; but the nature of the operations, and the nutritional condition of the subjects, were not stated.

In contrast to neonates and children undergoing cardiac surgery, there have been no reports on the use of indirect calorimetry to ascertain how 'general' surgery might affect metabolic rate in children, and whether this response may differ from that in the adult. Following trauma, the energy expenditure of children increases, broadly in line with the severity of injury (Winthrop *et al.*, 1987b).

It was therefore against a background of relatively little published data that, in the second half of the 1980s, the group in Newcastle upon Tyne set out to undertake a comprehensive study of the metabolic and endocrine responses to surgery in children. Much of the metabolic data is easily accessible (Ward Platt *et al.*, 1990) but some of the endocrine information is less so (Ward Platt, 1988). The remainder of this chapter concentrates on these data and their implications.

We studied 46 children aged from 1 month to 10 years undergoing a wide range of operations (Table 9.1), and graded the severity of surgery using the Oxford Surgical Stress Score (SSS: Anand & Aynsley-Green, 1988). By standardising the anaesthetic (nitrous oxide/oxygen/halothane), we were able to separate the effects of the ages of the children and the severity of the surgery they underwent in the analysis with minimal

Table 9.1. *Operations classified as minor and major according to the Oxford Surgical Stress Score (SSS)*

Minor (SSS ≤ 5)	Major (SSS ≥ 6)
Inguinal herniotomy	Nephrectomy
Orchidopexy	Pyeloplasty
Repair of tracheo-oesophageal fistula (cervical approach)	Abdominoperineal pull-through
Trimming anal mucosa	Correction of malrotation of the gut
Repair of hypospadias	Closure of colostomy
Reconstruction of penis	Pyelolithotomy
Meatotomy	Repair of diaphragmatic eventration
Excision of lump in neck	Resection of ileum
Excision of dermoid cyst	Fundoplication
Dilatation of oesophagus	Reimplantation of ureters

Source: From Anand & Aynsley-Green (1988).

risk of confounding by other variables – although that remains a constant risk in an essentially observational study.

The metabolic responses of the children (Ward Platt *et al.*, 1990) can be summarised as follows. We were able to demonstrate increases in concentrations of glucose, lactate, pyruvate, free fatty acids and ketones in association with surgery, and the concentrations at the end of surgery were significantly correlated with the Surgical Stress Score of the operation. Because glucose was not infused during the operation, the absolute increase in circulating concentrations of glucose was not particularly large, but mild hyperglycaemia was sustained for longer in the older children. An unexpected finding was that, in spite of the study protocol, children received widely varying doses of morphine in their premedication. When this was taken into account in a multiple regression analysis, the morphine dose (which varied between 150 and 320 μg/kg) was found to account for as much variance in glucose concentrations at the end of surgery as the Surgical Stress Score, but had no independent effect on concentrations of other major intermediary metabolities.

The gluconeogenic substrates lactate, pyruvate, alanine and glycerol share the same metabolic fate (recycling to form glucose) and can usefully be considered together as the sum of their molar concentrations. An interesting pattern emerged which appeared to be unique to childhood: concentrations of total gluconeogenic substrates (TGNS) increased from baseline values to a peak at the end of surgery, then fell to levels considerably below baseline values from 12 hours after the operation and remained low at 48 hours (Figure 9.2). Both the magnitude to the peak, and the fall below baseline, were found to be in direct relation to the Surgical Stress Score. As the timing

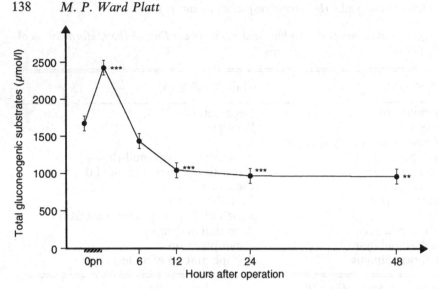

Figure 9.2. The effect of major surgery on blood concentrations of total gluconeogenic substrates in children. *** $P < 0.001$, ** $P < 0.01$ with respect to preoperative values. Mean $\pm$ SEM.

of the peak corresponded to the maximum neuroendocrine response, it is tempting to postulate a direct relation between the two. The subsequent fall in concentration took place in the absence of continuing endocrine drive, and it may be that changes in hepatic metabolism, possibly mediated by cytokine drive, could have been responsible for this. Certainly, this pattern of change in gluconeogenic substrate concentrations is seen in neither neonates nor adults (Ward Platt et al., 1990).

We were interested in defining whether there were any patterns in the metabolic or endocrine responses which could be related to the ages of the children, other than the small effect in relation to glucose referred to above. Only patterns of insulin, adrenaline and prolactin concentrations displayed some variation with age. After major surgery, the insulin:glucose ratio in older children was higher and did not return to baseline levels over the 48 hours after operation, while younger children had lower values which fall considerably after a peak 6 hours after operation (Ward Platt et al., 1990). Older children also had a greater and more prolonged increase in the insulin:glucagon ratio (Figure 9.3).

Glucagon concentrations (Table 9.2) did not change significantly, regardless of age, which contrasts with the findings in adults (Russell et al., 1975) and preterm neonates (Anand et al., 1987). In view of the substantial increases in concentrations of cortisol and adrenaline, it was surprising that plasma glucagon concentrations were unaffected even by major surgery in children, because in adults glucagon appears to be an important stress hormone, acting synergistically with cortisol and adrenaline to main-

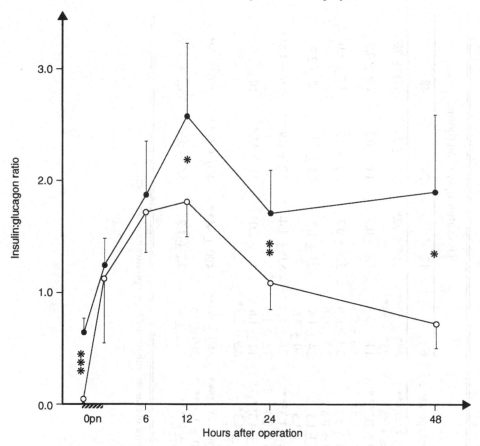

Figure 9.3. Effect of major surgery on insulin: glucagon ratios in young (< 5 years) and older children (≥ 5 years). Mean ± SEM. *$P < 0.05$, ** $P < 0.01$, *** $P < 0.001$.

tain high circulating concentrations of glucose (Bessey *et al.*, 1984). On the other hand, glucagon concentrations have been found to be greatly elevated after cardiac surgery in infants (Milne *et al.*, 1986; Anand *et al.*, 1990). It seems, therefore, reasonable to conclude that glucagon is not an important stress hormone in infants and children, except under conditions of severe surgical stress.

Preoperative serum insulin concentrations were very low, some below the detection limit of the assay (1 mU/l), and correlated with the ages of the children (Kendall's $\tau = 0.47$, $P < 0.001$). As preoperative insulin concentrations, and insulin:glucose ratios, tend to be higher in older children (being closely related to body weight), this probably reflects the ontogeny of endocrine pancreatic function in childhood. In spite of the absence of a glucose infusion perioperatively, mean plasma insulin

Table 9.2. *Concentrations of counterregulatory hormones in association with major (a) and minor (b) surgery in children*

| | | Preoperative | Postoperative | Time after operation (hours) | | | |
				6	12	24	48
Cortisol (nmol/l)	a	322 ± 39	866 ± 48***	683 ± 57***	510 ± 72*	389 ± 57	471 ± 70**
	b	190 ± 21	308 ± 78	452 ± 58**			
Adrenaline (nmol/l)	a	1.6 ± 0.5	3.9 ± 0.7***	1.8 ± 0.3	1.2 ± 0.3	1.0 ± 0.2	1.0 ± 0.2
	b	1.2 ± 0.4	3.9 ± 0.5	1.5 ± 0.4			
Noradrenaline (nmol/l)	a	4.4 ± 0.4	4.0 ± 0.5	3.3 ± 0.3	3.3 ± 0.3	3.5 ± 0.3	3.7 ± 1.0
	b	3.5 ± 0.5	3.9 ± 0.8	3.3 ± 0.6			
Glucagon (pmol/l)	a	24 ± 1.4	26 ± 1.5	24 ± 1.4	23 ± 1.7	23 ± 1.6	27 ± 3.2
	b	28 ± 1.0	26 ± 1.5	30 ± 3.8			
Insulin (mU/l)	a	1.5 ± 0.4	5.4 ± 1.3***	7.6 ± 1.0***	8.0 ± 1.4***	5.2 ± 0.9***	5.9 ± 1.8**
	b	0.8 ± 0.5	1.5 ± 0.4	2.6 ± 1.0			
Growth Hormone (mU/l)	a	12 ± 3.3	28 ± 4.3**	12 ± 1.6	16 ± 2.0*	21 ± 4.9*	10 ± 1.9
	b	5.7 ± 2.6	15 ± 4.3*	8.9 ± 3.1*			
Prolactin (mU/l)	a	910 ± 140	1330 ± 144***	480 ± 50**	490 ± 45**	420 ± 50**	210 ± 70*
	b	520 ± 79	970 ± 140**	260 ± 65			
Beta-endorphin (pmol/l)	a	9.5 ± 1.2	83 ± 12***	17.5 ± 42	7.7 ± 1.2	5.6 ± 0.7	7.2 ± 0.9

Means ± standard errors of the mean. Statistical significance of changes with respect to preoperative concentrations:
*** $P < 0.001$, ** $P < 0.01$, * $P < 0.05$.

concentrations increased as a consequence of surgery and achieved a peak 12 hours after operation, concentrations at the end of the operation being higher after major than minor surgery. A similar response was also found in the neonate (Anand *et al.*, 1985b), but adults showed very little change in insulin concentrations around the time of surgery (Håkanson *et al.*,1985), although there may be an increase in insulin concentrations 24 hours after surgery (Russell *et al.*, 1975).

Although insulin does not behave as a 'stress hormone' in the adult, it does in children, and it seems that the converse is true of glucagon. As the chief characteristic of the actions of the stress hormones in adult studies is that they are catabolic, it is of particular interest that the stress response in childhood should have a strong anabolic component, the evidence for which is the behaviour of the insulin:glucose and insulin:glucagon ratios. Furthermore, these parameters show a substantial change with age during the prepubertal years.

The higher insulin:glucose and insulin:glucagon ratios might have been expected to lead the postoperative hyperglycaemia to return to normal more quickly in older children, but in fact the opposite is true: older children have a more prolonged postoperative elevation in blood glucose concentrations than young ones (Ward Platt *et al.*, 1990). This suggests that during childhood there is a progressive development of relative insulin insensitivity, compared with early infancy.

Major surgery resulted in an immediate increase in mean circulating concentrations of cortisol (Figure 9.4). Concentrations then returned towards preoperative values and were not significantly different from preoperative values at 24 hours after surgery. The pattern and magnitude of the observed changes were not related to the ages of the children. Plasma cortisol concentrations at the end of surgery were closely related to its severity as measured by the Oxford Surgical Stress Score (Figure 9.5).

Plasma cortisol concentrations in infants and children were higher at the end of major surgery than at any time thereafter, but were still significantly greater than preoperative values until 24 hours after surgery. In the adult, in contrast, maximum plasma cortisol concentrations appear not to be achieved until after the end of surgery (Nistrup Madsen *et al.*, 1977; Rutberg *et al.*, 1984; Lacoumenta *et al.*, 1986, 1987a).

We found significant elevations in plasma adrenaline concentrations as a result of major surgery (a mean increase of 2.3 nmol/l, Table 9.2), but the spread of values was wide. Postoperative plasma adrenaline concentrations correlated poorly but significantly with the surgical stress score (Kendall's $\tau = 0.29$, $P = 0.003$). Adrenaline concentrations returned to preoperative values more quickly in younger than in older children (Figure 9.6).

As with cortisol, peak values of adrenaline were comparable to those measured in adults undergoing major surgery; but in adults, circulating concentrations of

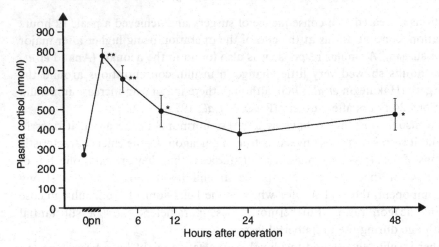
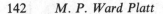

Figure 9.4. Effect of major surgery on concentrations of cortisol in children. Mean ± SEM. ** $P < 0.001$, * $P < 0.05$, with respect to preoperative values.

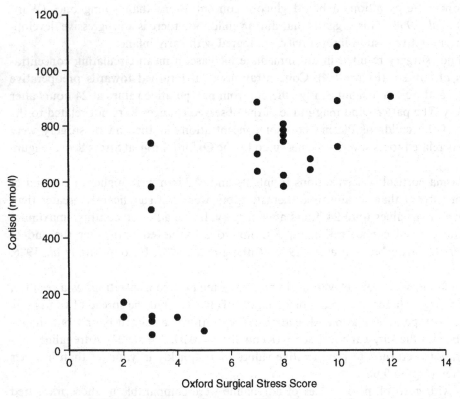

Figure 9.5. Relation between the Surgical Stress Score and circulating cortisol concentrations at the end of surgery.

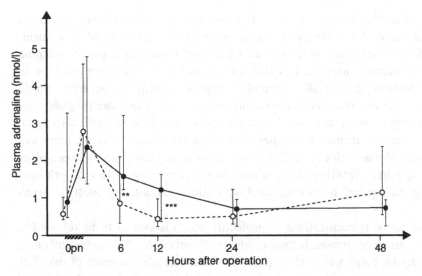

Figure 9.6. Effect of major surgery on concentrations of adrenaline in young (< 2.5 years; - - -) and older children (≥ 2.5 years; ———). Median and interquartile range. Group differences are significant: ** $P < 0.01$; *** $P < 0.001$.

adrenaline also appeared to achieve a later peak than in childhood, and returned to values not significantly different to preoperative concentrations within 12 hours of the end of surgery (Nistrup Madsen *et al.*, 1978; Rutberg *et al.*, 1984; Lacoumenta *et al.*, 1986).

In the neonate, plasma adrenaline concentrations increased acutely following major surgery with halothane anaesthesia, but were not significantly different to preoperative values 6 hours after surgery Anand *et al.* (1988). Although the severity of surgery in Anand's study (using the Oxford Surgical Stress Score) was comparable to that in our own, and the same assay in the same laboratory was used, the increase in adrenaline levels as a result of surgery was only of the order of 1 nmol/l, which suggests that even term neonates have a reduced ability to secrete adrenaline when compared with older children.

We were unable to demonstrate any significant changes in plasma noradrenaline concentrations, nor was there any difference between age groups or with severity of surgery. This contrasts with the findings in the neonate (Anand *et al.*, 1987, 1988), and possibly with the adult, although the data are conflicting (Nistrup Madsen, 1988; Rutberg *et al.*, 1984; Derbyshire & Smith, 1984). It is also different to the findings of Dupont *et al.* (1987) in children undergoing minor surgery. These differences, however, may reflect homeostatic responses to different degrees of intravascular volume loss rather than to intrinsic physiological differences between neonates, adults and children.

Growth hormone has long been known to be released in response to surgical stress in adults (Reier *et al.*, 1973; Wright & Johnston, 1975). Its measurement is problematical because of its pulsatile release, so that a 'baseline' value may appear to be quite high if sampling happens to coincide with a natural peak in plasma concentrations. In spite of this limitation, the overall pattern of mean growth hormone concentrations in children (Table 9.2) was reasonably consistent: concentrations increased significantly at the end of surgery when compared with preoperative values; but although mean postoperative concentrations were higher after major than minor surgery, there was no correlation with the Oxford Surgical Stress Score or any difference between older and younger children. Whether children tend to produce more or less growth hormone for a given surgical stress compared with adults cannot at present be determined.

We also measured concentrations of prolactin, which is known to be released in response to a variety of stresses, including surgery (Noel *et al.*, 1972; Anfilogoff *et al.*, 1987). Once again, there was a clear pattern of increase after surgery (Table 9.2); however, concentrations at the end of surgery not only correlated with the Surgical Stress Score but younger children had a significantly greater response, even when allowing for the Surgical Stress Scores (Figure 9.7). A subsequent study (Khilnani *et al.*, 1993) was not able to show any effect of age on prolactin concentrations at the end of surgery, but the wide variety of anaesthetic techniques and the heterogeneity of the operations preclude any firm conclusions from this work. The prolactin response to minor surgery in infants does not seem to be abolished by the use of epidural anaesthesia (Salerno *et al.*, 1989).

In adults, there are increased concentrations of β-endorphin following surgery (Lacoumenta *et al.*, 1987b), and in the infant undergoing cardiac surgery there is clear evidence that potent analgesia can abolish the β-endorphin response (Anand & Hickey, 1992). We measured β-endorphin concentrations in a subset of 19 patients over 1 year of age undergoing major surgery (Table 9.2), and showed a clear increase in mean concentrations at the end of surgery; however, even within this well-defined group of children, peak concentrations ranged from less than 20 pmol/l to over 170 pmol/l (Ward Platt *et al.*, 1989).

The Oxford Surgical Stress Score related well to concentrations of cortisol at the end of surgery, but less to concentrations of adrenaline. Adrenaline has a short plasma half-life, and it is probable that peak adrenaline concentrations occur during surgery rather than at the end of it, as it is during visceral manipulation that signs of adrenergic stimulation such as tachycardia and hypertension are maximal. Together with the evidence from metabolic changes, it would appear that the Oxford Surgical Stress Score gives a valid representation of the severity of surgery in infants and children, as in the neonate.

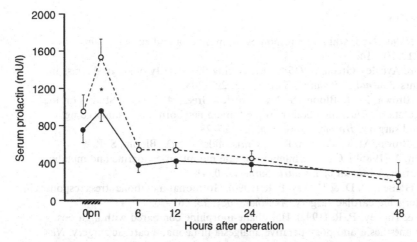

Figure 9.7. Effect of major surgery on centrations of prolactin in young (o - - - o, < 5 years') and older children (•—•≥5 years). Mean ± SEM. Group differences significant, * $P < 0.001$.

Conclusion

In summary, neonates, infants and children show a substantial stress response to surgery, and this response is generally of more rapid onset, and of shorter duration, than in the adult. The stress response can be manipulated by the choice of anaesthetic technique. Clear differences in the pattern of the adrenocortical and adrenal medullary responses to surgical stress are evident in preterm and term neonates, children and adults; yet the pattern in childhood is reasonably stable from 1 month to 10 years of age. The Oxford Surgical Stress Score appears to be a valid measure of operative stress in children; and children appear to have more anabolic drive than adults, which may partly account for their resilience in the face of major surgical procedures.

It appears that the ontogenetic changes in the neuroendocrine stress response are physiological rather than psychological in origin. It seems likely that with puberty, the pattern of the stress response may become more akin to that of the adult. Further studies of the endocrine and metabolic response to surgery in adolescents and young adults will be needed to confirm this.

Infants and prepubertal children show an unique pattern of metabolic and endocrine response to surgery. It follows that in other situations of injury the stress response of children will also be different from that of adults. As accidents and trauma remain the major cause of death and disability in the mid-childhood years, studies of the stress response after severe injuries in children will be necessary to allow management to be based on scientific fact rather than empirical extrapolation from knowledge gained in adults; and thus improve the outcome of childhood injury.

References

Anand, K. J. S. (1990). Neonatal stress responses to anesthesia and surgery. *Clinics in Perinatology*, **17**, 207–14.

Anand, K. J. S. & Aynsley-Green, A. (1988). Measuring the severity of surgical stress in newborn infants. *Journal of Pediatric Surgery*, **23**, 297–305.

Anand, K. J. S., Brown, M. J., Bloom, S. R. & Aynsley-Green, A. (1985a). Studies on the hormonal regulation of fuel metabolism in the human newborn infant undergoing anaesthesia and surgery. *Hormone Research*, **22**, 115–28.

Anand, K. J. S., Brown, M. J., Causon, R. C., Christofides, N. D., Bloom, S. R. & Aynsley-Green, A. (1985b). Can the human neonate mount an endocrine and metabolic response to surgery? *Journal of Pediatric Surgery*, **20**, 41–8.

Anand, K. J. S., Hansen, D. D. & Hickey, P. R. (1990). Hormonal-metabolic stress responses in neonates undergoing cardiac surgery. *Anesthesiology*, **73**, 661–70.

Anand, K. J. S. & Hickey, P. R. (1992). Halothane-morphine compared with high-dose sufentanil for anesthesia and postoperative analgesia in neonatal cardiac surgery. *New England Journal of Medicine*, **326**, 1–9.

Anand, K. J. S., Sippell, W. G. & Aynsley-Green, A. (1987). Randomised trial of fentanyl anaesthesia in preterm neonates undergoing surgery: effects on the stress response. *Lancet*, **1**, 62–6.

Anand, K. J. S., Sippell, W. G., Schofield, N. M. & Aynsley-Green, A. (1988). Does halothane anaesthesia decrease the metabolic and endocrine stress responses of newborn infants undergoing operation? *British Medical Journal*, **296**, 668–72.

Anfilogoff, R., Hale, P. J., Nattrass, M., Hammond, V. A. & Carter, J. C. (1987). Physiological response to parachute jumping. *British Medical Journal*, **295**, 415.

Benzing, G., Francis, P. D., Kaplan, S., Helmsworth, H. A. & Sperling, M. A. (1983). Glucose and insulin changes in infants and children undergoing hypothermic open-heart surgery. *American Journal of Cardiology*, **52**, 133–6.

Bessey, P. Q., Walters, J. M., Aoki, T. T. & Wilmore, D. W. (1984). Combined hormonal infusion simulates the metabolic response to injury. *Annals of Surgery*, **200**, 264–80.

Boninsegni, R., Salerno, R., Giannotti, P., Andreuccetti, T., Busoni, P., Santoro, S. & Forti, G. (1983). Effects of surgery and epidural or general anaesthesia on testosterone, 17-hydroxyprogesterone and cortisol plasma levels in prepubertal boys. *Journal of Steroid Biochemistry*, **19**, 1783–7.

Cathero, D. M., Forsyth, C. C. & Cameron, J. (1969). Adrenocortical response to stress in newborn infants. *Archives of Disease in Childhood*, **44**, 88–95.

Chwals, W. J., Fernandez, M. E., Jamie, A. C. & Charles, B. J. (1993). Relationship of metabolic indexes to postoperative mortality in surgical infants. *Journal of Pediatric Surgery*, **28**, 819–22.

Derbyshire, D. R. & Smith, G. (1984). Sympathoadrenal responses to anaesthesia and surgery. *British Journal of Anaesthesia*, **56**, 725–39.

Doerr, H. G., Versmold, H. T., Bidlingmaier, F. & Sippell, W. G. (1989). Adrenocortical steroids in small-for-gestational-age term infants during the early neonatal period. *Pediatric Research*, **25**, 115–18.

Dupont, D., Velin, P., Cabour, F., Candito, M. & Rives, E. (1987). Influence of caudal anesthesia on the secretion of catecholamines in children. *Annales Francaises d'Anesthesie et Reanimation*, **6**, 156–8.

Gebara, B. M. Gelmini, M. & Sarnaik, A. (1992). Oxygen consumption, energy expenditure, and substrate utilization after cardiac surgery in children. *Critical Care Medicine*, **20**, 1550–4.

Glover, V. & Giannokoulopoulos, X. (1995). Stress and pain in the fetus. In *Stress and Pain in Infancy and Childhood*, ed. A. Aynsley-Green, M. P. Ward Platt, A. Lloyd-Thomas, pp. 495–510. London: Baillière's Clinical Paediatrics.

Gouyet, I., Dubois, M.-C., Murat, I. & Saint-Maurice, C. (1993). Comparison of two anesthesia techniques on perioperative insulin response to i.v. glucose infusion in children. *Acta Anaesthesiologica Scandanavica*, **37**, 12–16.

Groner, J. I., Brown, M. F., Stallings, V. A., Ziegler, M. M. & O'Neill, J. A. Jr. (1989). Resting energy expenditure in children following major operations. *Journal of Pediatric Surgery*, **14**, 825–8.

Håkanson, E., Rutberg, H., Jorfeldt, L. & Mårtensson, J. (1985). Effects of the extradural administration of morphine or bupivacaine, on the metabolic response to upper abdominal surgery. *British Journal of Anaesthesia*, **57**, 394–9.

Hawdon, J. M. & Ward Platt, M. P. (1993). Metabolic adaptation in small for gestational age infants. *Archives of Disease in Childhood*, **68**, 262–8.

Hawdon, J. M., Ward Platt, M. P. & Aynsley-Green, A. (1992). Patterns of metabolic adaptation for preterm and term infants in the first neonatal week. *Archives of Disease in Childhood*, **67**, 357–65.

Hughes, D., Murphy, J. F., Dyas, J., Robinson, J. A., Riad-Fahmy, D. & Hughes, I. A. (1987). Blood spot glucocorticoid concentrations in ill preterm infants. *Archives of Disease in Childhood*, **62**, 1014–18.

Jones, M. O., Pierro, A., Hammond, P. & Lloyd, D. A. (1993). The metabolic response to operative stress in infants. *Journal of Pediatric Surgery*, **28**, 1258–63.

Jones, M. O., Pierro, A., Hashim, I. A., Shenkin, A. & Lloyd, D. A. (1994). Postoperative changes in resting energy expenditure and interleukin 6 level in infants. *British Journal of Surgery*, **81**, 536–8.

Jones, M. O., Pierro, A., Garlick, P. J., McNurlan, M. A., Donnell, S. C. & Lloyd, D. A. (1995a). Protein metabolism kinetics in neonates: effect of intravenous carbohydrate and fat. *Journal of Pediatric Surgery*, **30**, 458–62.

Jones, M. O., Pierro, A., Hammond, P. & Lloyd, D. A. (1995b). The effect of major operations on heart rate, respiratory rate, physical activity, temperature and respiratory gas exchange in infants. *European Journal of Pediatric Surgery*, **5**, 9–12.

Khilnani, P., Munoz, R., Salem, M., Gelb, C., Todres, I. D. & Chernow, B. (1993). Hormonal responses to surgical stress in children. *Journal of Pediatric Surgery*, **28**, 1–4.

Lacoumenta, S., Patterson, J. L., Burrin, J., Causon, R. C., Brown, M. J. & Hall, G. M. (1986). Effects of two differing halothane concentrations on the metabolic and endocrine responses to surgery. *British Journal of Anaesthesia*, **58**, 844–50.

Lacoumenta, S., Yeo, T. H., Burrin, J. M. & Hall, G. M. (1987a). Beta-endorphin infusion fails to modulate the hormonal and metabolic response to surgery. *Clinical Endocrinology*, **26**, 657–66.

Lacoumenta, S., Yeo, T. H., Burrin, J. M., Bloom, S. R., Patterson, J. L. & Hall, G. M. (1987b). Fentanyl and the beta-endorphin, ACTH and glucoregulatory hormonal response to surgery. *British Journal of Anaesthesia*, **59**, 713–20.

Lind, L. (1995). Metabolic gas exchange during different surgical procedures. *Anaesthesia*, **50**, 304–7.

Lopaschuk, G. D., Collins-Nakai, R., Olley, P. M., Montague, T. J., McNeil, G., Gayle, M., Penkoske, P. & Finegan, B. A. (1994). Plasma fatty acid levels in infants and adults after myocardial ischemia. *American Heart Journal*, **128**, 61–7.

Maekawa, N., Mikawa, K., Nishina, K. & Obara, H. (1993). Effects of 2-, 4- and 12-hour fasting intervals on preoperative gastric fluid pH and volume, and plasma glucose and lipid homeostasis in children. *Acta Anaesthesiologica Scandinavica*, **37**, 783–7.

Milne, E. M. G., Elliot, M. J., Pearson, D. T., Holden, M. P., Ørskov, O. & Alberti, K. G. M. M. (1986). The effect on intermediary metabolism of open-heart surgery with deep hypothermia and circulatory arrest in infants of less than 10 kilograms body weight. A preliminary study. *Perfusion*, **1**, 29–40.

Mitchell, I. M., Davies, P. S. W., Day, J. M. E., Pollocks, J. C. S., Jamieson, M. P. G., Wheatley, D. J., Bove, E. L. & Allen, B. S. (1994). Energy expenditure in children with congenital heart disease, before and after cardiac surgery. *Journal of Thoracic and Cardiovascular Surgery*, **107**, 374–80.

Murat, I., Walker, J., Esteve, C., Nahoul, K. & Saint-Maurice, C. (1988). Effect of lumbar epidural anaesthesia on plasma cortisol levels in children. *Canadian Journal of Anaesthesia*, **35**, 20–4.

Nilsson, K., Larsson, L. E., Andréasson, S. & Ekström-Jodal, B. (1984). Blood glucose concentrations during anaesthesia in children. *British Journal of Anaesthesia*, **56**, 375–9.

Nishina, K., Mikawa, K., Maekawa, N., Asano, M. & Obara, H. (1995). Effects of exogenous intravenous glucose on plasma glucose and lipid homeostasis in anesthetized infants. *Anesthesiology*, **83**, 258–63.

Nistrup Madsen, S., Brandt, M. R., Engquist, A., Badawi, I. & Kehlet, H. (1977). Inhibition of plasma cyclic AMP, glucose and cortisol response to surgery by epidural analgesia. *British Journal of Surgery*, **64**, 669–71.

Nistrup Madsen, S., Fog-Møller, F., Christiansen, C., Vester-Andersen, T. & Engquist, A. L. (1978). Cyclic AMP, adrenaline and noradrenaline in plasma during surgery. *British Journal of Surgery*, **65**, 191–3.

Noel, G. I., Suh, H. K., Stone, J. G. & Frantz, A. G. (1972). Human prolactin and growth hormone release during surgery and other conditions of stress. *Journal of Clinical Endocrinology and Metabolism*, **35**, 840–51.

Obara, H., Sugiyama, D., Maekawa, N., Hamatani, S., Tanaka, O., Chuma, R., Kitamura, S. & Iwai, S. (1984). Plasma cortisol levels in paediatric anaesthesia. *Canadian Anaesthetic Society Journal*, **31**, 24–47.

ó Nualláin, E. M., Puri, P. & Reen, D. J. (1993). Early induction of IL-1 receptor antagonist (IL-1Ra) in infants and children undergoing surgery. *Clinical and Experimental Immunology*, **93**, 218–22.

Puhakka, K., Rasanen, J., Leijala, M. & Peltola, K. (1993). Metabolic effects of corrective surgery in infants and children with congenital heart defects. *British Journal of Anaesthesia*, **70**, 149–53.

Puhakka, K., Rasanen, J., Leijala, M. & Peltola, K. (1994). Oxygen consumption following pediatric cardiac surgery. *Journal of Cardiothoracic and Vascular Anesthesia*, **8**, 642–8.

Ratcliffe, J. M., Elliott, M. J., Wyse, R. K. H., Hunter, S. & Alberti, K. G. M. M. (1986). The metabolic load of stored blood. Implications for major transfusions in infants. *Archives of Disease in Childhood*, **61**, 1208–14.

Ratcliffe, J. M., Wyse, R. K. H., Hunter, S., Alberti, K. G. M. M. & Elliott, M. J. (1988). The role of the priming fluid in the metabolic response to cardiopulmonary bypass in children of less than 15 kg body weight undergoing open-heart surgery. *Thoracic and Cardiovascular Surgery*, **36**, 65–74.

Redfern, N., Addison, G. M. & Meakin, G. (1986). Blood glucose in anaesthetised children. *Anaesthesia*, **41**, 272–5.

Reier, C. E., George, J. M. & Kilman, J. W. (1973). Cortisol and growth hormone response to surgical stress during morphine anesthesia. *Anesthesia and Analgesia*, **52**, 1003–10.

Ridley, P. D., Ratcliffe, J. M., Alberti, K. G. M. M. & Elliott, M. J. (1990). The metabolic consequences of a 'washed' cardiopulmonary bypass pump-priming fluid in children undergoing cardiac operations. *Journal of Thoracic and Cardiovascular Surgery*, **100**, 528–37.

Russell, R. C. G., Walker, C. J. & Bloom, S. R. (1975). Hyperglucagonaemia in the surgical patient. *British Medical Journal*, **1**, 10–12.

Rutberg, J., Håkanson, E., Anderberg, B., Jorfeldt, L., Mårtensson, J. & Schildt, B. (1984). Effects of the extradural administration of morphine, or bupivacaine, on the endocrine response to upper abdominal surgery. *British Journal of Anaesthesia*, **56**, 233–7.

Salerno, R., Forti, G., Busoni, P. & Casadio, C. (1989). Effects of surgery and general or epidural anesthesia on plasma levels of cortisol, growth hormone, and prolactin in infants under one year of age. *Journal of Endocrinological Investigation*, **12**, 617–21.

Shanbhogue, R. L. K. & Lloyd, D. A. (1992). Absence of hypermetabolism after operation in the newborn infant. *Journal of Parenteral and Enteral Nutrition*, **16**, 333–6.

Shanbhogue, R. L. K., Jackson, M. & Lloyd, D. A. (1991). Operation does not increase resting energy expenditure in the neonate. *Journal of Pediatric Surgery*, **16**, 578–80.

Sigurdsson, G., Lindahl, S. & Norden, N. (1982). Influence of premedication on plasma ACTH and cortisol concentrations in children during adenoidectomy. *British Journal of Anesthesia*, **54**, 1075–9.

Sigurdsson, G. H., Lindahl, S. G. E. & Norden, N. E. (1984). Catecholamine and endocrine response in children during halothane and enflurane anaesthesia for adenoidectomy. *Acta Anaesthesiologica Scandanavica*, **28**, 47–51.

Schmeling, D. J. & Coran, A. G. (1991). Hormonal and metabolic response to operative stress in the neonate. *Journal of Parenteral and Enteral Nutrition*, **15**, 215–38.

Severino Brandi, L., Oleggini, M., Lachi, S., Frediani, M., Bevilacqua, S., Mosca, F. & Ferrannini, E. (1988). Energy metabolism of surgical patients in the early postoperative period: a reappraisal. *Critical Care Medicine*, **16**, 18–22.

Stayer, S. A., Steven, J. M., Nicholson, S. C., Jobes, D. R., Stanley, C. & Baumgar, S. (1994). The metabolic effects of surface cooling neonates prior to cardiac surgery. *Anesthesia and Analgesia*, **79**, 834–9.

Stuart, A. G. & Ward Platt, M. P. (1995). The ontogeny of the metabolic and endocrine stress response to elective surgery. In *Stress and Pain in Infancy and Childhood*, ed. A. Aynsley-Green, M. P. Ward Platt and A. Lloyd-Thomas, pp. 529–46. London: Ballière's Clinical Paediatrics.

Sweed, Y., Puri, P. & Reen, D. J. (1992). Early induction of IL-6 in infants undergoing najor abdominal surgery. *Journal of Pediatric Surgery*, **27**, 1033–7.

Thomas, S., Murphy, J. F., Dyas, J., Ryalls, M. & Hughes, I. A. (1986). Response to ACTH in the newborn. *Archives of Disease in Childhood*, **61**, 57–60.

Tsang, T. M. & Tam, P. K. H. (1994). Cytokine response of neonates to surgery. *Journal of Pediatric Surgery*, **29**, 794–7.

Tulla, H., Takala, J., Alhava, E., Huttunen, H. & Kari, A. (1991). Hypermetabolism after coronary artery bypass. *Journal of Thoracic and Cardiovascular Surgery*, **101**, 598–600.

Voutilainen, R. & Miller, W. L. (1986). Developmental expression of genes for the steroidogenic enzymes P450SCC (20,22-desmolase), P450C17 (17 alpha hydroxylase/17,20-lyase), and P450C21 (21-hydroxylase) in the human fetus. *Journal of Clinical Endocrinology and Metabolism*, **63**, 1145–50.

Ward Platt, M. P. (1988). *The metabolic and endocrine responses to surgery in children*. MD Thesis, University of Bristol.

Ward Platt, M. P., Aynsley-Green, A. & Anand, K. J. S. (1990). The ontogeny of the stress response and its implications for pediatric practice. *Advances in Pain Research and Therapy*, **15**, 123–36.

Ward Platt, M. P., Tarbit, M. & Aynsley-Green, A. (1990). The effects of anesthesia and surgery on metabolic homeostasis in infancy and childhood. *Journal of Pediatric Surgery*, **25**, 472–8.

Ward Platt, M. P., Weddle, A. & Aynsley-Green, A. (1989). The effect of major surgery on plasma beta endorphin concentrations in children. *Journal of Pain and Symptom Management*, **4**, S8 (abstract).

Welborn, L. G., McGill, W. A., Hannallah, R. S., Nisselson, C. L., Ruttimann, U. E. & Hicks, J. M. (1986). Perioperative blood glucose concentrations in pediatric outpatients. *Anesthesiology*, **65**, 543–7.

Wood, M., Shand, D. G. & Wood, A. J. J. (1980). The sympathetic response to profound hypothermia and circulatory arrest in infants. *Canadian Anaesthetic Society Journal*, **27**, 125–31.

Winter, J. S. D. (1985). The adrenal cortex in the fetus and neonate. In *Adrenal Cortex*, ed. D. C. Anderson and J. S. D. Winter, pp. 32–56. London: Butterworths.

Winthrop, A. L., Filler, R. M., Smith, J. & Heim, T. (1989). Analysis of energy and macronutrient balance in the postoperative infant. *Journal of Pediatric Surgery*, **24**, 686–9.

Winthrop, A. L., Jones, P. J. H., Schoeller, D. A., Filler, M. M. & Heim, T. (1987a). Changes in the body composition of the surgical infant in the early postoperative period. *Journal of Pediatric Surgery*, **22**, 546–9.

Winthrop, A. L., Wesson, D. E., Pencharz, P. B., Jacobs, D. G., Heim, T. & Filler, R. M. (1987b). Injury severity, whole body protein turnover, and energy expenditure in pediatric trauma. *Journal of Pediatric Surgery*, **22**, 534–7.

Wright, P. D. & Johnston, I. D. A. (1975). The effect of surgical operation on growth hormone levels in plasma. *Surgery*, **77**, 479–86.

Yamashita, M., Wakayama, S., Matsuki, A., Kudo, M. & Oyama, T. (1982). Plasma catechomaline levels during extracorporeal circulation in children. *Canadian Anaesthetic Society Journal*, **29**, 126–9.

10

Head injury in children

P. M. SHARPLES

Importance of head injury

Head injury is the major single cause of mortality and acquired neurological morbidity among children in developed countries. It has important consequences not only for the injured children and their families but also for society as seriously brain injured children who survive represent a significant financial burden on health, education and social service budgets.

In North America, a population-based study by Kraus *et al.* (1986) found that 10 per 100 000 children aged between 1 and 14 years die each year as a result of trauma to the head. In the UK, the annual mortality rate from head injury in children aged over 1 year is 5.3 per 100 000 children (Sharples *et al.*, 1990a). The mortality rate from childhood head injury increases with age, head injury accounting for 15% of all deaths among children aged 1–15 years and 25% of all deaths aged 5–15 years. Boys are twice as likely as girls to sustain a fatal head injury.

Head injuries also account for a considerable proportion of paediatric admissions to hospital. The North American National Head and Spinal Cord Survey found the incidence of children aged 0–14 years admitted to hospital for head injury to be 230 per 100 000 children (Kalsbeek *et al.*, 1980), while in California, Kraus *et al.* (1986) reported a paediatric admission rate for head injury of 185 per 100 000 children. Admission figures are higher in the UK, where approximately 1 in 200 children each year is admitted to hospital with a head injury (Sharples *et al.*, 1990a).

Head injury is not only an important cause of childhood deaths and hospital admissions, but is also a major cause of neurological disability. In the study by Kraus *et al.* (1986), the severity of head injury among children admitted to hospital was classed as mild in 86%, moderate in 8% and severe in 6%. Significant disability occurred in 5% of survivors, giving a morbidity rate of 25 per 100 000 per annum. If these disability rates are applied to the UK, then approximately 3000 children acquire significant neurological morbidity each year as a consequence of head injury. In fact the true morbidity may be higher as significant levels of cognitive and behavioural morbidity have been reported in children considered to have made a good recovery following head injury (Klonoff *et al.*, 1977; Casey *et al.*, 1986).

Although it is often suggested in the literature that outcome in head injured children is better than in head injured adults, there is evidence to suggest that in fact the reverse may be the case, with young children being most vulnerable of all to developing long-term disability following head injury (Filley *et al.*, 1987).

Using the conservative estimate of approximately 3000 children in the UK acquiring disability each year following head injury, the long-term cost to the UK economy can be estimated as being of the order of £840 million per annum. If the number of head injured children with long-term problems is in fact greater than this, then the cost to society will be proportionately higher. There is thus a powerful financial as well as humanitarian argument for reducing childhood disability following head injury by preventing head injuries and by optimising the management of the injured.

Prevention of head injury

Approaches to accident prevention can be divided into three groups, namely primary, secondary and tertiary prevention. Primary prevention aims to prevent the accident occurring, secondary prevention aims to prevent the subject being injured and tertiary prevention aims to ensure the optimal treatment of injury to promote recovery with minimal disability. Both acute management and rehabilitation therapy are forms of tertiary prevention.

Primary and secondary preventive measures need to be based on local epidemiological information. In North America (Kraus *et al.*, 1990) and the UK (Sharples *et al.*, 1990b), road traffic accidents (RTAs) are the main cause of paediatric head injury, followed by falls; however, most children injured in RTAs in North America are injured as occupants of motor vehicles, whereas in the UK the majority of children injured in RTAs are injured as pedestrians (Craft *et al.*, 1972; Sharples *et al.*, 1990b).

Several studies have demonstrated a correlation between the incidence of childhood accidents and socioeconomic deprivation. Our study of all fatal accidents involving head injuries in children in the Northern health region showed that the mortality rate from childhood pedestrian RTAs was 40 times higher in the most deprived areas of the region compared with the most affluent areas (Sharples *et al.*, 1990b). Children were often injured while playing unsupervised in the street after school.

The clustering of serious injuries in deprived areas makes targeting of preventive measures possible. Children often behave in a unsafe fashion in traffic (Sandels, 1974), which is not surprising in view of the fact that children aged under 12 years have developmental difficulties coping with traffic. Road safety campaigns aimed at children are therefore likely to be of limited value. The alternative approach, altering the environment to make it safer for children, could be achieved by legislation to make drivers drive more safely, and by engineering and town planning measures which reduce the amount of traffic to which children are exposed. Paediatricians have an important role in the prevention of childhood disability from head injury, not only by optimising its medical management, but also by acting as advocates for preventive measures.

Management of head injury

If primary and secondary preventive measures are unsuccessful, medical management aims to ensure that recovery from the head injury is as complete as possible. This involves providing the optimal environment for recovery from primary (impact) brain damage while preventing the occurrence of secondary brain damage, which occurs after injury.

Primary brain damage is the direct result of the impact and comprises two types of lesion; contusions and diffuse axonal injury.

1. Contusions occur on the crests of the gyri of the cerebral cortex, especially on the undersurface of the frontal lobes and around the temporal pole. They may cause focal neurological signs, especially if followed by oedema and local ischaemia, and scarring from contusions may result in post traumatic epilepsy.
2. Diffuse axonal injury (DAI) is a widespread lesion of the white matter, thought to result from shearing forces, which has a particular predilection for the corpus callosum and upper brain stem (Adams *et al.*, 1982). It is only since the use of appropriate stains for nerve processes that the importance of DAI as a mechanism of primary brain damage has been fully appreciated as there may be little evidence of it radiologically or at post-mortem. Loss of consciousness after head injury may be due to DAI, a brief period of unconsciousness reflecting a mild injury.

Secondary brain damage is the result of complications occurring after head injury and is potentially preventable. More than 90% of fatally head injured patients show neuropathological evidence of diffuse hypoxic-ischaemic damage and many have hippocampal damage due to compression secondary to raised intracranial pressure (ICP) (Graham *et al.*, 1978). The potential importance of secondary complications is also illustrated by reports of patients who talked after a head injury, indicating that the primary brain injury was not overwhelming, yet subsequently died (Reilly *et al.*, 1975; Jeffreys & Jones, 1981). Secondary complications can not only result in death after head injury but also lead to neurological disability in survivors (Miller & Becker, 1982).

Secondary brain damage after head injury can be due to intracranial or extracranial factors (Table 10.1). These produce brain damage either by causing cerebral hypoxia-ischaemia and/or by causing increased ICP, which leads to compression and brain shift. The development of an intracranial haematoma is the most frequent secondary complication, while others include brain swelling, poorly controlled epilepsy, meningitis, hypoxia and hypotension.

Bleeding inside the skull leads to the development of a clot, either between the skull and meninges (extradural haematoma) or beneath the dura (intradural haematoma). Intradural haematomas may be subdural, intracerebral or a combination of the two. As the skull is a rigid box, the development of a volume-occupying lesion, such as an intracranial haematoma or brain swelling will have to be compensated for by a decrease in the volume of another intracranial component, such as cerebrospinal fluid or cerebral blood volume. Once these compensatory mechanisms are exhausted, further increases in the volume of the intracranial lesion will result in raised ICP.

If ICP rises beyond a critical level, then brain shift across the tentorium and/or the foramen magnum occurs, compressing important structures. Tentorial herniation compresses the oculomotor nerve leading to ptosis, pupillary dilatation and impaired medial gaze. It also distorts the brainstem, producing mid-brain dysfunction and decerebrate rigidity. In tonsillar herniation the medulla and cerebellar tonsils are extruded through the foramen magnum, compressing the medulla. This produces vasomotor and respiratory disturbances and may cause respiratory arrest and death.

Avoidable factors

The main aim of the acute management of head injured patients is the prevention of secondary complications. Despite this, studies of the management of head injured patients who died after admission to hospital have indicated that approximately half had potentially avoidable secondary complications that probably contributed to death (Miller et al., 1978; Mendelow et al., 1979; Jeffreys & Jones, 1981). Most of these patients were adults, but recent evidence indicates that the incidence of potentially avoidable secondary complications in children is similar.

Our study of head injury children dying during 1979–86 demonstrated that avoidable factors possibly or probably contributing to death occurred in 81 (32%) of the 255 children (Table 10.2) (Sharples et al., 1990a). Potentially avoidable factors occurred in 27 (22%) of the 125 children who died before admission to hospital and in 54 (42%) of the 130 who died after hospital admission. Of the avoidable factors occurring in children after admission to hospital, 36 occurred at district general hospitals, 11 during

Table 10.1. *Causes of secondary brain damage after head injury*

Intracranial	Extracranial
Intracranial haematoma	Airways obstruction or respiratory failure
Brain swelling	Hypotension
Meningitis	
Hydrocephalus	
Subarachnoid haemorrhage	

transfer from a district hospital to a regional neurosurgical centre and 46 at a regional neurosurgical centre.

Organisation and delivery of acute care

The finding that one-third of all proportions of deaths from childhood head injury are associated with potentially avoidable factors emphasises the importance of delivering optimal care, before and after admission to hospital.

Studies from the USA have suggested that advanced prehospital care can appreciably reduce deaths following severe head injury (Baxt & Moody, 1987). Our study showed that of the head injured children who died before admission to hospital, those who had aspirated blood or vomit died with significantly milder injuries than those who had not aspirated, implying that better management of the airways might have prevented some deaths. Such data have led to the employment of paramedics to provide prehospital care for severely injured patients, with the aim of reducing deaths from respiratory obstruction or blood loss from extracranial injuries.

Once a head injured child has reached hospital, it is necessary to decide whether admission is required. This is straightforward in the case of severely head injured children, but is more difficult in the case of those who appear to have been mildly injured. Hospital admission may be disturbing to a child, often proves unnecessary and is expensive. The object of admitting mildly head injured children is to permit secondary complications, in particular intracranial haematomata or brain swelling, to be detected and treated immediately. If large numbers of children are admitted who do not develop secondary complications, doctors may be lulled into a false sense of security and may discharge patients who deserve observation.

Teasdale *et al.* (1990) have demonstrated that the presence of a skull fracture and/or change in conscious level permits identification of subgroups of head injured children with widely differing degrees of risk for an intracranial haematoma. Their results suggest that the absolute risk of intracranial haematoma is one in 12 for a child in

Table 10.2. *Summary of avoidable factors probably or possibly contributing to death in children with head injury*

	Before admission		Talked and died	After admission		
	Talked and died	Aspiration and respiratory arrest		Aspiration and respiratory arrest	Associated injury	Intracranial haematoma
Number of children	3	25	21	35	13	24
Median age (years)	10	11	9	7	9	9
Age range (years)	7–15	0.5–15	2–15	0.1–15	1–15	0.1–15
Median ISS*	16	25.0	9.0	25.0	48.0	22.5
ISS* range	—	9.0–66.0	4.0–48.0	4.0–59.0	41.0–59.0	16.0–59.0

*ISS: Injury Severity Score
Source: Baker & O'Neill (1976)

coma with a skull fracture, one in 157 a fully conscious child with a skull fracture, and one in 12 559 for a fully conscious child without a skull fracture. Priority thus needs to be given to admitting children who have sustained a skull fracture.

Although the presence of a skull fracture is an important factor to take into account when deciding whether to admit a child to hospital following a head injury, an expanding intracranial haematoma is not the only cause of secondary deterioration in conscious level. Other causes in children include seizures and raised ICP secondary to cerebral swelling (Bruce *et al.*, 1981; Snoek *et al.*, 1984).

Secondary cerebral swelling in children often represents a benign transient syndrome with spontaneous full recovery, but sometimes it progresses to severe and uncontrollable brain swelling leading to death (Aldrich *et al.*, 1992). The pathophysiological basis of this swelling remains unknown, although it has been suggested that it represents an increase in cerebral blood volume (Bruce *et al.*, 1981).

A study by Sainsbury & Sibert (1984) suggested the risk of a child with an apparently mild head injury who is symptom-free 6 hours after injury developing an extradural haematoma is minimal. Until the predictive factors for secondary cerebral swelling in children have been established, however, it may be prudent to observe head injured children in hospital for longer than this.

Conscious level is the best indicator of whether a severe head injury has been sustained, or if a secondary complication is developing. In adult patients and older children this is routinely monitored using the Glasgow Coma Score (GCS). Most workers regard a GCS of ≤ 8 shortly after injury as indicating a severe head injury, a GCS of 9–12 as indicating a moderately severe injury, and a GCS of 13–15 as indicating a mild injury. A progressive deterioration in conscious level after head injury suggests that a secondary complication is developing.

The original Glasgow Coma Score is unsuitable for use in young children because of the weight given to the verbal response. A number of alternative coma scales have been devised. Some of these are modifications of the Glasgow Score (Simpson & Reilly, 1982; James & Trauner, 1985). Of these, the James and Trauner method (Table 10.3) has the advantage of summing to the same number as the original Glasgow Score, facilitating communication between paediatricians and doctors from other specialties. It has been shown to be associated with good inter- and intraobserver reliability (W. Whitehouse, personal communication).

To reduce the occurrence of medically avoidable factors, several hospitals and health regions have tried to standardise the management of head injured children by producing guidelines for optimal treatment. The guidelines produced and used in the Northern health region are illustrated in Table 10.4. These were based on the guidelines produced for use in adult patients by a Group of Neurosurgeons (1984).

It is now recognised that interhospital transfer of comatose patients is potentially hazardous. A recent study (Gentleman & Jennett, 1990) has also demonstrated the

Table 10.3. *Comparison of the original Glasgow Coma Score with the adaptation proposed by James and Trauner*

Activity	Best response	Score
Original Glasgow Coma Score[a]		
Eye opening	Spontaneous	4
	To verbal stimuli	3
	To pain	2
	None	1
Verbal	Orientated	5
	Confused	4
	Inappropriate words	3
	Non-specific sounds	2
	None	1
Motor	Follows commands	6
	Localises pain	5
	Withdraws to pain	4
	Flexion to pain	3
	Extension to pain	2
	None	1
Adaptation to infants[b]		
Eye opening	Spontaneous	4
	To speech	3
	To pain	2
	None	1
Verbal	Coos, babbles	5
	Irritable cries	4
	Cries to pain	3
	Moans to pain	2
	None	1
Motor	Normal spontaneous movement	6
	Localises pain	5
	Withdraws in response to pain	4
	Abnormal flexion	3
	Abnormal extension	2
	None	1

[a] Teasdale & Jennett (1974)
[b] James & Trauner (1985)

potential hazards associated with transport within hospitals, emphasising the importance of preserving adequate oxygenation and cardiovascular stability at all times.

Neurointensive care

More than 90% of fatally head injured adults and children have histological evidence to suggest that ischaemic brain damage and/or raised intracranial pressure occurred in life (Graham *et al.*, 1989). The aims of neurointensive care are therefore twofold: (1) to prevent secondary ischaemic brain damage by ensuring an adequate cerebral blood flow (CBF) for cerebral metabolic needs, and (2) to ensure that ICP does not rise to levels at which cerebral herniation may occur.

Intracranial pressure

Intracranial volume consists of three minimally compressible compartments: neural tissue (80–90% of the volume), cerebrospinal fluid (CSF) (5–10%) and blood (5–10%). Any increase in volume of one constituent must be compensated by equal reduction in volume of another, otherwise ICP rises. Once compensatory mechanisms are exhausted, further increases in volume lead to an exponential steep rise in ICP.

Although cerebral blood volume is a relatively small component of the intracranial contents it is the most easily manipulated by therapeutic measures. Reduction in $PaCO_2$, or an increase in arterial oxygen content, both result in a reduction in cerebral blood flow (CBF) by increasing cerebrovascular resistance.

Raised ICP after head injury can be caused by an expanding space-occupying intracranial haematoma, brain swelling or, occasionally, hydrocephalus. Brain swelling can occur as a result of an increase in cerebral blood volume (engorgement) or an increase in brain water (cerebral oedema). There is a well recognised association between elevated ICP and increased mortality and morbidity (Narayan *et al.*, 1982).

Raised ICP can have two adverse consequences: brain shift and cerebral ischaemia. Cerebral ischaemia may occur because of blood vessel compression during brain shift or as a result of global reduction of CBF.

The factors controlling CBF are cerebral perfusion pressure (CPP) (systemic arterial pressure (SAP) minus ICP) and cerebrovascular resistance. Falls in SAP, or rises in ICP, will reduce CPP. In a healthy brain, changes in CPP over the approximate range 50–150 mmHg will be offset by compensatory changes in cerebrovascular resistance, ensuring that CBF is maintained at an appropriate level to meet metabolic requirements (pressure autoregulation) (Figure 10.1). If CPP falls below the lower autoregulatory limit, further cerebral vasodilatation cannot occur and CBF falls.

If pressure autoregulation is impaired, as it may be after a severe head injury, then CBF may be directly related to CPP at all levels of CPP. In this situation, any fall in

Table 10.4. *Northern region guidelines for the management of head injury*

IN ALL CASES DIAGNOSIS AND INITIAL TREATMENT OF SERIOUS
EXTRACRANIAL INJURIES TAKES PRIORITY OVER INVESTIGATION
AND TRANSFER TO NEUROSURGERY

Initial assessment

Airway	Clear and maintain a patent airway
	Control cervical spine until injury exclusion
Breathing	Oxygen 100% by mask (then blood gases)
	Intubate if airway obstructed, threatened or after aspiration
	Exclude tension/open pneumothorax clinically and treat if present[a]
	Indications for ventilation include:
	Cyanosis or oxygen saturation $< 90\%$
	$PaO_2 < 60\,mmHg\,(< 8\,kPA)$
	$PaCO_2 > 45\,mmHg\,(> 6\,kPA)$ or $< 30\,mmHg\,(< 4\,kPA)$
	Not obeying commands AND not localising to a painfaul stimulus
Circulation	Commence IV infusion
	Assess degree of shock and transfuse as appropriate for age/weight (shock in infants may follow intracranial blood loss)
	Record pulse, BP and respiratory rate
	Control external haemorrhage by direct pressure and immobilise fractures
	Exclude occult haemorrhage (chest/abdomen/pelvis/lower limbs)
Disability	Record pupils, consciousness on Glasgow Coma Scale (appropriate for age) and limb motor responses
Examination	All clothing should be removed
	Seek senior advice (children below 5 years of age are particularly difficult to assess and paediatric advice should be sought after initial assessment and resuscitation)

Criteria for skull radiography after recent head injury

Skull radiograph not necessary if immediate indication for CT scan is present
Clinical judgement is necessary but the following criteria are helpful:

1 Loss of consciousness or amnesia suspected at any time
2 Neurological symptoms or signs (including headache and/or vomiting)
3 Cerebrospinal fluid or blood from the nose or ear
4 Suspected penetrating injury)
5 Scalp bruising or laceration (to bone or $> 5\,cm$ long)
6 Falls from a height ($> 60\,cm$) or onto a hard surface
7 Suspected non-accidental injury
8 Tense fontanelle
9 Inadequate history

Criteria for admission to hospital
1 Confusion or any other depression of the level of consciousness at the time of examination (< 5 years AT ANY TIME FOLLOWING INJURY)
2 Skull fracture
3 Neurological symptoms or signs even if minor, particularly in children (e.g. headache or vomiting)
4 Other medical conditions (e.g. coagulation disorders)
5 Difficulty in assessing the patient (e.g. suspected drugs/glue/alcohol/non-accidental injury)

Patients sent home should be accompanied by a responsible adult who should receive written advice to return immediately if there is a deterioration

Criteria for consultation with a neurosurgical unit

1 Deterioration in level of consciousness or other neurological signs
2 Confusion or coma continuing after adequate resuscitation
3 Tense fontanelle
4 Skull fracture
5 Sutural diastasis
6 Compound depressed fractures of the skull
7 Suspected fracture of skull base

Transfer to neurosurgical unit
1 Consultation process to be completed and recorded
2 Personnel able to insert or reposition endotracheal tube and to initiate or maintain ventilation
3 Ensure adequate IV access and fluid to maintain systolic BP appropriate for age
4 Adequate notes, trauma charts and radiographs to accompany patient
5 Observations should be continued during transfer

---

[a] Adequate lateral cervical spine and chest radiography to be performed after resusciation.
IV: intravenous; BP: blood pressure; CT: computed tomography.

CPP will lead to a fall in CBF, rendering the patient very vulnerable to secondary ischaemic brain damage.

The critical levels of ICP and CPP associated with brain shift and cerebral ischaemia have not been definitely identified, particularly in children. Most workers currently regarded ICP > 20 mmHg as significantly elevated and requiring treatment (Miller *et al.*, 1981). Recent evidence, however, suggests that the clinically 'critical' level of ICP may be much lower than previously thought (Saul & Ducker, 1982), a report by Marshall *et al.* (1983), suggesting that brain herniation can occur sometimes at pressures only slightly above normal.

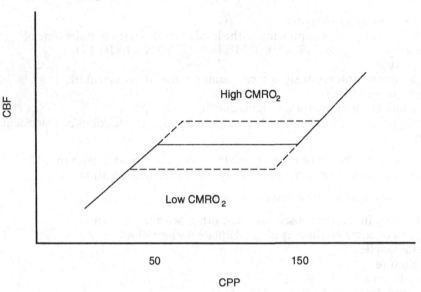

Figure 10.1. Diagrammatic representation of the relation between cerebral perfusion pressure (CPP) and cerebral blood flow (CBF) at various levels of cerebral metabolic rate (CMRO$_2$). The baseline of CBF is 'set' at a relatively low or high level in relation to metabolic rate. Within the normal range of pressure autoregulation, approximately 50–150 mmHg, changes in CPP are counterbalanced by changes in cerebrovascular resistance, maintaining CBF constant at a level to meet cerebral metabolic demands.

Cerebral blood flow and metabolism

A number of workers have measured CBF in head injured patients, using the Kety Schmidt method or the xenon-133 technique. Despite the histological evidence that ischaemic brain damage occurs in more than 90% of fatally head injured patients, most studies did not show cerebral ischaemia. CBF results varied widely, from abnormally low values to hyperperfusion, but very low values (< 20 ml/g per minute) were rarely seen and there was no clear evidence of a relation between low CBF and poor neurological outcome (Bruce *et al.*, 1973; Enevoldsen *et al.*, 1976; Obrist *et al.*, 1984). Pressure autoregulation was defective in some patients but most workers failed to demonstrate a relation between impaired pressure autoregulation and poor outcome (Tabaddor *et al.*, 1973; Fieschi *et al.*, 1974; Overgaard, & Tweed, 1974; Enevoldsen & Jensen, 1978).

It is difficult to assess the adequacy of CBF for cerebral metabolic needs without some measure of cerebral metabolism, which was obtained in some studies by measuring the arterio–jugular venous oxygen content difference (AJVDO$_2$), an indicator of brain oxygen extraction. The cerebral metabolic rate for oxygen ($CMRO_2$) can be calculated from global CBF and $AJVDO_2$ ($CMRO_2 = CBF \times AJVDO_2$).

If CBF is appropriately matched (coupled) to cerebral metabolism, the $AJVDO_2$ remains constant. If the normal coupling of CBF to cerebral metabolism is disturbed, however, and CBF becomes insufficient for metabolic needs, the brain extracts more oxygen from arterial blood, and the $AJVDO_2$ increases. If the normal coupling is disturbed, and CBF becomes excessive for cerebral metabolic requirements, then brain extracts less oxygen, and the $AJVDO_2$ falls (Obrist *et al.*, 1984).

Most studies of comatose head injured patients have reported normal or low $AJDVDO_2$ results, suggesting that cerebral blood flow is adequate or even excessive for cerebral metabolic needs. As the $AJVDO_2$ is a measure of global rather than regional oxygen extraction, a normal $AJVDO_2$ does not exclude focal cerebral ischaemia. Regional differences in CBF in head injured patients are usually minor (Obrist *et al.*, 1984; Messeter *et al.*, 1986); however, although one recent study has suggested that sometimes significant regional differences may occur (Marion *et al.*, 1991).

There is an apparent paradox between the almost universal histological evidence of ischaemic brain damage in fatally head injured patients and the results of clinical physiological studies, which suggest that cerebral ischaemia rarely occurs after head injury. This paradox could be explained, however, if ischaemic brain damage occurs very soon after head injury. Bouma *et al.* (1991) have reported low CBF and high $AJVDO_2$ values in the first 8 hours after head injury, with CBF rising and $AJVDO_2$ falling over time. These data suggest that head injured patients may be particularly vulnerable to ischaemic damage shortly after injury, highlighting the importance of good prehospital care and early resuscitation.

Cerebral blood flow and metabolism in severely head injured children

Until recently, there has been controversy about the changes in CBF and metabolism which occur following severe head injury in children, and the relation between these and ICP. Obrist *et al.* (1979) and Zimmermann *et al.* (1978) first reported an increased incidence of diffuse brain swelling in children and adolescents compared with older subjects, and suggested that age was an important factor in determining the pathophysiological response to head injury. This hypothesis was further developed by Bruce *et al.* (1979, 1981) who reported normal or elevated CBF results in six head injured patients, aged 14–21 years, who had the radiological appearance of diffuse cerebral swelling. These findings led them to conclude that in children raised ICP is usually due to vasodilation and increased CBF, rather than to cerebral oedema. They recommend that comatose head injured children should be electively ventilated to reduce CBF and thereby prevent ICP becoming elevated, and that mannitol should be avoided in case it increased cerebral blood flow, and thereby increased ICP.

Although the recommendations of Bruce and colleagues have been repeated in review articles (Pascucci, 1988), more recent research has not supported their hypothesis. Muizelaar *et al.* (1989a, b) performed 72 measurements of cerebral blood flow in 32 severely head injured patients aged 3–18 years using the inhalational or intravenous xenon-133 method. Elevated CBF was found to be uncommon and high ICP was not associated with high CBF.

The findings of Muizelaar and colleagues are in keeping with the results of our own study (Sharples *et al.*, 1995a, b) in which a modification of the Kety Schmidt technique (Sharples *et al.*, 1991) was used to perform a total of 151 measurements of CBF, $AJVDO_2$ and $CMRO_2$ in 21 comatose head injured children. CBF values tended to be low, with 116 of 150 (77%) lying below the mean CBF value reported in normal children and only 9 of 150 (6%) being at or above the upper limit of the normal range. Elevated ICP (> 20 mmHg) was associated with elevated CBF on only three occasions, while overall there was a significant inverse relation between ICP and CBF.

The evidence that elevated CBF (absolute cerebral hyperemia) is uncommon in severely head injured children has important therapeutic implications. First, there no longer seems any need to avoid the use of mannitol in these patients. Second, if CBF is not elevated, hyperventilation to reduce CBF in order to reduce ICP might result in cerebral ischaemia.

Muizelaar *et al.* (1989a) concluded that CBF in head injured children was always excessive for metabolic demands (relative cerebral hyperemia) even though the values were rarely elevated above normal. In view of this, they agreed with Bruce and colleagues that vigorous hyperventilation is safe in comatose head injured children, being unlikely to result in cerebral ischaemia.

Like Muizelaar and colleagues, we found that most of the $AJVDO_2$ results in our population of severely head injured children fell within or below the normal range, which suggests adequate CBF for metabolic needs (Figure 10.2). Indeed, only three $AJVDO_2$ values were above the upper limit of the normal range, suggesting actual or incipient cerebral ischaemia. In our study repeated measurements of CBF and $AVDO_2$ were made in individual children, a mean of seven measurements being performed in each child. The results demonstrated a fall in $AJVDO_2$ over time, similar to that reported by Bouma *et al.* (1991). $CMRO_2$ also fell over time. These results suggest that therapeutic measures designed to reduce intracranial pressure by lowering CBF, such as hyperventilation, should be used with caution in children, as well as adults, in the first 24 hours after injury.

Experimental studies in animals by Langfitt *et al.* (1965, 1966) led to the suggestion that in brain injured subjects the cerebral circulation might be 'vasospastic' with severely impaired responsivity to normal physiological control mechanisms. This concept of 'vasospastic paralysis' was cited by Bruce and colleagues to account for the normal or elevated CBF which they reported in head injured children. The two recent

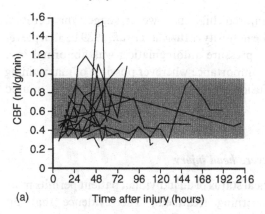

(a)

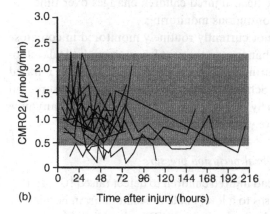

(b)

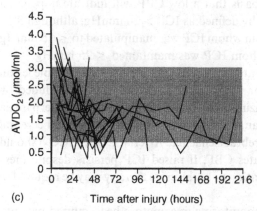

(c)

Figure 10.2. Relation between time after injury and cerebral blood flow (CBF) (a), cerebral metabolic rate for oxygen (CMRO$_2$) (b) and arterio–jugular venous oxygen difference (AJVDO$_2$) (c) in 21 severely head injured children, age 2–16 years. The shaded part of each graph represents the range reported in normal children by Settergen *et al.* (1980).

major studies of CBF in severely head injured children, however, suggest that cerebral autoregulation to pressure is intact in the majority (Muzielaar *et al.*, 1989 b; Sharples *et al.*, 1995 b). In both studies, however, pressure autoregulation was abnormal in a significant proportion, emphasising the importance wherever possible of maintaining adequate systemic and cerebral perfusion pressures in all severely head injured children.

Physiological monitoring in severe head injury

Information about the pathophysiological status of an individual patient permits more rational decisions to be made concerning treatment. The evidence that the pathophysiological status of comatose head injured children changes over time emphasises the importance of serial or continuous monitoring.

CBF and cerebral metabolism are not currently routinely monitored in comatose patients, although this situation may change over the next few years with the development of bedside techniques for measuring CBF, such as SPECT scanning, infrared spectroscopy and the adapted Kety Schmidt technique. Intracranial pressure and cerebral perfusion pressure are routinely monitored in most centres and many now monitor AJVDO$_2$ or jugular venous oxygen saturation.

Intracranial pressure and cerebral perfusion pressure

Monitoring of ICP is widely used in head injured children to detect raised ICP, so that treatment can be instituted before it rises to a level liable to result in brain herniation. CPP is also often monitored, on the basis that a low CPP will indicate impending cerebral ischaemia. Raised ICP is usually defined as ICP > 20 mmHg, although Saul & Ducker (1982) reported that patients in whom ICP was manipulated to ≤ 15 mmHg had a better outcome than those in whom ICP was maintained ≤ 25 mmHg.

Raised ICP should first prompt a hunt for the cause. A surgically remediable lesion such as an intracranial haematoma or hydrocephalus should first be excluded by computed tomography (CT) scan. Seizure activity should be treated, hyperpyrexia corrected and adequate sedation and analgesia assured, to prevent elevated cerebral metabolic rate and increased risk of cerebral ischaemia. Arterial CO$_2$ ($PaCO_2$) should be checked, since raised $PaCO_2$ elevates CBF. If raised ICP persists despite these measures, diuretic therapy, hyperventilation or barbiturate therapy may be required to normalise ICP (Langfitt, 1986).

Despite the widespread use of ICP monitoring in comatose head injured patients, there is still controversy about its role and about the vigour with which raised ICP should be treated in the absence of a surgically treatable lesion (Narayan *et al.*, 1982). Although many studies have demonstrated a relationship between raised ICP and poor outcome, this does not necessarily mean that reducing ICP will improve outcome as both ICP and outcome may simply both be reflections of the severity of primary impact damage (Eisenberg *et al.*, 1988).

Studies of head injured adults and children have demonstrated an association between low CPP and poor outcome (McGraw *et al.*, 1986; Tsutsumi *et al.*, 1986; Sharples, 1995) and clinical studies of children with acute non-traumatic encephalopathies have also shown a correlation between low CPP and poor neurological outcome (Barzilay *et al.*, 1988; Tasker *et al.*, 1988). Some workers have taken these findings to indicate a causal relation and between low CPP and poor outcome and have attempted to define the minimum CPP which must be maintained to ensure adequate CBF for metabolic requirements and prevent secondary ischaemic damage. Studies have not led to a consensus regarding the critical CPP for children, with various authors proposing that CPPs ranging from 30 to 70 mmHg must be maintained.

In patients in whom pressure autoregulation is impaired, CBF will be directly related to CPP at all levels of CPP, a situation described as the 'pressure passive circulation'. In this situation, CPP would need to be maintained at a relatively high level to achieve normal CBF, whereas patients with intact pressure autoregulation would be able to maintain CBF at a level appropriate for metabolic needs unless CPP fell below the lower limit of the range for pressure autoregulation. The lower limit of the autoregulatory range is usually accepted as being 50 mmHg in adults but may be lower in young children.

Few studies relating CPP to neurological outcome have related CPP directly to CBF or cerebral oxygen delivery. As cerebral metabolic rate is usually reduced in comatose patients, a low level of CBF may nevertheless be sufficient to meet the brain's reduced metabolic requirements; the association between low CPP and poor outcome may simply be a consequence of elevated ICP, and low CPP acting as a marker of a profound neurological insult. Until this issue is further clarified, however, it is probably appropriate to aim to maintain CPP above the lower limit of the adult autoregulatory range (50 mmHg), in severely head injured children.

Some workers have recently recommended that CPP in severely head injured patients should be routinely maintained at relatively high levels (70–80 mmHg) (Rosner & Daughton, 1990). This recommendation is based on the 'vasodilatory cascade' hypothesis, which assumes pressure autoregulation to be preserved in most comatose head injured patients. If pressure autoregulation is preserved, then a fall in CPP acts as a stimulus to vasodilation. Rosner & Daughton proposed that this vasodilation results in an increase in cerebral blood volume, leading to a rise in ICP and a further fall in CPP, and that this cycle will continue, with progressively increasing ICP, until maximal cerebral vasodilation has occurred. They suggest that routinely maintaining a high CPP would reverse the vasodilatory cascade and thus lower ICP fall.

Although pressure autoregulation appears to be preserved in the majority of severely head injured children, it is impaired in a significant minority (Muzielaar et al., 1989b; Sharples et al., 1995b). Therapeutically elevating systemic blood pressure to produce a high CPP could be potentially dangerous in such patients as raising the arterial blood pressure might increase CBF and thus increase ICP. Such a treatment protocol should probably only be applied if intact pressure autoregulation has been demonstrated.

Despite the above caveats, monitoring ICP and CPP has the undoubted advantage of providing early warning of changes in a patient's condition and preventing inappropriate treatments, designed to lower elevated ICP, from being applied blindly. It also provides information about the underlying pathophysiology and, particularly if used in combination with new methods of monitoring CBF and cerebral metabolism, may indicate the most appropriate therapy in individual cases.

Arterio–jugular venous oxygen difference ($AJVDO_2$)

In comatose head injured patients, cerebral metabolic rate is often depressed. CBF may therefore be sufficient for cerebral metabolic requirements, despite being lower than normal. Information concerning CBF alone is thus insufficient to indicate whether a patient is at risk of sustaining ischaemic brain damage.

It has been suggested that regular measurements of the $AJVDO_2$, or continuous measurements of internal jugular bulb oxygen saturation ($SJVDO_2$), would provide as a guide to the balance between CBF and cerebral metabolism (Robertson et al., 1989: Sheinberg et al., 1992). A normal $AJVDO_2$ or $SJVDO_2$ indicates appropriate matching of CBF and cerebral metabolic rate, a high $AJVDO_2$ or $SJVDO_2$ suggests impending cerebral ischaemia and a low $AJVDO_2$ or $SJVDO_2$ indicates cerebral hyperaemia. The normal value for $SJVDO_2$ is of the order of 50% (Sheinberg et al., 1992), while in children, the normal value for $AJVDO_2$ is 2.2 mmol/ml (Sharples et al., 1991).

Workers who have tried using the fibreoptic catheter oximetry to continuously monitor $SJVDO_2$ (Cruz et al., 1990; Sheinberg et al., 1992) have noted that rapid fluctuations, which are often artefactual, tend to limit its usefulness. Despite this, their results suggest that episodes of cerebral ischaemia do occur in head injured patients receiving intensive care, although the overall incidence is probably not high. In the future, continuous monitoring of cerebral oxygenation will probably be routinely used to supplement continuous monitoring of CPP.

Biochemical and molecular consequences of head injury

Despite the suggestion that ischaemic brain damage occurs in the first few hours after severe head injury, studies in animals have not shown unequivocal evidence of early cerebral ischaemia after head injury (Unterberg et al., 1988; Povlishock, 1989). An alternative explanation for the apparent discrepancy between the very high incidence of 'ischaemic' brain damage observed in histological studies of fatally head injured patients and the low incidence of cerebral ischaemia observed in clinical studies is that neuronal loss after head injury is due to primary cellular dysfunction rather than to a shortage of oxygen or glucose (Sharples *et al.*, 1995a). It is now increasingly appreciated that traumatic brain injury triggers a cascade of biochemical and molecular 'autodestructive' events which lead to further brain damage and that therapeutic intervention in this cascade may improve outcome (Faden & Salzman, 1992).

Recent experimental studies indicate that the biochemical response to head injury evolves over time (Hovda *et al.*, 1991; Yoshino *et al.*, 1991). These data, in conjunction with the clinical evidence of a progressive change in the pathophysiological response to severe head injury (Sharples *et al.*, 1995a) suggest that there may be a 'window of opportunity' during which secondary brain damage is potentially preventable.

The observation that $CMRO_2$ may be initially normal in comatose head injured children (Sharples *et al.*, 1995a), is in accordance with experimental evidence that brain injury can be accompanied by normal or increased levels of cerebral metabolic activity (Hovda *et al.*, 1991; Yoshino *et al.*, 1991, Kuroda *et al.*, 1992). Kuroda proposed that the glucose hypermetabolism observed in their subjects was due to the release of excitotoxic amino acids, an hypothesis supported by studies demonstrating increased extracellular levels of glutamate and aspartate in head injured subjects (Faden *et al.*, 1989; Katayma *et al.*, 1990).

It is now believed that after head injury glutamate acts on the *N*-methyl-D-aspartate receptors to cause a massive increase in intracellular free calcium to occur after central nervous system injury (Choi, 1987) which in turn induces uncontrolled activation of Ca^{2+} stimulated enzymes, such as phospholipase, proteases and endonucleases (Okiyama *et al.*, 1992). The excess activation of these enzymes may result in the generation of active and potentially toxic metabolites, including lysophospholipids, arachidonic acid, prostaglandins, leukotrienes, thromboxanes and oxygen free radicals and lead to oedema (Baethmann *et al.*, 1989), mitochondrial dysfunction (Yang *et al.*, 1985), disruption of cytoskeletal networks and the breakdown of the nuclear membrane (Polvishock *et al.*, 1989). Such processes would lead to neuronal dysfunction, a fall in cerebral metabolic rate and, ultimately, neuronal loss.

Greater understanding of the nature of the biochemical events underlying secondary brain damage will lead to new approaches to treatment. Clinical trials of excitatory amino acid blocking agents and free radical scavengers are already in progress in severely head injured adult patients.

In addition to the biochemical events which may lead to secondary brain damage following severe head injury, there is increasing interest in the role of immunological and molecular events. Outside the central nervous system, mononuclear phagocytes migrate to areas of injured tissue, engulf debris and secrete a variety of cytotoxic agents, and there is now evidence that mononuclear phagocytes also mediate tissue response to injury in the central nervous system (Giulian & Robertson, 1990; Melton *et al.*, 1994). This is not surprising as a number of toxic agents implicated in the pathogenesis of traumatic and ischaemic brain injury are released by activated mononuclear phagocytes (free radicals, nitric oxide, proteases, leukotrienes, cytokines) (Dawson *et al.*, 1991).

The cytotoxic effects of mononuclear phagocytes are almost certainly mediated, at least in part, by cytokines, including interleukin 1 beta (IL-1 beta), which may also be produced from neurons and glial cells. IL-1 beta has been demonstrated to be produced in increased concentrations in the brain following head injury (Giulian & Lachman, 1985; Taupin *et al.*, 1993; Melton *et al.*, 1994) and there is evidence that it acts as an important mediator of destructive processes (Toulmond & Rothwell, 1995). Some of the destructive effects of IL-1 beta may be due to its effect on the synthesis of beta amyloid protein and amyloid precursor protein (Yankner *et al.*, 1990), which have been shown to be produced shortly after head injury (Roberts *et al.*, 1991; Melton *et al.*, 1994).

In addition to their potential for mediating destructive processes, cytokines, including IL-1 beta, may play an important part in reparative processes by inducing production of neurotrophins, particularly nerve growth factor (NGF) (Brennerman *et al.*, 1992). Upregulation of NGF mRNA has recently been reported after experimental head injury (Yang *et al.*, 1995) and the intraventricular infusion of NGF has been shown to improve cognitive outcome in experimentally head injured rats (Sinson *et al.*, 1995). These findings have led a number of workers to hypothesise that the intraventricular infusion of NGF may have the potential to improve outcome in severely head injured patients.

Interest in the role of cytokines and growth factors in the pathophysiology of severe head injury has gone hand in hand with a revision of the concept that primary traumatic injury is necessarily immediate and irreversible. It is now hypothesised that even diffuse axonal injury evolves over time and may be amenable to treatment with neurotrophic factors (Steward & Jane, 1989). Much research at present is concentrated on defining the biochemical, immunological and molecular events which occur following head injury in order to devise therapies which reverse destructive processes and enhance reparative ones.

References

Adams, J. H., Graham, D. I., Murray, L. S. & Scott, G. (1982). Diffuse axonal injury due to non-missile injury in humans: an analysis of 45 cases. *Ann Neurol*, **12**, 557–63.
Baethmann, A., Maier-Hauff, K., Schurer, L. *et al.* (1989). Release of glutamate and free fatty acids in vasogenic oedema. *J Neurosurg*, **70**, 578–91.

Baker, S. P. & O'Neill, B. (1976). The injury severity score: an update. *J. Trauma*, **16**, 882–5.

Barzilay, Z., Augarten, A., Sagy, M. *et al.* (1988). Variables affecting outcome from severe brain injury in children. Intensive Care Med, **14**, 417–21.

Baxt, W. G. & Moody, P. (1987). The impact of advanced prehospital emergency care on the mortality of severely brain-injured patients. *J Trauma*, **27**, 365–9.

Bouma, G. J., Muzielaar, J. P., Choi, S. C., Newlon, P. G. & Young, H. F. (1991). Cerebral circulation and metabolism after severe traumatic brain injury: the elusive role of ischaemia. *J Neurosurg*, **75**, 685–93.

Brennerman, D. E., Schultzberg, M., Bartfai, T. & Gozes, I. (1992). Cytokine regulation of neuronal survival. *J Neurochem*, **58**, 454–60.

Bruce, D. A., Alavi, A., Bilaniuk, L. *et al.* (1981). Diffuse cerebral swelling following head injuries in children; the syndrome of 'malignant brain oedema'. *J Neurosurg*, **54**, 170–8.

Bruce, D. A., Langfitt, T. A., Miller, J. D. *et al.* (1973). Regional cerebral blood flow, intracranial pressure, and brain metabolism in comatose patients. *J Neurosurg*, **38**, 131–44.

Bruce, D. A., Raphaely, R. C., Goldberg, A. I. *et al.* (1979). Pathophysiology, treatment and outcome following severe head injury in children. *Child's Brain*, **5**, 174–91.

Casey, R., Ludwig, S. & McCormick, M. C. (1986). Morbidity following minor head trauma in children. *Pediatrics*, **78**, 497–502.

Choi, D. W. (1987). Ionic dependence of glutamate neurotoxicity. *J. Neurosci*, **7**, 369–79.

Craft, A. W., Shaw, D. A. & Cartlidge, N. E. (1972). Head injuries in children. *Br Med J*, **4**, 200–3.

Cruz, J., Milner, M. E., Allen, S. J., Alves, W. M. & Gennarelli, T. S. (1990). Continuous monitoring of cerebral oxygenation in acute brain injury: injection of mannitol during hyperventilation. *J Neurosurg*, **73**, 725–30.

Dawson, V. L., Dawson, T. M., London, E. D. *et al.* (1991). Nitric oxide mediates glutamate neurotoxicity in primary cortical culture. *Proc Natl Acad Sci USA*, **88**, 6368–71.

Eisenberg, H. M., Frankowski, R. F., Contant, C. F. *et al.* (1988). High-dose barbiturate control of elevated intracranial pressure in patients with severe head injury. *J Neurosurg*, **69**, 15–23.

Enevoldsen, E. M., Gold, G., Jensen, F. T. *et al.* (1976). Dynamic changes in regional CBF, intraventricular pressure, CSF pH and lactate levels during the acute phase of head injury. *J Neurosurg*, **44**, 191–214.

Enevoldsen, E. M. & Jensen, F. T. Autoregulation and CO_2 responses of cerebral blood flow in patients with acute severe head injury. *J Neurosurg*, **48**, 689–703.

Faden, A. I., Demediuk, P., Panter, S. & Vink, R. (1989). The role of excitatory amino acids and NMDA receptors in traumatic brain injury. *Science*, **244**, 798–800.

Faden, A. I. & Salzman, S. (1992). Pharmacological strategies in CNS trauma. *Trends Pharmacol Sci*, **13**, 29–35.

Fieschi, C., Battistini, N. Beduschi, A. *et al.* (1974). Regional cerebral blood flow and intraventricular pressure in acute head injuries. *J Neurol Neurosurg Psychiatry*, **37**, 1378–8.

Filley, C. M., Cranberg, L. D., Alexander, M. F. & Hart, E. J. (1987). Neurobehavioural outcome after closed head injury in children and adolescents. *Arch Neurol*, **44**, 194–8.

Gentleman, D. & Jennett, B. (1990). Audit of transfer of unconscious head injured patients to a neurosurgical unit. *Lancet*, **335**, 330–4.

Giulian, D. & Lachman, L. (1985). Interleukin-1 stimulation of astroglial proliferation after brain injury. *Science*, **228**, 497–9.

Giulian, D. & Robertson, C. (1990). Inhibition of mononuclear phagocytes reduces ischaemic injury in the spinal cord. *Ann Neurol*, **27**, 33–42.

Graham, D. I., Adams, H. J. & Doyle, D. (1978). Ischaemic damage in fatal non-missile head injuries. *J Neurol Sci*, **39**, 213–34.

Graham, D. I., Ford, I., Hume Adams, J. H. *et al.* (1989). Fatal head injury in children. *J Clin Pathol*, **42**, 18–22.

Group of Neurosurgeons. (1984). Guidelines for initial management after head injury in adults. *Br Med J*, **288**, 983–5.

Hovda, D. A., Yoshino, A., Katayma, T. & Becker, D. P. (1991). Diffuse prolonged depression of oxidative metabolism following concussive brain injury in the rat: a cytochrome oxidase histochemistry study. *Brain Res*, **567**, 1–10.

James, H. E. & Trauner, D. A. (1985). The Glasgow Coma Scale. In: *Brain Insults in Infants and Children*, ed. H. E. James, N. G. Anas & R. M. Perkin, pp. 179–82. London: Grune & Stratton.

Jeffreys, R. V. & Jones, J. J. (1981). Avoidable factors contributing to the death of head injury patients in general hospitals in Mersey region. *Lancet*, **2**, 459–61.

Kalsbeek, W. D., McLaurin, R. L., Harris, B. S. H. III *et al.* (1980). The National Head and Spinal Cord Injury Survey: major findings. *Journal of Neurosurgery*.

Katayama, Y., Becker, D. P., Tamura, T. & Hovda, D. A. (1990). Massive increases in extracellular potassium and the indiscriminate release of glutamate following concussive brain injury. *J Neurosurg*, **73**, 889–900.

Klonoff, H., Low, R. D. & Clark, C. (1977). Head injuries in children: a prospective five year follow-up. *J Neurol Neurosurg Psychiatry*, **40**, 1211.

Kraus, J. F., Fife, D., Cox, P., Ramstein, K. & Conroy, C. (1986). Incidence, severity and external cause of pediatric brain injury. *AJDC*, **140**, 687–93.

Kraus, J. F., Fife, D. & Conroy, C. (1987). Pediatric brain injuries: the nature, clinical course and early outcomes: a defined United States population. *Pediatrics*, **79**, 501–7.

Kraus, J. F., Rock, A. & Hemyari, P. (1990). Brain injuries among infants, children, adolescents and young adults. *AJDC*, **144**, 684–91.

Kuroda, Y., Inglis, F. M., Miller, J. D. *et al.*, (1992). Transient glucose hypermetabolism after acute subdural haematoma in the rat. *J Neurosurg*, **76**, 471–7.

Langfitt, T. W. (1986). Raised ICP in head injury, its significance, causes and therapy. In: *Intracranial Pressure VI*, ed. J. D. Miller, G. M. Teasdale, J. O. Rowan *et al.*, pp. 789–94. Berlin: Springer.

Langfitt, T. W., Tannenbaum, H. M. & Kassell, N. F. (1966). The etiology of acute brain swelling following experimental brain injury. *J Neurosurg*, **24**, 47–56.

Langfitt, T. W., Weinstein, J. D. & Kassell, N. F. (1965). Cerebral vasomotor paralysis produced by intracranial hypertension. *Neurology*, **15**, 622–41.

Lewelt, W., Jenkins, L. W. & Miller, J. D. (1980). Autoregulation of cerebral blood flow after experimental fluid percussion injury of the brain. *J Neurosurg*, **53**, 500–11.

McGraw, C., Shields, C. B., Gamel, J. W. & Greenberg, R. A. (1986). Impact of cerebral perfusion pressure on survival following trauma. In: Intracranial Pressure VI, ed. J. D. Miller, G. M. Teasdale, J. O. Rowan, S. L. Galbraith & A. D. Mendelow, pp. 667–70. New York: Springer.

Marion, D. W., Darby, J. & Yonas, H. (1991). Acute regional cerebral blood flow changes caused by severe head injuries. *J Neurosurg*, **74**, 407–14.

Marshall, L. F., Barba, D., Toole, B. M. *et al.* (1983). The oval pupil: clinical significance and relationship to intracranial hypertension. *J. Neurosurg*, **58**, 566–8.

Melton, L., Hillhouse, E. W., Gunn, A. J., Candy, J. & Sharples, P. M. (1994). Changes in interleukin 1 beta and amyloid precursor protein after traumatic brain injury in the rat. *J Neuroimmunol*, **54**, 182.

Mendelow, A. D., Karmi, M. Z., Paul, K. S., Fuller, G. A. G. & Gillingham, F. J. (1979). Extradural haematoma: effect of delayed treatment. *Br Med J*, **1**, 1240–2.

Messeter, K., Nordstrom, C. H., Sundbarg, G. *et al.* (1986). Cerebral haemodynamics in patients with acute severe head trauma. *J Neurosurg*, **64**, 231–7.

Miller, J. D. (1985). Head injury and brain ischaemia – implications for therapy. *Br J Anaesth*, **57**, 120–9.

Miller, J. D. & Becker, D. P. (1982). Secondary insults to the injured brain. *JR Coll Surg Edinb*, **27**, 292–8.

Miller, J. D., Sweet, R. C., Narayan, R. & Becker, D. P. (1978). Early insults to the injured brain. *JAMA*, **24**, 439–42.

Miller, J. D., Butterworth, J. F., Gudeman, S. K. *et al.* (1981). Further experience in the management of severe head injury. *J Neurosurg*, **54**, 289–99.

Morray, J. P., Tyler, D. C., Jones, T. K., Stuntz, J. T. & Lemire, R. L. (1984). Coma scale for use in brain injured children. *Crit Care Med*, **12**, 1018–20.

Muizelaar, J. P., Marmarou, A., DeSalles, A. A. F. *et al.* (1989a). Cerebral blood flow and metabolism in severely head injured children. Part 1. Relationship with GCS score, outcome, ICP and PVI. *J Neurosurg*, **71**, 63–71.

Muizelaar, J. P., Ward, J. D., Marmarou, A., Newlon, P. G. & Wachi, A. (1989b). Cerebral blood flow and metabolism in severely head injured children. Part 2. Autoregulation. *J Neurosurg*, **71**, 72–6.

Narayan, R. K., Kishore, P. R. S., Becker, D. P. *et al.* (1982). Intracranial pressure; to monitor or not to monitor? *J Neurosurg*, **56**, 650–9.

Obrist, W. D., Gennarelli, T. A., Segawa, H., Dolinskas, C. A. & Langfitt, T. W. (1979). Relation of cerebral blood flow to neurological status and outcome in head-injured patients. *J Neurosurg*, **51**, 292–300.

Obrist, W. D., Langfitt, T. W., Jaggi, J. L., Cruz, J. *et al.* (1984). Cerebral blood flow and metabolism in comatose patients with acute head injury. Relationship to intracranial hypertension. *J Neurosurg*, **61**, 241–53.

Okimaya, K., Smith, D. H., Thomas, M. J. & McIntosh, T. K. (1992). Evaluation of a novel calcium channel blocker, (S)-emopamil, on regional cerebral edema and neurobehavioural function after experimental brain injury. *J Neurosurg*, **77**, 607–15.

Overgaard, J. & Tweed, W. A. (1974). Cerebral circulation after head injury. Part 1. Cerebral blood flow and its regulation after closed head injury and emphasis on clinical correlations. *J Neurosurg*, **41**, 531–41.

Overgaard, J., Mosdal, C., Tweed, W. A. (1981). Cerebral circulation after head injury. Part 3. Does reduced cerebral blood flow determine recovery of brain function after blunt head injury? *J Neurosurg*, **55**, 63–74.

Pascucci, R. C. (1988). Head trauma in the child. *Intensive Care Med*, **14**, 185–95.

Povlishock, J. T. (1989). Experimental studies of head injury. In: *Textbook of Head Injury*, ed. D. P. Becker & S. K. Gudeman. Philadelphia: WB Saunders Company, 1989; 437–50.

Reilly, P. L., Graham, D. I., Adams, J. H. & Jennett, B. (1975). Patients with head injury who talk and die. *Lancet*, **2**, 375–7.

Roberts, G. W., Gentleman, S. M., Lynch, A. & Graham, D. I. (1991). Beta A4 amyloid protein deposition in brain after head trauma. *Lancet*, **338**, 1422–3.

Robertson, C. S., Narayan, R. K., Gokaslan, Z. L. *et al.* (1989). Cerebral arteriovenous oxygen difference as an estimate of cerebral blood flow in head injured patients. *J Neurosurg*, **70**, 222–30.

Rosner, M. J. & Daughton, S. (1980). Cerebral perfusion pressure management in head injury. *J Neurosurg*, **30**, 933–41.

Rutter, M., Chadwick, O., Shaffer, D. *et al.* (1980). A prospective study of children with head injuries. I. Design and methods. *Psychol Med*, **10**, 633–45.

Sainsbury, C. P. Q. & Sibert, J. R. (1984). How long do we need to observe head injuries in hospital? *Arch Dis Child*, **59**, 856–9.

Sandels, S. (1974). An overall view of children in traffic. In: *Children, the Environment and Accidents*, ed. R. H. Jackson, pp. 29–7. Tunbridge Wells: Pitman Medical.

Saul, T. G. & Ducker, T. B. (1982). Effect of intracranial pressure monitoring and aggressive treatment on mortality in severe head injury. *J Neurosurg*, **56**, 498–503.

Settergen, G., Linblad, B. S. & Persson, B. (1980). Cerebral blood flow and exchange of oxygen, glucose and ketone bodies, lactate, pyruvate and amino acids in anaesthetised children. *Acta Paediatr Scand*, **69**, 457–65.

Sharples, P. M. (1995). *Reducing mortality and morbidity from head injury in children*. PhD Thesis, Newcastle, University of Newcastle upon Tyne.

Sharples, P. M., Storey, A., Aynsley-Green, A. & Eyre, J. A. (1990a). Avoidable factors contributing to the death of children with head injury. *Br Med J*, **300**, 87–91.

Sharples, P. M., Storey, A., Aynsley-Green, A. & Eyre, J. A. (1990b). Causes of fatal childhood accidents involving head injury in the Northern region 1979–86. *Br Med J*, **301**, 1193–7.

Sharples, P. M., Stuart, A. G., Aynsley-Green, A. *et al.* (1991). A practical method of serial bedside measurement of cerebral blood flow and metabolism during neurointensive care. *Arch Dis Child*, **66**, 1326–32.

Sharples, P. M., Stuart, A. G., Matthews, D., Aynsley-Green, A. & Eyre, J. A. (1995a). Cerebral blood flow and metabolism in severely head injured children. Part 1. Relationship to age, Glasgow Coma Score, intracranial pressure, time after injury and outcome. *J Neurol Neurosurg Psychiat*, **58**, 145–52.

Sharples, P. M., Matthews, D. & Eyre, J. A. (1995b). Cerebral blood flow and metabolism in severely head injured children. Part 2. Determinants of cerebrovascular resistance. *J Neurol Neurosurg Psychiat*, **58**, 152–9.

Sheinberg, M., Kanter, M. J., Robertson, C. S. *et al.* (1992). Continuous monitoring of jugular venous oxygen saturation in head injured patients. *J. Neurosurg*, **76**, 212–17.

Siesjo, B. K. (1988). Historical overview. Calcium, ischaemia, and death of brain cells. *Ann NY Acad Sci*, **522**, 638–61.

Simpson, D. & Reily, P. (1982). Paediatric coma scale. *Lancet*, **2**, 450.

Sinson, G., Voddi, M. & McIntosh, T. (1995). Nerve growth factor administration attentuates cognitive but not neurobehavioural motor dysfunction or hippocampal cell loss following fluid percussion injury in rats. *J Neurochem*, **65**, 2209–16.

Snoek, J. W., Minderhoud, J. N. & Wilnink, J. S. (1984). Delayed deterioration following mild head injury in children. *Brain*, **107**, 15–36.

Steward, O. & Jane, J. A. (1989). Repair and reorganisation of neuronal connections following CNS trauma. In: *Textbook of Head Injury*, ed. D. P. Becker & S. K. Gudeman, pp. 466–506. Philadelphia: W. B. Saunders Company.

Tabaddor, K., Bhushan, C., Pevsner, P. H. & Walker, A. E. (1973). Prognostic value of cerebral blood flow (CBF) and cerebral metabolic rate of oxygen (CMRO$_2$) in acute head trauma. *J Trauma*, **12**, 1053–5.

Tasker, R. C., Matthew, D. J., Helms, P., Dinwiddie, R. & Boyd, S. (1988). Monitoring in non-traumatic coma. Part I. Invasive intracranial measurements. *Arch Dis Child*, **63**, 888–94.

Taupin, V., Toulmand, S., Benavides, J. & Zavala, F. (1993). Increase in IL-6, IL-1 and TNF levels in rat brain following traumatic lesion. Incidence with pre- and post-traumatic treatment with Ro5 4864, a peripheral-type (p site) benzodiazepine ligand. *J Neuroimmunol*, **42**, 177–85.

Teasdale, G. & Jennett, B. (1974). Assessment of coma and impaired consciousness. *Lancet*, **2**, 81–4.

Teasdale, G. A., Murray, G., Anderson, E. *et al.* (1990). Risks of acute traumatic intracranial haematoma in children and adults: implications for managing head injuries. *Br Med J*, **300**, 363–7.

Toulmond, S. & Rothwell, N. J. (1995). Interleukin-1 receptor antagonist inhibits neuronal damage caused by fluid percussion injury in the rat. *Brain Res*, **671**, 261–6.

Tasutsumi, H., Ide, K., Mizutani, T. *et al.* (1986). The relationship between intracranial pressure, cerebral perfusion pressure and outcome in head injured patients; the critical level of cerebral perfusion pressure. In: *Intracranial Pressure VI*, ed. J. D. Miller, G. M. Teasdale, J. O. Rowan, S. L. Galbraith & A. D. Mendelow, pp. 661–6. New York: Springer.

Unterberg, A. W., Andersen, B. J., Clarke, G. D. & Maramrou, A. (1988). Cerebral energy metabolism following fluid-percussion brain injury in cats. *J Neurosurg*, **68**, 594–600.

Yang, M. S., DeWitt, D. S., Becker, D. P. *et al.* (1985). Regional brain metabolite levels following mild experimental injury in the cat. *J Neurosurg*, **1**, 297–311.

Yang, K., Mu, X. S., Xue, J. J., Perez-Polo, J. R. & Hayes, R. L. (1995). Regional and temporal profiles of c-fos and nerve growth factor mRNA expression in rat brain after lateral cortical impact injury. *J Neurosci Res*, **42**, 571–8.

Yankner, B. A., Duffy, L. K. & Kirschner, D. A. (1990). Neurotrophic and neurotoxic effects of amyloid beta protein; reversal by tachykinin neuropeptides. *Science*, **250**, 279–82.

Yoshino, A. Hovda, D. A., Kawamata, T., Katayama, Y. & Becker, D. P. (1991). Dynamic changes in local glucose utilisation following a fluid percussion injury: evidence of a hyper- and subsequently hypometabolic state. *Brain Res*, **561**, 106–19.

Zimmerman, R. A., Bilaniuk, L. T., Bruce, D. *et al.* (1978). Computer tomography of pediatric head trauma: acute cerebral swelling. *Radiology*, **126**, 403–40.

11

Near drowning

D. BOHN

Epidemiology

With increasing popularity of recreational activities involving water, submersion injury and its consequences have become a major public health problem in certain parts of the world. The impression that the paediatric age group is particularly at risk is confirmed by the fact that drowning is one of the three leading causes of accidental death in children. There are several published epidemiological surveys reporting incidences of drowning or submersion accidents in children requiring hospitalisation which vary from 20 per 100 000 of population in the USA (Wintemute, 1990), 6.2 per 100 000 in Australia (Pitt & Balanda, 1991) and 1.5 per 100 000 in the UK (Kemp & Sibert, 1992). In the USA alone there are 2000 deaths annually from drowning in children (Wintemute *et al.*, 1987) and in a single year (1989) in England and Wales there were 306 submersion incidents involving admission to hospital in children less than 15 years of age, 149 of whom died (Kemp & Sibert, 1992). When age and sex are examined as factors there are obvious bimodal peaks, one at less than 5 years of age, which represents one-third of all drownings, and the second in the adolescent age group, with a preponderance of males in all age groups. The incidence of drowning also varies with geographical area, climate and socioeconomic conditions, as reflected in the number of private swimming pools and warmer climates, with their attendant increases in the length of the 'swimming' season (Wintemute *et al.*, 1987). In the USA in the three-state combination of California, Arizona and Florida drowning is the leading cause of death in children under 5 years of age. Residential pools account for up to 80% of toddler drowning accidents and in the under 5 year old age group a swimming pool is 14 times more likely to kill a child than a motor vehicle. A survey of accidental death in children in the state of Florida, which has a long coastline and a high density of swimming pools, showed that 38% of fatalities were due to motor vehicle accidents and 32% were due to near drowning (Rowe *et al.*, 1977). Apart from this mortality, it has been estimated that for every fatality there are up to four near drowning accidents, where

176

the victim has been rescued and successfully resuscitated. The greatest risk to the small child is in a household with a newly acquired pool where lessons in safety are frequently learned the hard way (Wintemute *et al.*, 1991). Several studies have emphasised the importance of adequate pool fencing in substantially reducing the mortality in the at risk group and in New Zealand this has recently been mandated by legislation (Hassell, 1989). Apart from private swimming pools, bathtub submersion accidents remain the second most common form of drowning in the under 2 year old age group. This type of incident always raises the possibility of non-accidental injury which, in one study, was confirmed in 10% of cases (Kemp *et al.*, 1994). Outside this age group children at greatest risk from bathtub drownings are those with epilepsy (Diekema *et al.*, 1993; Kemp & Sibert, 1993).

With the more widespread knowledge and teaching of cardiopulmonary resuscitation (CPR) techniques, many more victims of drowning accidents are now surviving the original submersion incident only to be left with devastating neurological injuries as the result of prolonged cerebral hypoxia. Unfortunately as many of these victims are children, the consequence that the family is then faced with is the prospect of caring for a severely brain damaged child with the likelihood that he or she may survive for many years, requiring constant medical care with major economic costs. It is important therefore that every effort should be made to improve resuscitation and treatment techniques both in hospital and in the pre-hospital environment in order to try and improve the substantial morbidity and mortality in near drowning.

Pathophysiological changes following submersion

The immediate sequence of events that occur immediately after a submersion accident have been the subject of considerable speculation in the medical literature. Much of this has centred on the importance of the 'diving reflex' in protecting against cerebral hypoxia, the amount of fluid aspiration during submersion and the concept of 'dry drowning' and whether there are important physiological differences between salt and fresh water drowning. Many of the conclusions have been based on either experiments in anaesthetised animals with direct flooding of the lungs with water or deductions from post-mortem studies in humans. The reality is that pathophysiological changes that occur during and immediately after a near drowning accident vary according to the circumstances in which the submersion occurs. The enthuasiasm for the use of cerebral protection regimens over the past decade has tended to obscure the fact that near drowning is more than just a problem of cerebral hypoxia but is in reality a global hypoxic insult, which frequently results in multiple organ damage, with the brunt of the damage taken by the central nervous system and the lungs. The pathophysiological changes in near drowning should therefore be considered as a global hypoxic insult, which may be complicated by hypothermia, and the pathophysiological changes considered according to the effect on the principal systems involved.

Cardiorespiratory effects of submersion

The cardiorespiratory changes seen in near-drowning depend on whether the accident results in immediate submersion or there is immersion (maintainance of flotation). In the former, the commonest scenario in infant and toddler accidents in swimming pools and bathtubs, the onset of hypoxia is immediate. Immersion followed by drowning is exclusive to older children and adults, is seen in boating and swimming accidents and frequently involves salt water.

Immediately following immersion or submersion there is frequently a reflex brady-cardia which is commonly seen with facial immersion in cold water. This, together with prolonged breath-holding and shunting of blood flow from the periphery to the core, are part of the so-called 'diving reflex' by which diving mammals maintain cerebral oxygenation and survive prolonged periods in an hypoxic environment (Elsner et al., 1966). This mechanism is frequently invoked to explain some of the dramatic survivals seen in children with prolonged submersions in hypothermic conditions. Studies on breath holding in humans performed by Hayward et al. (1984) would suggest that this mechanism is unlikely. They have shown that the maximum breath hold in children under experimental conditions is less than 20 seconds and that this is reduced in cold water. Furthermore, they have shown that the magnitude of the reflex bradycardia is the same in adults and children (Ramey et al., 1987). In fact both facial immersion in water and breath holding result in similar degrees of bradycardia (Paulev et al., 1990). A much more likely explanation for this preservation of brain function is rapid core cooling and this issue will be dealt with in greater detail in the section on submersion hypothermia.

Following submersion it is likely that spontaneous respiratory efforts will continue for around 60 seconds. This conclusion is based on an animal study performed in 1951 on resuscitation in unanaesthetised drowned dogs (Fainer et al., 1951) in which the investigators found that the acute cardiorespiratory changes following submersion could be divided into three phases (Figure 11.1). In stage one which lasted for an average of 71 seconds respiration continued while blood pressure and heart rate increased; this was followed by apnoea and falling blood pressure (stage 2) which lasted another 60 seconds and then a final phase when there was a precipitous fall in blood pressure to zero (stage 3 average duration 130 seconds). The total time from initial submersion to total cardiac arrest in this study was a mean of 262 seconds. The findings of this probably are a much closer approximate to what actually happens during human submersion accidents than the subsequent studies performed on anaes-

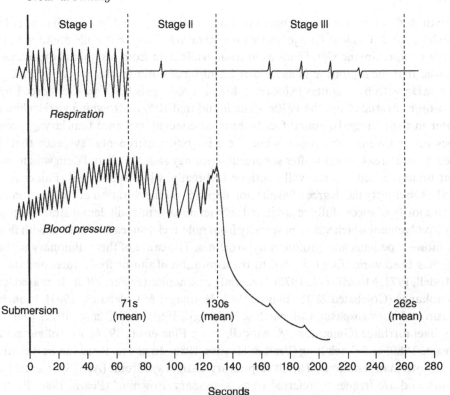

Figure 11.1. Cardiorespiratory changes associated with submersion in experimental animals. IV: intravenous; CPR: cardiopulmonary resuscitation; ETT: endotracheal tube. From Fainer *et al.*, *J. Appl. Physiol.*, 1951. Reproduced with permission.

thetised animals, although one would prefer the ethics of the latter. In fact these data agree substantially with studies on asphyxia (without drowning) in anaesthetised animals which showed that the heart rate and blood pressure increase in the first minute before decreasing and that PaO_2 falls to around 20 mmHg (2.7 kpa) by the time that circulatory collapse and cardiac arrest occurs at around 10 minutes (Kristoffersen *et al.*, 1967). A more recent study on drowning involving anaesthetised dogs showed that following 4 minutes of submersion all animals were profoundly bradycardic and hypotensive with a PaO_2 of less than 20 mmHg (2.7 kpa) (Conn *et al.*, 1995).

Submersion victims will also aspirate water into the lungs, although the actual amount is not precisely known but has been extrapolated from animal experiments and human post-mortem studies and has been used to draw a distinction between 'dry' and 'wet' drowning. Some authorities suggest that up to 10% of drowning victims do not aspirate water because they develop laryngospasm. This conclusion is based on a human study of 91 resuscitated near drowning victims reported by Modell *et al.* (1976) which showed 10% had PaO_2 of more than 80 mmHg (10.4 kpa) while breathing 21% oxygen, indicating no significant aspiration, while data from his animal experiments showed that the aspiration of as little as 2.2 ml/kg of water results in a fall in PaO_2 to 60 mmHg within 3 minutes (Modell & Moya, 1966). This belief was reinforced by a post-mortem study from the 1930s which found that 10% of drowning victims had no water in their lungs. In actual fact there is no concrete evidence that laryngospasm does occur during submersion while there is good experimental evidence that the breath hold breaks shortly after submersion (Ramey *et al.*, 1987) and data which show that unaesthetised animals will continue to breathe while submerged (Fainer *et al.*, 1951). Obviously the degree of aspiration depends on the duration of submersion and the majority of successfully resuscitated submersion victims will demonstrate pulmonary involvement which varies in severity from mild tachypnoea to a patient with florid pulmonary oedema and profound hypoxaemia. The cause of this pulmonary pathology has been variously attributed to the aspiration of salt or fresh water and debris (Modell, 1971; Modell *et al.*, 1976), bacterial pneumonitis (Fuller, 1963), decreased lung compliance (Colebatch & Halmagyi, 1961; Halmagyi & Colebatch, 1961), bronchospasm and laryngospasm (Colebatch & Halmagyi, 1961; Modell *et al.*, 1972), pulmonary haemorrhage (Giammona & Modell, 1967; Fine *et al.*, 1974), loss of surfactant (Pearn, 1980) and shock lung (Pratt & Haynes, 1986). In fact all these can be described as various manifestations of adult respiratory distress syndrome (ARDS) or acute lung injury and are frequently referred to as 'secondary drowning' (Pearn, 1980; Pratt & Haynes, 1986), as symptoms may not manifest themselves until many hours after the event. Certainly significant lung damage may occur with the aspiration of relatively trivial amounts of water. One of the theories advanced for the development of ARDS following near drowning is loss of surfactant due to aspiration. Giammona & Modell (1967) in an experimental drowning study were able to produce a surfactant-depleted lung in dogs who aspirated distilled water. In this model normal saline and sea water lesions were less severe than distilled water lesions. Whether this results in any clinically relevant difference in the frequency of the development of ARDS between salt and fresh water drownings is difficult to determine. Modell *et al.* (1976) in their series of 91 consecutive near drowning victims, 27 of which were salt water, found that 77% had abnormal chest radiographic findings, which varied from isolated infiltrates to massive bilateral oedema. A recent review by Simcock (1986) of 130 near drownings from the UK, 93 of which were in salt water, showed that while 50% had evidence of aspiration only one patient actually died from acute respiratory failure.

The theory that there are important differences between the aspiration of salt and fresh water in terms of the effect on circulating red cells and serum electrolytes is largely of academic interest. Swann & Spafford (1951) were able to show in experimental animals that large volumes of fresh water lung lavage resulted in absorption of this hypotonic fluid into the circulation. Furthermore, this led to extensive haemolysis and ventricular fibrillation because of potassium release. Modell & Davis (1969) have shown a considerable degree of hyponatraemia and haemolysis in post-mortem blood samples taken from fresh water drowning victims in contrast to salt water drowning; however, these differences disappear following resuscitation. They were also unable to demonstrate a difference in either haemoglobin or electrolyte values between the salt water and some fresh water drownings (Modell *et al.*, 1976).

Although there has been a tendency in the past to consider the pulmonary changes in near drowning as a straightforward aspiration, the sequence of events that occurs within the lung following a submersion accident are now more complex and are common to all other forms of ARDS. In this instance, it is the aspiration of water into the lungs which results in intrapulmonary sequestration of polymorphonuclear leucocytes (PMNs), damage to the pulmonary capillary endothelial membrane, leak of protein-rich oedema fluid into the interstitial space and eventually flooding of the alveoli. Pathologically this is referred to as the exudative phase of ARDS (Shapiro & Cane, 1981; Rinaldo & Rogers, 1982). In the early phases of this acute lung injury, the only clinical manifestation may be a slight increase in respiratory rate and hypoxaemia because of a fall in lung compliance and a decrease in functional residual capacity (FRC) as the lung loses its elastic properties. This process may be reversible with appropriate treatment in milder immersion accidents, or go on to develop into the proliferative phase where there is disruption and damage to epithelial cells, hyaline membrane formation and fibroblast proliferation. In the most severe cases this may result in the development of pulmonary fibrosis where high inspired oxygen levels and large amounts of positive and expiratory pressure (PEEP) are required to maintain oxygenation (Glauser & Smith, 1975) (Chapter 8).

Central nervous system injury

The central nervous system is obviously the most susceptible to damage in any form of hypoxia. In the normal brain the energy substrate required for the preservation of neuronal function is provided by adenosine triphosphate (ATP), the generation of which is fuelled by both oxygen and glucose. In the event of either a reduction in supply, as in progressive hypoxia, or complete failure in delivery, as occurs in circulatory arrest, there is a rapid depletion of ATP stores and neuronal damage. Neuronal cells do have a limited ability to maintain ATP levels by anaerobic glycolysis with cerebral blood flow levels as low as 30% of normal (Hossmann, 1983), but below this level there is a rapid accumulation of lactate which is partly responsible for the development of ischaemic cellular oedema. The precipitous fall in high energy compound levels results in turn in the breakdown of the cells' ability to maintain the normal gradients between intracellular and extracellular sodium and potassium ions resulting in a intracellular influx of Na^+ and efflux of K^+. This in turn leads to the cells and mitochondria absorbing water and swelling. There is a well established window of 4–6 minutes before irreversible neuronal damage occurs in the presence of complete interruption of oxygen supply to the brain under normothermic conditions (Weinberger et al., 1940; Heymans, 1950); although there is preservation of high energy metabolic activity, enzymatic functions and action potentials even after 60 minutes of total anoxia (Hossmann & Kleiheies, 1973). There is a secondary phase of injury even after the hypoxia is corrected or the circulation restored which has been the focus of much research and therapeutic endeavour over the past 10 years. It has recently become clear that one of the principal mediators of posthypoxic/ischaemic injury is calcium ion (Ca^{2+}) which is normally required for the preservation of cell membrane integrity. In hypoxic/ischaemic injury Ca^{2+} influx has been noted in neuronal (Harris et al., 1981) as well as cardiac and smooth muscle cells (Naylor et al., 1979). This sudden influx of Ca^{2+} results in the activation of destructive proteases and phospholipases. Enzymic reactions in turn wreak havoc with intracellular membrane stability and metabolism.

While this chain of events occurs rapidly in the situation of either reduced or absent organ perfusion or hypoxia, the cycle is not interrupted or reversed by simply restoring perfusion. There is an ongoing period of cell injury that occurs during the re-establishment of the circulation which is frequently referred to as the 'reperfusion injury' and is common to all forms of hypoxic/ischaemic cellular injury, whether it be neuronal, cardiac, pulmonary or renal. The key role played by Ca^{2+} in this reperfusion injury has now been well established, which in turn has led to the considerable recent interest in the potential use of calcium channel blockers in posthypoxic cerebral injury (White et al., 1983; Deshpande & Wieloch, 1986). Even with restoration of an adequate circulation there will be a prolonged period of cerebral hypoperfusion despite the fact that the mean systemic pressure perfusing the cerebral circulation has returned to normal. Winegar (et al., 1983) have shown that cerebral cortical flow approaches zero 90 minutes after reperfusion following a 20 minute cardiac arrest. Furthermore, this state of hypoperfusion is maintained for up to 18 hours after circulatory arrest, while at the same time there was no change in intracranial pressure (ICP). Posthypoxic cellular injury will also trip the cyclo-oxygenase pathway of the arachidonic acid cascade, producing the vasoactive compounds thromboxane and the leukotrienes (Pichard, 1981), thromboxane in particular being intensely vasoconstrictive. The other major cytotoxic products of ischaemic injury are the free oxygen radicals. These are the byproducts of high energy metabolism which will attack the cell if the normal defence mechanisms, which consists of enzymes and free radical scavengers, fail (McCord, 1985). The role of toxic oxygen radicals in cellular injury has been most clearly defined in the lung in ARDS or acute lung injury, where they have been identified as one of the principal causes of ongoing pulmonary damage (Deneke & Fanburg, 1980; Rinaldo & Rogers, 1982; Davis *et al.*, 1983; Tate & Repine, 1983). This serves to underscore the fact that there is a unifying concept in all forms of hypoxic/ischaemic cellular injury. The cycle of events that begins with ATP depletion on through K^+ efflux, cellular edema, reperfusion injury with Ca^{2+} influx through the tripping of the arachidonic acid cascade and the release of toxic oxygen radicals, is common to all organs.

The central nervous system injury in near drowning is analagous to asphyxiation, where the heart will continue to circulate blood to the brain that is becoming increasingly desaturated, so that there is an ongoing cerebral insult even before the circulation ceases altogether. In this period if the victim is rescued there is a chance that with onsite CPR effective circulation and oxygen to the brain will be restored. If not and the period of submersion extends beyond the point of circulatory arrest the outlook is very much worse, except in the setting of hypothermia. The temperature of the water at the time of the accident has a profound influence on the ability of the brain to withstand hypoxia. It is now becoming increasingly clear that near drownings which occur in icy (less than 5 °C) water conditions have a much more favourable prognosis for cerebral recovery compared with those that occur in warm water pools. There are now many well-documented cases in the medical literature where full neurological recovery has been associated with prolonged submersion times (Kvittengern & Naess, 1963; De Villata *et al.*, 1973; Hunt, 1974; Siebke *et al.*, 1975; Montes & Conn, 1980; Sekar *et al.*, 1980; Young *et al.*, 1980; Bolte *et al.*, 1988; Biggart & Bohn, 1990). In each instance the core temperature shortly after rescue was less than 30 °C; indeed there seems to be a fairly well-defined cutoff point at around 30 °C above which the prognosis for neurological recovery with prolonged submersion becomes considerably worse. It has been known since the experiments of Bigelow in 1950 that the brain's ability to withstand periods of hypoxia is considerably increased by hypothermia (Bigelow *et al.*, 1950). This phenomenon is used to advantage during the repair of complex congenital heart lesions in newborn infants where periods of complete circulatory arrest can be tolerated for up to 60 minutes without neurological sequelae with brain temperatures as low as 12 °C. Although some authorities have suggested that the 'diving reflex' is responsible for these remarkable recoveries (Keatinge, 1969; Gooden, 1972) it is far more likely that it is the rapid core cooling seen in submersion in children that is responsible for the preservation of brain function.

Immersion and submersion hypothermia

Many incidents of near drowning, particularly in high latitudes where water temperatures are cooler, are associated with accidental hypothermia. The degree of hypothermia and the rapidity of onset will depend on whether the victim is submerged or merely immersed. Older children or adolescents may be able to maintain floatation until, with the onset of hypothermia, the victim may become increasingly confused, disorientated, stuporous and will finally drown following loss of consciousness. The rapidity of onset of these stages of hypothermia will depend mainly on the water temperature but to a lesser extent on factors such as the amount of adipose tissue, type of clothing and victim's activity while immersed. In freezing water even an excellent swimmer cannot expect to survive more than a few minutes before severe hypothermia and drowning ensue. At the opposite end of the scale, a skilful swimmer could be expected to survive indefinitely in water above a temperature of 20°C without developing hypothermia, until drowning following exhaustion (Keatinge, 1969). In high latitudes, sea and lake temperatures seldom rise above 15°C, even in summer months, so in this environment hypothermia is a frequent accompaniment to near drowning accidents.

Profound physiological changes occur following immersion in cold water (less than 15°C) which have important implications for the individual's ability to survive the incident (Figure 11.2). Immediately on immersion there may be a precipitous rise in arterial blood pressure. Goode (1976) has recorded a blood pressure of over 200 mmHg in a healthy subject suddenly immersed to the neck in cold water. LeBlanc (1976) has shown mean increases of 30–40 mmHg in systolic pressure when either the face or the limbs are immersed in water at 4°C. At the same time, facial immersion causes a reflex bradycardia, the afferent limb of which is the trigeminal nerve and which is independent of baroreceptor function. On the other hand, immersion of a limb into cold water produces a reflex sympathetic discharge, resulting in an increase in heart rate.

The other area where there are major and immediate changes on contact with cold water is the respiratory system. There is a near instantaneous increase in minute ventilation due to the onset of an involuntary hyperventilation. This may result in an increase in minute ventilation of up to 90 litres/minute in adults for the first few breaths (Cooper, 1976). There is an immediate reduction in $PaCO_2$ and a decrease in cerebral blood flow commensurate with the increase in minute ventilation. The duration of this response varies from individual to individual. Human volunteers may continue to hyperventilate for up to 10 minutes in water at 16°C while in other subjects ventilation returns to normal within 3 minutes in water at 8°C. The magnitude of this respiratory response also depends on the amount of clothing worn by the immersion victim, with gasping and hyperventilation subsiding more quickly when the subject is fully clothed.

Following the immediate cardiorespiratory responses to immersion in a hypothermic environment, a more gradual adaptation takes place which depends on the duration of immersion, the water temperature, insulation factors that may decrease heat loss and to some extent the behaviour of the immersion victim. As the core temperature decreases to between 36 and 33°C, the body will attempt to defend the victim against further heat loss and restore normothermia by peripheral vasoconstriction which results in shunting of blood from the periphery to the core. Cardiac output

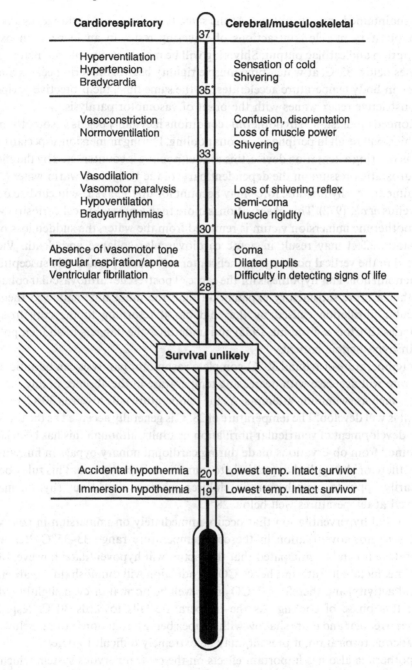

Cardiorespiratory		Cerebral/musculoskeletal
	37°	
Hyperventilation Hypertension Bradycardia		Sensation of cold Shivering
	35°	
Vasoconstriction Normoventilation		Confusion, disorientation Loss of muscle power Shivering
	33°	
Vasodilation Vasomotor paralysis Hypoventilation Bradyarrhythmias		Loss of shivering reflex Semi-coma Muscle rigidity
	30°	
Absence of vasomotor tone Irregular respiration/apneoa Ventricular fibrillation		Coma Dilated pupils Difficulty in detecting signs of life
	28°	
	Survival unlikely	
Accidental hypothermia	20°	Lowest temp. Intact survivor
Immersion hypothermia	19°	Lowest temp. Intact survivor

Figure 11.2. Pathophysiological changes that occur with cooling in immersion and accidental hypothermia.

will be maintained, initially at least. At the same time shivering thermogenesis begins. The involuntary muscle contractions of shivering result in an increase in oxygen consumption and cardiac output. Shivering will be maintained until core temperature decreases below 33°C, at which time muscle rigidity begins. Shivering ceases and the decrease in body temperature accelerates. At the same time, the protective peripheral vasoconstrictive reflex wanes with the onset of vasomotor paralysis.

Prolonged immersion in hypothermic conditions inevitably begets vasomotor paralysis, which will result in peripheral venous pooling. During immersion, especially if the victim is wearing a floatation device, this venous pooling is counteracted by the effect of the hydrostatic pressure on the dependent parts of the body. In a warm water (25°C) environment, this hydrostatic force may account for up to 35% rise in cardiac output (Arborelius *et al.*, 1972). This observation is more than a physiological curiosity. When the hypothermic immersion victim is removed from the water, the sudden loss of this hydrostatic effect may result in acute cardiovascular collapse and death. Victims extracted in the vertical position (e.g. helicopter rescue) are particularly susceptible to this phenomenon. This hypothesis for the cause of postrescue cardiovascular collapse is altogether a more satisfactory explanation than the more time-hallowed theory of ventricular fibrillation caused by the cold blood returning to the core from the peripheries (Burton & Foholm, 1955) and underlines the dangers of sudden position shifts in hypothermic patients.

At a temperature of around 30°C, complete vasomotor paralysis can be anticipated. Heart rate will decrease with decreasing temperature in the absence of any vigorous activity, such as swimming attempts. As the temperature falls towards 30°C, bradyarrhythmias will develop. The temperature of 28°C is generally accepted as the threshold for the development of ventricular fibrillation in adults, although this has been largely determined from observations made during cardiopulmonary bypass in humans and cannot therefore be applied as precisely to immersion hypothermia. This rule does not necessarily apply to hypothermia in children where a slow sinus rhythm may be preserved at temperatures well below 28°C.

The initial hyperventilation that occurs immediately on immersion in cold water subsides to normoventilation in the core temperature range 33–35°C. Below this temperature it can be anticipated that the victim will hypoventilate; however, at the same time, metabolic rate and hence CO_2 production will diminish (in the absence of physical activity) and therefore $PaCO_2$ may well be normal or even slightly reduced during this phase of cooling. As the temperature falls towards 30°C, respiration becomes irregular and more shallow with apnoea being a common feature. Below 30°C spontaneous respiration, if present, may be extremely difficult to detect.

Hypothermia also has important effects on the central nervous system which may result in a delayed drowning. As body temperature decreases below 35°C, the victim becomes increasingly confused and disorientated and may result in irrational decisions being made, such as discarding clothing, which further lessen the chances of survival. Below 33 °C, a victim becomes semi-comatose and can no longer maintain his head clear of the water. A substantial number will die from asphyxia and aspiration at this time. At core temperatures of 30 °C it may be difficult to distinguish between hypothermia and death as frank coma supervenes. Pupil responses are unreliable, as they may become fixed and dilated under severely hypothermic conditions. Below a temperature of 30 °C, in an adult, the chances for full recovery with intact cerebral function are poor, although there are reports of full recovery at temperatures as low as 20 °C in accidental hypothermia following exposure (Althaus *et al.*, 1982). The same criteria do not apply to children, however, where full recovery following submersion near drowning accidents have been reported with temperatures as low as 19 °C (Bolte *et al.*, 1988).

The rate of cooling with immersion hypothermia depends on many factors, not the least of which is the temperature of the water. In the human, there is a balance between heat production generated by metabolism and exercise and heat loss to the environment. Normally, when humans are exposed to a thermally hostile environment, behavioural and physiological adaptation occurs which reduces the heat loss, e.g. adding clothing and increased exercise will tend to reduce the degree of cooling. Clothing will provide insulating properties in accidental hypothermia, as warm air is trapped between layers. Obviously, these same rules do not apply in hypothermic immersion accidents. The victim is frequently inadequately clad in the first place, and even when clothing is worn, its insulating properties are greatly reduced when wet. Despite this, clothing should always be retained following immersion as it has been estimated that the rate of heat loss can be reduced by 50% in such circumstances.

Exercise will also greatly increase heat loss during immersion as this tends to increase blood flow to muscles and thereby accelerate the rate of cooling. Also, during swimming attempts, movements of the arms and legs tend to expose areas of high vascular supply near the skin surface, such as the groins and axillae. The standard teaching is not to try and swim for the shore, unless it is within easy reach, and to minimise the heat loss by adopting the Heat Escape Lessening Position (HELP), a tucked position, with the arms by the sides and the legs drawn up (Collis, 1976). In warm water (less than 20 °C) the immersion victim may well be able to maintain normal body temperature with exercise, as the heat production in this instance will balance the heat loss. Keatinge (1969) has produced survival charts for water at various temperatures, which would suggest that in water greater than 20 °C the victim's survival is limited only by his capacity to stay afloat, whereas at 10 °C the maximum time limit before succumbing to hypotheremia and drowning is around 3 hours.

Finally, the rate of cooling will be profoundly affected by the amount of adipose tissue and the body surface area. The tall, thin person will lose heat much more rapidly than the short, fat individual. The issue of surface area highlights the important differences in cooling between adults and children. Children, with a large surface area to weight ratio, will cool faster. This has important implications in the prognosis for cerebral recovery from hypothermic near drowning incidents in children, where the rapidity of cooling means that core temperature drops quickly and this undoubtedly confers some degree of cerebral protection during the hypoxia of submersion and helps to explain some of the remarkable recoveries seen after prolonged submersion in children. The core cooling in this situation is so rapid as cannot be accounted for by surface cooling alone and recent studies in animals have shown that the aspiration of cold water (less than 5°C) sets up a counter-current exchange mechanism within the lung which accounts for a temperature decrease of up to 8°C within 2 minutes of submersion (Conn *et al.*, 1995).

Resuscitation from near drowning

Near drowning provided one of the most fertile grounds for the pioneering work in cardiopulmonary resuscitation. In the 18th century, drowning became a great public issue in Europe and it was in 1740 that the Paris Academy of Sciences first recommended mouth-to-mouth resuscitation for the newly drowned victim. In 1744, Tossach first described the successful use of the technique in a human. It is worth noting how quickly this lesson was forgotten, for 20 years later in 1783 this was supplanted when DeHaen described a technique for manual ventilation of the lungs which consisted of chest pressure combined with arm lift. Ten years later positive pressure ventilation using a bellows or piston device was recommended for resuscitation. It took almost 200 years for mouth-to-mouth resuscitation to be rediscovered in the 1970s. In the meantime, various methods for artificial ventilation were tried and discarded, including in the introduction of tank respirators in the late 19th century. In 1876, a manually operated tank respirator designed by Woillez so impressed the city fathers of Paris that they proposed that a number should be strategically placed along the banks of the river Seine for assisted respiration of drowning victims! Up until the mid 1960s, the Shafer and Neilson manual methods of assisted respiration were still advocated for drowning victims. Even though the successful use of closed chest cardiac massage was first described in 1885 by Koenig, this again was forgotten and it was not until 1960 that Kouwenhoven first combined closed chest massage and mouth-to-mouth for resuscitation. Medical science had at last a technique for immediate resuscitation of the apparently dead after a near-drowning accident.

Resuscitation at the scene

As there is now a widespread knowledge of techniques of cardiopulmonary resuscitation, most submersion victims will arrive at a medical facility having had some sort of resuscitation attempted. The time honoured ABCs (Airway, Breathing and Circulation) of resuscitation should be applied at the scene. If the victim makes no respiratory effort following clearing of the airway, mouth-to-mouth ventilation should be started immediately, which will often result in the resumption of spontaneous respiration, if the immersion period has been of short duration. If no pulses are palpable, chest compressions should be started. CPR should not be attempted until the victim has been removed from the water, as it is completely ineffective and puts the rescuers at risk. If the victim is severely hypothermic, peripheral pulses may be difficult or impossible to detect, but when in doubt, CPR should be started. The reported dangers of causing the hypothermic victim's heart to fibrillate with chest compressions are greatly exaggerated. The victim should be removed as quickly as possible to a hospital, with CPR continued in transit.

If vital signs return within the initial resuscitation manoeuvres, the patient should be wrapped in clothing or blankets to minimise further heat loss and evacuated to a hospital, with care taken to avoid sudden positional changes, which may cause haemodynamic instability in the hypothermic patient.

The most difficult dilemma that faces the on-site rescuer is whether to initiate CPR in the apparently lifeless prolonged submersion victim, especially in the presence of hypothermia. There is no absolute rule in such circumstances but as a general principle, if the victim has been submerged for less than 1 hour in hypothermic (icy) conditions, CPR should be started and the decision on whether to continue deferred until the patient reaches hospital. In normothermic near drowning accidents submersion times of greater than 10 minutes are not associated with normal neurological recovery. Reported submersion times from parents or other witnesses are notoriously unreliable. Quan & Kinder (1992) in a series that addressed predictors that could be used to determine survival following aggressive on site resuscitation following submersion in non-icy water found that there were no neurologically intact survivors in children who had been submerged for more than 10 minutes and who did not have return of a perfusing cardiac rhythm within 25 minutes.

Resuscitation in the Emergency department

Techniques and duration of resuscitation depend on whether the victim is hypothermic and whether vital signs are present or absent at the time of arrival. If there is no palpable pulse without chest compression on admission to the Emergency department, CPR should be continued according to standard advanced cardiac life support (ACLS) and paediatric advanced cardiac life support protocols (Advanced Paediatric Life Support, 1993). The importance of administering 100% oxygen to all near drowning victims, even if they have regained consciousness cannot be over emphasised. Hasan *et al.* (1971), in a series of 36 near drowning victims found that the mean PaO_2 was 55 mmHg, even when breathing supplemental oxygen. Unrecognised and untreated hypoxaemia can change a minor hypoxic insult into devastating cerebral damage.

Rectal temperature should be measured with a low reading rectal thermometer, even if the drowning occurred in warm water. Children in particular have the ability to cool rapidly even following a relatively short immersion in non-hypothermic conditions. A brief neurological assessment should be made to evaluate the level of coma, with particular note being made of abnormal movements such as decerebrate or decorticate posturing, or seizure activity. Those patients that exhibit these abnormal findings, or fail to regain consciousness, should be intubated and mildly hyperventilated to a $PaCO_2$ of around 35 mmHg. The other invariable finding in near drowning is the presence of a metabolic acidosis with a pH of 7.2 or less consistent throughout most published series (Kruss *et al.*, 1979; Modell *et al.*, 1980; Frates, 1981; Biggart & Bohn, 1990; Quan *et al.*, 1990). Successful outcomes have been reported with initial pHs of < 7.0. Consequently, with the likelihood of acidosis and hypoxaemia being present, it is mandatory to obtain arterial blood gases as soon as possible. Empiric treatment of the acidaemia with bicarbonate is appropriate if there is a delay in obtaining blood gas analysis. Although there is currently some debate about the use of bicarbonate therapy during cardiac arrest in adults, there is no doubt that paediatric patients require relatively large doses for resuscitation (Advanced Paediatric Life Support, 1993).

Severe asphyxia will frequently result in sequestration of large amounts of fluid from the intravascular space, the so-called 'leaky capillary syndrome'. Replacement of these third space losses will frequently necessitate that large amounts of colloid be given in the initial resuscitation period in order to obtain an adequate systemic and cerebral perfusion pressure. Failure to respond to intravascular replacement (20 ml/kg) of colloid, should be an indication to start inotropes.

Acidaemia will tend to antagonise the effect of catecholamine drugs, as will hypothermia, although a study has shown that dopamine will increase cardiac output even under hypothermic conditions (Nicodemus *et al.*, 1981). Even with the best of resuscitation it is unlikely that sinus rhythm and cardiac output can be restored in the patient with a fibrillating heart and a core temperature of less than 30°C. Therefore a rewarming protocol should be commenced in hypothermic patients. The choice of rewarming technique depends on the degree of hypothermia and to some extent on whether the circulation is intact.

Rewarming techniques

The modes of rewarming can be divided into those that use the body's own endogenous heat production or the application of external or internal heat sources to raise body temperature, and whether rewarming is rapid or slow.

Passive rewarming is achieved by the prevention of excessive heat loss. The patient is placed in an ambient temperature of 21–23 °C and covered with warm blankets. The technique relies on the patient's ability to raise body temperature by endogenous heat production while at the same time minimising further heat losses to the environment. The respiratory tract evaporative losses can be minimised by breathing warmed humidified oxygen (40–45 °C) and intravenous fluid infusions are warmed by passage through a heating coil. For passive rewarming to be effective it is essential that the shivering mechanism be preserved. Below 30 °C shivering is suppressed and little benefit is gained by slow passive rewarming at these temperatures. The temperature increase using this technique is about 1 °C per hour (Edsall, 1980).

Active rewarming relies on heat transfer from an exogenous heat source to the patient through the skin or via the core. In the former this may take the form of external surface rewarming by heated water mattress or a radiant heat source. This technique is useful in mild hypothermia (32–35 °C) but care must be exercised with the use of all topical heating as thermal injury to the skin is a real possibility. Meticulous attention to maintaining an adequate circulating volume and oxygenation are crucial during rewarming as the onset of vasodilation is accompanied by major fluid shifts which may lead to cardiovascular collapse and death.

Active core rewarming is the most rapid and efficient of all rewarming techniques as heat is delivered in close proximity to the central circulation. Methods of active core rewarming include: (1) airway rewarming, (2) warmed intravenous fluids, (3) peritoneal dialysis with warmed dialysate fluid, (4) gastric lavage, (5) colonic lavage, (6) bladder irrigation, (7) mediastinal and pleural lavage, and (8) partial cardiopulmonary bypass. Of all forms of active core rewarming, the most accessible and least invasive is through heating the inspired gas delivered by an endotracheal tube. Increasing the temperature of the inspired gas to 40–45 °C with high relative humidity is an efficient method of increasing temperature. By exposing the extensive capillary network of the pulmonary vascular bed to humidified heated gases this technique will reduce the net heat loss from the respiratory tract to zero. Humidification of the respiratory tract will also have beneficial effects on mucociliary transport. If a heated water bath humidifier is unavailable a condenser humidifier (Swedish nose) or a Waters cannister will provide heating of inspired gases in the intubated patient. The condenser humidifier is simply a gauze screen which allows expired water vapour to condense. The moisture then evaporates and warms the inspired gases. The efficiency of this device for the conservation of temperature and the reduction of respiratory tract heat loss has been demonstrated in the operating room environment (Steward, 1976). A Waters cannister which was formerly used for CO_2 absorption of exhaled gases during anaesthesia is also useful for airway rewarming. The CO_2- soda lime reaction produces heat which then raises the temperature of the inspired gases. While neither device is as efficient in the hypothermic patient as heated water bath humidifiers they are readily portable and ideal for resuscitation in the field or during patient transport. Lloyd (1973) has described a portable version of the Waters cannister complete with mask and breathing circuit for use in the field. In unintubated, spontaneously breathing patients raising the temperature of the oxygen delivered by mask will also have a beneficial effect on core temperature, although it will be less efficient when compared with that delivered by an endotracheal tube.

There are several reports in the literature of central core rewarming by the irrigation of body cavities and the gastrointestinal tract (Linton & Ledingham, 1966; Coughlin, 1973; Johnson, 1977; Soung et al., 1977; Jessen & Hagelsten, 1978; Ledingham & Mone, 1978; Reuler & Parker, 1978; Ledingham & Mone, 1980; Ledingham et al., 1980; Miller et al., 1980; Mahajan et al., 1981; Schissler et al., 1981). Rewarming the peritoneum and abdominal organs with rapid exchanges of warmed peritoneal dialysis fluid has proven successful in resuscitating severely hypothermic victims. The described technique is to use isotonic dialysate with 1.5% dextrose warmed to 45–50°C with exchanges every 40 minutes (Johnson, 1977). Temperature rises of up to 2°C per hour have been reported using this approach. Careful monitoring of serum potassium and blood sugar is necessary, as hyperglycaemia and hypokalaemia may occur with rapid fluid exchanges.

Heat may also be transferred to the body by intragastric or intracolonic infusions of warm fluid which will indirectly transfer heat to the core. There are several reports of the use of intragastric lavage techniques in the literature, commonly combined with peritoneal dialysis (Reuler & Parker, 1978; Miller et al., 1980) and Ledingham et al. (1980) has described a modified Senstaken tube with a continuous flushing system for lavage of the oesophagus and stomach. Colonic rewarming is technically more difficult as the proper positioning of the tube is uncertain and there is always the possibility of damage to the colonic mucosa. Direct warming of the heart and mediastinum through a thoracotomy has been described (Coughlin, 1973; Althaus et al., 1982). A less invasive but equally effective method is direct blood rewarming using a partial cardiopulmonary bypass and a heat exchanger. There are now several case reports of the successful use of this technique in severe non-immersion hypothermic accidents associated with cardiac arrest (Towne et al., 1972; Truscott et al., 1973; Wickstrom et al., 1976; Althaus et al., 1982). Partial bypass is typically established from femoral or iliac veins to femoral artery. Wickstrom et al. (1976) has described three cases with ventricular fibrillation and temperatures less than 25°C who were rewarmed to normal temperatures in less than 1 hour, two of whom survived without sequelae. Althaus et al. (1982) described a truly remarkable series of successful resuscitations using partial bypass in three adult avalanche victims. All had core temperatures of less than 25°C and were in ventricular fibrillation and yet survived intact, even though one in particular had been buried for 5 hours.

There is little doubt that partial cardiopulmonary bypass is the 'Rolls Royce' of rewarming techniques and is the most rapid and effective method of rewarming the arrested patient. The technique is invasive, does require heparinisation and can only be carried out in large centres where the equipment and personnel are available. Although there have been some remarkable recoveries using this technique in severe accidental hypothermia, the outcome is less likely to be successful in submersion hypothermia because of the timing of cerebral hypoxia in relation to cooling. The two situations are not comparable as the 'dry' hypothermia victim cools gradually before the hypoxic insult, while the cerebral insult is instantaneous and frequently devastating in near drowning. Having said that, Bolte *et al.* (1988) has reported full neurological recovery where extracorporeal rewarming used in the resuscitation of a 2.5-year-old child who was submerged for 66 minutes in freezing water and had a core temperature of 19 °C at the time of rescue and Letsou *et al.* (1992) reported two children submerged for more than 30 minutes with temperatures of less than 25 °C who made good neurological recoveries.

Choice of rewarming technique

Despite an improvement in diagnosis and treatment of hypothermia in the past decade there is still debate in the medical literature whether rewarming should be by the slow passive technique or by the rapid active technique. Proponents of the slow passive technique advocate its use as it causes the least haemodynamic disturbance and fluid shifts and cite an increased incidence of 'afterdrop' and cardiac arrhythmias during rapid active rewarming (Emslie-Smith, 1958; Eruehan, 1960; Duguid *et al.*, 1961; Savard *et al.*, 1985). Most of the negative experiences with rapid active rewarming were in the late 1950s and early 1960s when resuscitation as we know it was in the earlier phases of development and little was understood about fluid shifts associated with hypothermia. Most of the deaths that occurred could be more properly ascribed to the unmasking of hypovolaemia and hypoxaemia during rewarming.

There has recently been a more critical look at the theory of 'afterdrop' causing further core cooling and cardiac standstill during rewarming. The theory is based on the suggestion that the periphery dilates during rewarming and there is a return of cold blood to the core which causes further central cooling and cardiac rhythm disturbance. Savard *et al.* (1985) has shown, however, that the 'afterdrop' in core temperature precedes peripheral dilation in human volunteers exposed to hypothermia and, furthermore, at the time of maximal peripheral dilation, core temperature has already started to rise. There seems little reason, therefore, to advocate the use of slow passive rewarming for anything but mildly hypothermic patients. There is now a considerable body of evidence, albeit often anecdotal, to support the use of rapid active rewarming in serious hypothermic injury and several large series attest to the successful use of the technique where heart beat and cardiac output are maintained (O'Keefe, 1977; Leding-ham & Mone, 1978; Edsall, 1980; Miller *et al.*, 1980). In the situation where there is no spontaneous circulation body temperature *must* be increased by active core rewarm-ing. The current recommendations are that passive external rewarming be used in mild hypothermia (32–35°C), rapid active rewarming at temperatures below this, and rapid internal core rewarming be used in every instance in which there is no circulation (Advanced Paediatric Life Support, 1993). The current recommendations for rewarm-ing are summarised in Figure 11.3.

Duration of resuscitation

Perhaps the most difficult decision facing the physician in the emergency department is how long resuscitation efforts should be continued in the presence of no cardiac output, especially when hypothermia is present. The publicity given to some remark-able recoveries in children who have survived intact following prolonged hypothermic immersion accidents has led to some very protracted resuscitation efforts lasting

Hypothermia 33-36°C

- Warm IV fluids
- Warm blankets
- Heated water matress
- Heated, humidified oxygen

Hypothermia < 33°C

Intact circulation

- Warm IV fluids
- Heated humidified gases by ETT
- Peritoneal lavage
- Gastric/rectal lavage

No circulation

- CPR
- Warm IV fluids
- Heated humindified gases by ETT
- Peritoneal lavage
- Gastric/rectal lavage
- Extracorporeal rewarming

Figure 11.3. Rewarming protocal for immersion or accidental hypothermia. The approach depends on the degree of hypothermia and the presence or absence of a circulation.

several hours. The problem is compounded by the fact that there is some difficulty in distinguishing between death and hypothermia at less than 30 °C. CPR and rewarming are continued, therefore, until either a temperature of less than 33 °C is established, at which stage resuscitation is abandoned if there is no cardiac output, or until a sinus rhythm is restored.

Unfortunately there is no easy answer to this dilemma. A review of the literature reveals that the longest period of submersion associated with intact survival is now 66 minutes (Bolte *et al.*, 1988) and that this was associated with a core temperature of 19 °C in a child (Table 11.1). There is therefore a rational basis for pursuing aggressive resuscitation in children following a hypothermic submersion of 60 minutes duration who have been submerged in very cold water, as there have been successful outcomes following hypothermic arrests with periods of CPR greater than 2 hours. It should be borne in mind that these are isolated case reports and only the dramatic recoveries get published rather than the heroic failures. We hold to the view that failure to increase core temperature after 60 minutes of appropriate rewarming and resuscitation techniques probably truly indicates death.

In contrast, the prognosis for intact survival in paediatric victims of warm water drowning who present to the emergency room with absent vital signs is worse than hypothermic submersion. The outcome is probably as bad as from any other form of hypoxic cardiac arrest as victims uniformly remain dead or survive with devastating neurological damage (Nichter & Everett, 1989; Biggart & Bohn, 1990). The decision on the duration of CPR should be made in light of knowledge of the fact that although it may be possible with aggressive resuscitation to restore a sinus rhythm, the outcome is likely to be a severely brain damaged patient. The results of prolonged resuscitation in this group of patients would not justify continuing with CPR for more than 20 minutes.

Inhospital treatment of near drowning

As a rule all patients who have suffered a submersion accident, even if relatively trivial, should be admitted to hospital for a minimum of 24 hours observation. At the end of this period, those patients who have had a relatively brief submersion and who are neurologically normal with no respiratory symptoms may be discharged. The treatment of more severe near drowning accidents is based on the severity of the cerebral hypoxic insult and the degree of pulmonary damage. A neurological assessment based on the level of consciousness should be made following resuscitation. Those patients with posturing movements, seizures or persistent coma should be admitted to the intensive care unit and electively ventilated mechanically for at least 24 hours, as these abnormalities indicate a significant hypoxic insult. Also, any patient who regains

Table 11.1. *Intact neurological survival associated with prolonged submersion*

Reference	Temperature (°C)	Age (years)	Submersion time (min)	Duration of CPR
Siebke (1975)	24	5	40	1.75 hours
Kvittengen (1963)	24	5	22	2.5 hours
Hunt (1974)	27	5	30	2. hours
Young (1974)	27	7	15	2.5 hours
De Villata (1973)	28	16	—	1 hour
Sekar (1980)	29	23	25	45 min
Bolte (1988)	19	2.5	66	2 hours

CPR: cardiopulmonary resuscitation.

consciousness following resuscitation but who has signs of pulmonary oedema with a significant degree of ARDS (tachypnoea, cyanosis, grunting, etc.) should be admitted to the intensive care unit for 24 hours ventilation. Those with lesser degrees of pulmonary involvement (mild ARDS) may only require diuresis and monitoring of blood gases, without the necessity for ventilation.

Treatment of the secondary organ damage following near drowning

The principal objective in the treatment of near drowning is to minimise the secondary effects of the initial hypoxic damage to the principal organs at risk, namely the brain, lungs, myocardium and renal system, and to treat complications such as hypoxia and hypotension which would cause further injury to these already damaged organs.

Over the past 20 years there has been considerable interest in and enthusiasm for therapeutic measures aimed at attenuating posthypoxic cerebral damage. These measures were heralded by the introduction into clinical medicine of ICP monitoring, when for the first time the physician could actually measure changes associated with diagnostic and therapeutic interventions. Principal among these therapies were high dose barbiturate therapy and induced hypothermia.

Barbiturate therapy

The stimulus for the introduction of high dose barbiturate therapy into the treatment of cerebral hypoxia came from animal studies which reported both reductions in ICP and improved outcome following both global and regional hypoxia when barbiturate therapy was started before, during or after the insult (Yatsu *et al.*, 1972; Smith *et al.*,

1974; Michenfelder *et al.*, 1976; Bleyaert *et al.*, 1978; Lafferty *et al.*, 1978). This led to the widespread use of barbiturates in humans for the treatment of various forms of cerebral injury, including near drowning (Shapiro *et al.*, 1974; Conn *et al.*, 1978; Rockoff *et al.*,1979; Montes & Conn, 1980; Dean & McComb, 1981; Oakes *et al.*, 1982; Pfenninger & Sutter, 1982; Bruce *et al.*, 1983). Although initial results suggested an increased survival following their introduction, no randomised trials were ever carried out and most series only compared their results with historical controls. More recent studies have now shown that although barbiturates clearly are able to reduce raised ICP, their use in near drowning has not led to an increase in the number of neurologically intact survivors (Bruce *et al.*, 1983; Bohn *et al.*, 1986; Nussbaum & Maggi, 1988).

Therapeutic hypothermia

About the same time as barbiturate therapy was introduced therapeutic hypothermia began to be used for the treatment of posthypoxic cerebral oedema. It had been known for 30 years that surface cooling to temperatures of around 30°C would increase the ischaemia time in both cardiac and neurosurgical procedures. With the advent of ICP monitoring it could be demonstrated that in both experimental and clinical hypoxic cerebral damage ICP could be reduced, both with and without barbiturates. This, together with reports of astonishing recoveries following hypothermic near drowning accidents led to the seemingly logical conclusion that extension of hypothermia into the postrescue period could reduce the severity of secondary brain injury. Although initial results were encouraging, subsequent experience was similar to the barbiturate story, namely that while ICP could be reduced the number of neurologically intact survivors did not increase (Oakes *et al.*, 1982; Sarnaik *et al.*, 1985; Bohn *et al.*, 1986; Nussbaum & Maggi, 1988). For this reason, and because it has been shown that the use of hypothermia may result in an increase in morbidity in terms of the number of life-threatening bacterial infections (Frewin *et al.*, 1982; Bohn *et al.*, 1986), most centres have abandoned the use of therapeutic hypothermia.

Intracranial pressure monitoring

More recently the role of ICP monitoring in the treatment of near drowning has also been called into question. In a study of 20 children who suffered severe near drowning accidents and who had ICP monitoring, Dean & McComb (1981) have shown that when ICP was greater than 20 mmHg despite hyperventilation, diuresis and high dose barbiturate therapy the outcome was either death or severe neurological injury. In all only six patients had satisfactory control of ICP and yet two of these died and one had severe neurological damage. Nussbaum & Maggi (1988) have also found that ICP was greater than 20 mmHg in eight of ten children who died following near drowning accidents despite vigorous attempts to maintain it below this level. These results led some authors to question the value of ICP monitoring (Dean & McComb, 1981; Rogers, 1985; Biggart & Bohn, 1990), as a normal ICP by no means guarantees an intact survivor, and a persistently raised ICP frequently results in either death or devastating neurological sequelae. Intracranial hypertension may be a useful marker of cerebral injury but we should be careful to distinguish between efforts to reduce the ICP number on the one hand and producing an intact survivor on the other.

We have learned from ICP monitoring that certain preventable factors increase ICP (e.g. hypercarbia, hypoxia, hyperthermia, seizures). When these factors are identified and treated outcome will improve. Other therapies such as barbiturates and hypothermia while reducing ICP do not improve outcome, and monitoring of ICP becomes largely academic. In a recent retrospective review of neurological outcomes following near drowning accidents we found that mortality and morbidity were unchanged in a 5-year period since ICP monitoring and the use of barbiturates and hypothemia to control cerebral swelling was removed from the protocol for the management of these patients (Biggart & Bohn, 1990).

Near drowning treatment protocol

The current treatment protocol for near drowning is based on the attempt to decrease secondary cerebral injury factors and the treatment of pulmonary complications, which can both aggravate cerebral injury and lead to death from hypoxaemia.

Treatment of cerebral injury

The treatment of the hypoxic cerebral insult in near drowning consists of avoiding factors that will increase cerebral oedema in the already injured brain. These include overhydration, seizures, hyperthermia, hypercarbia and hypoxia. Consequently, those patients who remain comatose after resuscitation from near drowning are treated with a protocol consisting of the following:

1. Hyperventilation to a $PaCO_2$ 35 mmHg; where the patient is exhibiting abnormal posturing movements, muscle relaxants should be used to ablate presumed rises in ICP.
2. The maintenance of oxygenation: a PaO_2 of more than 90 mmHg with PEEP > 5 cm H_2O if the F_iO_2 requirement is above 0.5.
3. The maintenance of cerebral perfusion pressure: a mean systemic pressure (MAP) more than 50 mmHg is necessary in order to provide an adequate

cerebral perfusion pressure. In the event that MAP remains less than 50 mmHg, dopamine 5–20 μg/kg per minute should be started.

4. Free water restriction to 30% normal maintenance fluid for the first 24 hours with diuretics added to treat pulmonary oedema or to avoid a positive fluid balance.

5. The treatment of seizure activity with phenobarbitone 5–10 mg/kg per day up to a dose of 20 mg/kg per day if seizures are intractable.

6. The maintenance of normothermia: strict attention to the avoidance of a rise in temperature in the first 24–48 hours (above 37°C). Increases in temperature above this will aggravate cerebral injury and should be treated with paralysis and surface cooling.

This regimen should be maintained for 24 hours at the end of which a repeat neurological assessment should be made with specific note made of the depth of coma and the presence of abnormal movements. Those patients who show an improvement in neurological findings should be weaned from the respirator over a 24–48 hour period depending on the degree of cerebral insult and the extent of pulmonary involvement. Those patients who remain persistently comatose, especially with flaccidity or abnormal posturing movements should have an electroencephalogram (EEG) and evoked potentials to establish baseline cerebral activity. If the EEG is performed sooner, i.e. immediately after resuscitation, the result may be misleading as cerebral activity is frequently very depressed following prolonged hypoxia, especially when associated with hypothermia. In the event that the patient remains persistently comatose, treatment should be continued for a further 24 hours and the assessment repeated before a decision should be made to discontinue aggressive support. Somatosensory evoked potentials (SEP) and brainstem auditory evoked responses provide useful information on neurological outcome with bilaterally absent SEPs indicating persistent vegetative survival (Goodwin *et al.*, 1991; Fisher *et al.*, 1992,. Beca *et al.*, 1995).

Treatment of pulmonary complications

Immersion accidents are frequently accompanied by the development of ARDS triggered by the aspiration of water into the lungs. This may vary in degree from relatively trivial involvement with minimal respiratory symptoms, such as a slight increase in respiratory rate and a slightly increased alveolar to arterial oxygen difference (A– aDO$_2$), to florid pulmonary oedema with profound hypoxaemia and opacification of the lungs seen on radiographs. Fortunately, most minor immersion incidents fall into the former category and are the pathological equivalent of the beginning of the exudative phase of early ARDS. Good response to diuretics and fluid restriction is expected. At the other end of the scale of severity, the degree of acute lung injury may require positive pressure ventilation with high peak airway pressures and high levels of PEEP (up to 20 cm H_2O). This is the pathological equivalent of a florid exudative phase of ARDS, which may eventually evolve into the proliferative phase with damage to epithelial cells, dense hyaline membrane formation, the invasion of fibroblasts and the development of pulmonary fibrosis (Glauser & Smith, 1975). Death may result from progressive hypoxaemia. Although pulmonary aspiration is the trigger for the development of ARDS, hypoxic damage to multiple organs and sepsis may contribute significantly to the ongoing acute lung injury. It is now well established that oxygen therapy plays a major role in the development of ARDS through the generation of toxic oxygen radicals (Frank, 1985). The same principles of treatment apply to the treatment of pulmonary involvement in near drowning as in any other form of ARDS, namely to attempt to maintain an arterial saturation of more than 90% (PaO_2 of more than 60 mmHg) with an FiO_2 of less than 0.5 using the lowest peak inspiratory pressure possible. The major underlying mechanical change in ARDS is a decrease in lung compliance and functional residual capacity (FRC). This 'stiffening' of the lung caused by filling of the interstitial space with a protein rich exudative fluid can be reversed by the application of PEEP, which will result in the recruitment of lost lung volume and a rise in FRC. With respect to PEEP, the objective is to apply sufficient PEEP to increase the PaO_2 to reduce the FiO_2 less than 0.5 and simultaneously avoiding haemodynamic compromise (so called best PEEP) (Suter & Fairly, 1975). Septic complications should be identified and vigorously treated as septicaemia, a common problem in near drowning, will maintain the cycle of lung injury. More recently the successful use of extracorporeal membrane oxygenation (ECMO) for the treatment of ARDS secondary to near drowning has been reported (O'Rourke *et al.*, 1993) although this only addresses the issue of the reversal of the pulmonary rather than the cerebral injury. The majority of those patients with severe hypoxaemia which cannot be managed with conventional ventilation also have irreversible cerebral injury (Bohn *et al.*, 1986).

Infectious complications of near drowning

There is a high incidence of septic complications following severe near drowning accidents which may manifest as either a pneumonitis or septicaemia. Bacterial invasion may come from a variety of sources. In the first instance, the victim may inhale a significant quantity of water which may be contaminated by a variety of usually non-pathogenic organisms. There may also be severe ischaemic damage to the gut mucosa resulting in bloody diarrhoea, following severe asphyxia in near drowning. Loss of integrity of the gastrointestinal tract may result in bacterial invasion and septicaemia. In addition, there has been recent conclusive evidence to show that hypothermia itself may result in diminished immunity to bacterial invasion in the hypoxic host. Bohn *et al.* (1986) have found a high incidence of life-threatening septicaemia in hypothermic near drowning victims associated with marked reductions in the number of circulating polymorphonuclear leukocytes (PMNs); indeed septicaemia combined with hypoxia was the most frequent cause of death in this series, although all the patients that died had severe cerebral hypoxia. In a series of animal experiments, the same group have shown that under hypothermic conditions (30 °C) there is a reduction not only in circulating PMNs, but also in production and release by the bone marrow (Biggar *et al.*, 1983, 1984). Near drowning victims, especially those who are hypothermic, are greatly at risk for developing septic complications both from external invading organisms and also from nosocomial infections and autoinfection from their normally non-pathogenic bacteria. Oakes *et al.* (1982) have reported a 40% incidence of positive sputum cultures in 40 near drowning victims despite the use of prophylactic antibiotics. Our policy has not been to routinely use antibiotic prophylaxis, but to identify septic events by daily cultures of sputum, urine and blood and then to treat with the appropriate antibiotic.

Outcome

With improved on site resuscitation and advances in intensive care management, there has been an increase in the number of near drowning victims who survive both with and without neurological sequelae. There are only three possible outcomes from drowning: death, survival with severe neurological damage and intact survival. Very few, if any, children seem to survive with mild neurological deficits except in hypothermic submersion accidents (Bell *et al.*, 1985); however, reliable statistics on outcome following submersion accidents are difficult to interpret. Published figures for bad outcome (deaths or severe neurological damage) vary from 6 to 100% (Hasan *et al.*, 1971; Hunter & Whitehouse, 1974; Peterson, 1977; Conn *et al.*, 1978; Kruss *et al.*, 1979; Pearn *et al.*, 1979; Modell *et al.*, 1980; Montes & Conn, 1980; Dean & Kaufman, 1981; Dean & McComb, 1981; Frates, 1981; Pfenninger & Sutter, 1982; Oakes *et al.*, 1982; Jacobsen *et al.*, 1983; Bell *et al.*, 1985; Frewin *et al.*, 1985; Nichter & Everett, 1989; Biggart & Bohn, 1990; Quan *et al.*, 1990; Quan & Kinder, 1992). As the incidence of devastating neurological deficit, especially in children, tends to be very high it is important that prognostic factors be used to identify poor quality survivors as early as possible after resuscitation in order that aggressive support may be discontinued.

The principal prognostic factor affecting outcome prior to resuscitation in the drowning victim without vital signs is the water temperature. There is no doubt that the victim of a hypothermic immersion (water temperature less than 5 °C), especially a child, has a higher chance of surviving intact than the near drowning victim from the warm water backyard pool. The medical literature contains reports of prolonged submersion times of up to 40 minutes associated with intact survival. For this reason alone it is worthwhile pursuing a course of aggressive resuscitation in hypothermic near drowning. The details of successful resuscitations of hypothermic (less than 30°C core temperature) near drownings with intact survival are given in Table 11.1.

The other variable that may influence outcome in the pre-hospital period is the adequacy of on site resuscitation. Many victims who are rescued following brief (less than 5 minute) submersion will be cyanotic and apnoeic but with a preserved spontaneous heart beat which may be difficult to palpate because of profound bradycardia. Efficient CPR will frequently result in the return of a palpable pulse and spontaneous respiration, which will make all the difference to the outcome. The series published by Quan have shown that in non-icy water drownings where advanced life support resuscitation is rapidly available on site, good outcomes can be achieved in children without vital signs if the duration of submersion is less 10 minutes (Quan *et al.*, 1990; Quan & Kinder, 1992). Nussbaum (1985) in a series of warm water drownings found that estimated submersion times of less than 9 minutes were associated with a higher incidence of good outcomes. Although the duration of submersion is obviously important in determining outcome the observer estimates of the time elapsed tends to be rather inaccurate. Frates (1981) reviewed pre-hospital prognostic factors and correlated these with outcome using multivariant analysis. The 'best' correlation with poor outcome was fixed dilated pupils on admission, followed by persistent coma and the absence of vital signs on admission. In warm water drownings he was unable to show any statistical relation between duration of submersion and survival.

When attempting to judge the prognosis following resuscitation one should attempt to separate neurological and non-neurological assessment of prognostic indicators, although these overlap to some extent. The non-neurological assessment should include complications such as the severity of the lung injury and hypoxaemia which in the worst cases may result in the death of a neurologically intact survivor. One should also be alert to the fact that a considerable number of near drowning victims have co-incident diseases or trauma that may have been the underlying cause for the submersion accident. A published series of near drowning accidents in adults has shown that 50% have a significant medical history that may have contributed to the accident (Hunter & Whitehouse, 1974). Principal among these are seizure disorders, cervical spine injuries from diving into shallow water and drug and alcohol abuse (Table 11.2).

The assessment of prognosis for neurological outcome after resuscitation has proved more difficult. Some accurate method of assessing cerebral damage in these patients after the restoration of cardiac output is important not only to determine subsequent treatment but also to evaluate the efficacy of cerebral protection protocols. Factors that would indicate a poor prognosis are the absence of spontaneous respir-

Table 11.2. *Co-incident diseases and precipitating causes for near drowning accidents*

Head injuries
Air embolism
Cervical spine injuries
Cardiovascular disease
Seizure disorders
Drug and alcohol abuse
Hypoglycaemia
Child abuse

ation, except in the presence of hypothermia. Jacobsen *et al.* (1983) have reported a 100% mortality in children where spontaneous respiration has not returned following resuscitation. Lavelle & Shaw (1993) found that unreactive pupils in the emergency room and a Glasgow Coma Score (GCS) of 5 or less on arrival in the intensive care unit indicated a poor prognosis. Both Modell (Modell *et al.*, 1980) and Conn (Conn & Barker, 1984) have devised a scoring system based on whether the patients are awake (A), have a blunted sensorium (B), or are comatose (C) following resuscitation. In Modell's series those patients in group A have 100% survival, while mortality increases to 10% in group B and 34% in group C. Orlowski (1979) has devised a scoring system for paediatric near drowning victims using patient age, initial pH, submersion time, pupillary response and the effectiveness of resuscitation. Although these scoring systems may be a helpful guide in determining prognosis in the immediate postresuscitation period, we feel that a more definitive estimate can be made after a period of 12–24 hours has elapsed, when the continuation of a comatose state indicates a poor prognosis.

The near drowning victim who remains in coma without spontaneous limb movements who is exhibiting abnormal brainstem function 24 hours after the accident will have a poor neurological outcome (Bratton *et al.*, 1994). A modification of the Glasgow coma score has become a widely accepted criterion for evaluating neurological injury (Dean & Kaufman, 1981; Jacobsen *et al.*, 1983), a GCS of 5 or less being associated with a greater than 80% mortality in Dean's series (Dean & Kaufman, 1981). Abnormal posturing or seizure activity in the immediate postresuscitation period do not necessarily indicate a poor prognosis. In a review of 49 near drowning incidents in children, Bell *et al.* (1985) found that the presence of any motor activity was associated with a significantly greater incidence of intact survival. If posturing movements persist or recur after the first 12–24 hours, however, there is a high probability of severe brain damage. Similarly, flaccidity and fixed dilated pupils are associated with a high mortality. In Bell's series reactive pupils at the time of admission discriminated between fatalities and intact survivors but could not distinguish intact and vegetative survivors (Bell *et al.*, 1985). Caution should be exercised in interpreting pupillary responses in the immediate postresuscitation period as hypothermia may cause dilatation of pupils.

There is general agreement that the absence of a heart beat on admission to hospital is a universally poor prognostic sign. The finding of asystole in the emergency room is invariably associated with death or persistent vegetative state (Nichter & Everett, 1989; Biggart & Bohn, 1990; Lavelle & Shaw, 1993), the exception being made where the victim is hypothermic (less than 33 °C) following submersion in icy (less than 5 °C) water. Nichter & Everett (1989) have shown a universally bad outcome in near drowning victims who present without a perfusing cardiac rhythm in the emergency room. Biggart's series of 27 victims presenting to the emergency room without spontaneous circulation contained only three intact survivors (Biggart & Bohn, 1990). All three were hypothermic (less than 33 °C). An important distinction must be drawn between victims who are hypothermic because of prolonged submersion and cardiac arrest in warm water, who have a bad prognosis, while those who are hypothermic because of submersion in cold water, where there is the possibility of a good recovery.

References

Advanced Pediatric Life Support (1993). Published by The American Academy of Pediatrics and The American College of Emergency Physicians, 2nd edn.

Althaus, U., Aeberhard, P., Schupbach, P., Nachbur, B. H. & Mishlemann, W. (1982). Management of profound accidental hypothermia with cardiorespiratory arrest. *Annals of Surgery*, **195**, 492–5.

Arborelius, M., Balldin, U. I., Lilja, B. & Lundgren, C. E. (1972). Haemodynamic changes in men during immersion in head above water. *Aerospace Medicine*, **43**, 592–8.

Beca, J., Cox, P. N., Taylor, M. J., Bohn, D., Butt, W. & Barker, G. (1995). Somatosensory evoked potentials for prediction of outcome in acute severe brain injury. *Journal of Pediatrics*, **126**, 44–9.

Bell, T. S., Ellenberg, L. & McComb, J. G. (1985). Neuropsychological outcome after pediatric near drowning. *Neurosurgery*, **17**, 604–8.

Bigelow, W. G., Lindsay, W. K. & Greenwood, W. F. (1950). Hypothermia: its possible role in cardiac surgery. Investigation of factors governing survival in dogs at low temperatures. *Annals of Surgery*, **132**, 849–66.

Biggart, M. & Bohn, D. (1990). The influence of hypothermia on outcome following near-drowning accidents in children. *Journal of Pediatrics*, **117**, 179–83.

Biggar, W. D., Bohn, D. J., Kent, G., Barker, C. & Hamilton, C. (1983). Neutrophil circulation and release from bone marrow during hypothermia. *Infection & Immunology*, **40**, 708–12.

Biggar, W. D., Bohn, D. J., Kent, G., Barker, C. & Hamilton, C. (1984). Neutrophil migration in vitro and in vivo during hypothermia. *Infection & Immunology*, **46**, 857–9.

Bleyaert, Al, Nemoto, E. M., Safar, P., Stezoski, S. W., Michell, J. J., Moossy, J. & Roa, G. R. (1978). Thiopental amelioration of brain damage after global ischaemia in monkeys. *Anesthesiology*, **49**, 390–8.

Bohn, D. J., Biggar, W. D., Smith, C. R., Conn, A. W. & Barker, G. A. (1986). Influence of hypothermia, barbiturate therapy, and intracranial pressure monitoring on morbidity and mortality after near drowning. *Critical Care Medicine*, **14**, 529–34.

Bolte, R. G., Black, P. G., Bowers, R. S., Thorne, J. K. & Corneli, H. M. (1988). The use of extracorporeal rewarming in a child submerged for 66 minutes. *Journal of the American Medical Association*, **260**, 377–9.

Bratton, S. L., Jardine, D. S., Morray, J. P. (1994). Serial neurological examinations after near drowning and outcome. *Journal of Pediatric Adolescent Medicine*, **148**, 167–70.

Bruce, D. A., Schut, L. & Sutton, L. N. (1983). Brain resuscitation in children: fact or fantasy? *Concepts in Pediatric Neurosurgery*, **4**, 219–29.

Burton, A. C. & Foholm, O. G. (1955). *Man In a Cold Environment*. Edward Arnold, London.

Colebatch, H. J. H. & Halmagyi, D. F. J. (1961). Lung mechanics and resuscitation after fluid aspiration. *Journal of Applied Physiology*, **16**, 684–96.

Collis, M. L. (1976). Survival behaviour in cold water immersion. In *Proceedings of The Cold Water Symposium*. The Royal Life Saving Society of Canada, Toronto, pp. 25–7.

Conn, A. W. & Barker, G. A. (1984). Fresh water drowning and near-drowning: an update. *Canadian Anaesthetists Society Journal*, **31**, S38.

Conn, A. W., Edmonds, J. F. & Barker, G. A. (1978). Near drowning in cold fresh water: current treatment regimen. *Canadian Anaesthetists Society Journal*, **25**, 259–65.

Conn, A. W., Miyasaka, K., Katayama, M., Fujita, M. Orima, H., Barker, G. A. & Bohn, D. J. (1995). A canine study of cold water drowning in fresh versus salt water. *Critical Care Medicine*, **23**, 2029–37.

Cooper, K. E. (1976). Respiratory and thermal responses to cold water immersion. In *Proceedings of the Cold Water Symposium*. The Royal Life Saving Society of Canada, Toronto, pp. 23–4.

Coughlin, F. (1973). Heart warming procedure. *New England Journal of Medicine*, **288**, 326.

Davis, W. B., Rennard, S. I., Bitterman, P. B. & Crystal, R. G. (1983). Pulmonary oxygen toxicity: early reversible changes in human alveolar structures induced by hyperoxia. *New England Journal of Medicine*, **309**, 878–83.

De Villata, D., Barat, G., Peral, P. *et al.* (1973). Recovery from profound hypothermia with cardiac arrest after immersion. *British Medical Journal*, **2**, 394–5.

Dean, J. M. & Kaufman, N. D. (1981). Prognostic indicators in paediatric near drowning: the Glasgow coma scale. *Critical Care Medicine*, **9**, 536–9.

Dean, M. J. & McComb, J. G. (1981). Intracranial pressure monitoring in severe paediatric near drowning. *Neurosurgery*, **6**, 627–30.

Deneke, S. M. & Fanburg, G. L. (1980). Normobaric oxygen toxicity of the lung. *New England Journal of Medicine*, **303**, 76–86.

Deshpande, J. K. & Wieloch, T. (1986). Flunarizine, a calcium entry blocker, ameliorates ischaemic brain damage in the rat. *Anesthesiology*, **64**, 215–24.

Diekema, D. S., Quan, L. & Holt, V. L. (1993). Epilepsy as a risk factor for submersion injury in children. *Pediatrics*, **91**, 612–16.

Duguid, H., Simpson, R. G. & Stowers, J. M. (1961). Accidental hypothermia. *Lancet*, **2**, 1213–19.

Edsall, D. W. (1980). Treatment of hypothermia. *Journal of the American Medical Association*, **244**, 1902.

Elsner, R., Franklin, D. L., van Citters, R. L. & Kenney, D. W. (1966). Cardiovascular defence against asphyxia. *Science*, **153**, 941–7.

Emslie-Smith, D. (1958). Accidental hypothermia. A common condition with a pathognomic electrocardiography. *Lancet*, **2**, 492–5.

Eruehan, A. E. (1960). Accidental hypothermia. *Archives of Internal Medicine*, **106**, 218–29.

Fainer, D. C., Martin, C. G. & Ivy, A. C. (1951). Resuscitation of dogs from fresh water drowning. *Journal of Applied Physiology*, **3**, 417–26.

Fine, N. L., Myerson, D. A., Myerson, P. J. & Pagliaro, J. J. (1974). Near drowning presenting as the adult respiratory distress syndrome. *Chest*, **65**, 347–9.

Fisher, B., Peterson, B. & Hicks, G. (1992). Use of brainstem auditory-evoked response testing to assess neurologic outcome following near drowning in children. *Critical Care Medicine*, **20**, 578–85.

Frank, L. (1985). Oxidant injury to the pulmonary endothelium. In *The Pulmonary Circulation and Acute Lung Injury*, ed. S. A. Said, pp. 283–305. New York: Futura Publishing.

Frates, R. C. (1981). Analysis of predictive factors in the assessment of warm-water near drowning in children. *American Journal of Diseases of Childhood*, **135**, 1006–8.

Frewin, T. C., Sumabat, W. O., Han, V. K., Amacher, A. L., Del Maestro, R. F. & Sibbald, W. J. (1985). Cerebral resuscitation therapy in paediatric near drowning. *Journal of Pediatrics*, **106**, 615–17.

Frewin, T. C., Swedlow, D. B., Watcha, M., Raphaely, R. C., Godinez, R. I., Heiser, M. S., Kettrick, R. G. & Bruce, D. A. (1982). Outcome in Reye's syndrome with early pentobarbital coma and hypothermia. *Journal of Pediatrics*, **100**, 663–5.

Fuller, R. H. (1963). Drowning and the postimmersion syndrome; a clinico-pathological study. *Military Medicine*, **128**, 22–36.

Giammona, S. T. & Modell, J. H. (1967). Drowning by total immersion; effects on pulmonary surfactant of distilled water, isotonic saline and sea water. *American Journal of Disease in Childhood*, **114**, 612–16.

Glauser, F. L. & Smith, W. R. (1975). Pulmonary interstitial fibrosis following near drowning and exposure to short-term high oxygen concentrations. *Chest*, **68**, 373–5.

Goode, R. C. (1976). Acute responses to cold water. In *Proceedings of The Cold Water Symposium*. The Royal Life Saving Society of Canada, Toronto, pp. 19–22.

Gooden, B. A. (1972). Drowning and the diving reflex in man. *Medical Journal of Australia*, **2**, 583–7.

Goodwin, S. R., Friedman, W. A. & Bellefleur, M. (1991). Is it time to use evoked potentials to predict outcome in comatose children and adults? *Critical Care Medicine*, **19**, 518–24.

Halmagyi, D. F. J. & Colebatch, H. J. H. (1961). Ventilation and circulation after fluid aspiration. *Journal of Applied Physiology*, **16**, 35–40.

Harris, R. J., Symon, L., Bronston, N. M. *et al.* (1981). Changes in extracellular calcium activity in cerebral ischaemia. *Journal of Cerebral Blood Flow & Metabolism*, **1**, 203–9.

Hasan, S., Avery, W. G., Fabian, C. & Sackner, M. A. (1971). Near-drowning in humans: a report of 36 patients. *Chest*, **59**, 191–7.

Hassell, I. B. (1989). Thirty six consecutive under 5-year old domestic swimming pool drownings. *Australian Paediatric Journal*, **25**, 143–6.

Hayward, J. S., Hay, C., Matthews, B. R., Overweel, C. H. & Radford, D. D. (1984). Temperature effect on the human dive response in relation to cold water near-drowning.

Journal of Applied Physiology, **56**, 202–6.

Heymans, C. (1950). Survival and revival of nervous tissue after arrest of the circulation. *Physiology Review*, **30**, 375.

Hossmann, K. A. (1983). Neuronal survival and revival during and after cerebral ischaemia. *American Journal of Emergency Medicine*, **1**, 191–7.

Hossmann, K. A. & Kleiheies, P. (1973). Reversibility of ischaemic brain damage. *Archives of Neurology*, **20**, 375–84.

Hunt, P. K. (1974). Effect and treatment of the 'diving reflex'. *Canadian Medical Association Journal*, **111**, 1330–1.

Hunter, T. B. & Whitehouse, W. M. (1974). Fresh water drowning: radiological aspects. *Radiology*, **112**, 51–6.

Jacobsen, W. K., Mason, L. J., Briggs, B. A., Schneider, S. & Thompson, P. C. (1983). Correlation of spontaneous respiration and neurological damage in near drowning. *Critical Care Medicine*, **11**, 487–9.

Jessen, K. & Hagelsten, J. O. (1978). Peritoneal dialysis in the treatment of profound accidental hypothermia. *Avait Space Environmental Medicine*, **49**, 426–9.

Johnson, L. A. (1977). Accidental hypothermia: peritoneal dialysis. *Journal of the American College of Emergency Physicians*, **6**, 556–61.

Keatinge, W. (1969). *Survival in Cold Water*. Oxford: Blackwell Scientific Publications.

Kemp, A. M. & Sibert, J. R. (1992). Drowning and near-drowning in children in the United Kingdom: lessons for prevention. *British Medical Journal*, **304**, 1143–6.

Kemp, A. M. & Sibert, J. R. (1993). Epilepsy in children and the risk of drowning. *Archives of Disease in Childhood*, **68**, 684–5.

Kemp, A. M., Mott, A. M. & Sibert, J. R. (1994). Accidents and child abuse in bathtub submersions. *Archives of Disease in Childhood*, **70**, 435–8.

Kristoffersen, M. B., Rattenborg, C. C. & Holaday, D. A. (1967). Asphyxial death: the roles of acute anoxia, hypercarbia and acidosis. *Anesthesiology*, **28**, 488–97.

Kruss, S., Bergstrom, L., Suntarinen, T. & Hyvonen, R. (1979). The prognosis of near-drowned children. *Acta Pediatric Scandinavia*, **68**, 315–17.

Kvittengern, T. D. & Naess, A. (1963). Recovery from drowning in fresh water. *British Medical Journal*, **1**, 1315–17.

Lafferty, J. J. Kekyhah, M. M., Shapiro, H. M., van Horn, K. & Behar, M. G. (1978). Cerebral hypometabolism with deep pentobarbital anaesthesia and hypothermia. *Anesthesiology*, **49**, 159–64.

Lavelle, J. M. & Shaw, K. N. (1993). Near drowning: is emergency department cardiopulmonary resuscitation or intensive care unit cerebral resuscitation indicated? *Critical Care Medicine*, **21**, 368–73.

LeBlanc, J. (1976). Physiological changes in prolonged cold stress. In *Proceedings of The Cold Water Symposium*. The Royal Life Saving Society of Canada, Toronto, pp. 9–13.

Ledingham, I. McA. & Mone, J. G. (1978). Accidental hypothermia. *Lancet*, **1**, 391.

Ledingham, I. McA. & Mone, J. G. (1980). Treatment of accidental hypothermia: a prospective clinical study. *British Medical Journal*, **280**, 1102–5.

Ledingham, I. McA., Routh, G. S., Douglas, I. H. S. & MacDonald, A. M. (1980). Central rewarming system for the treatment of hypothermia. *Lancet*, **1**, 1168–9.

Letsou, G. V., Kopf, G. S., Elefteriades, J. A., Carter, J. E., Baldwin, J. C. & Hammond, G. L. (1992). Is cardiopulmonary bypass effective for treatment of hypothermic arrest due to drowning or exposure? *Archives of Surgery*, **127**, 525–8.

Linton, A. L. & Ledingham, I. McA. (1966). Severe hypothermia with barbiturate intoxication. *Lancet*, **1**, 24–6.

Lloyd, E. L. (1973). Accidental hypothermia treated by central rewarming through the airway. *British Journal of Anaesthesia*, **45**, 41–7.

Mahajan, S. L., Myers, T. J. & Baldini, M. G. (1981). Disseminated intravascular coagulation during rewarming following hypothermia. *Journal of the American Medical Association*, **245**, 2517–18.

McCord, J. M. (1985). Oxygen derived free radicals in postischemic tissue injury. *New England Journal of Medicine*, **312**, 159–63.

Michenfelder, J. D., Milde, J. H., Sundt, T. M. Jr (1976). Cerebral protection by barbiturate anesthaesia. *Archives of Neurology*, **33**, 345–50.

Miller, J. W., Danzl, D. F. & Thomas, D. M. (1980). Urban accidental hypothermia: 135 cases. *Annals of Emergency Medicine*, **9**, 456–61.

Modell, J. H. (1971). *Pathophysiology and Treatment of Drowning and Near Drowning*. Springfield, Illinois: Charles Thomas.

Modell, J. H. & Davis, J. H. (1969). Electrolyte changes in drowning victims. *Anesthesiology*, **30**, 414–20.

Modell, J. H., Graves, S. A. & Ketover, A. (1976). Clinical course of 91 consecutive near-drowning victims. *Chest*, **70**, 231–8.

Modell, J. H., Graves, S. A. & Kuch, E. J. (1980). Near drowning: correlation of level of consciousness and survival. *Canadian Anaesthetists Society Journal*, **27**, 211–15.

Modell, J. H., Kuck, E. J., Ruiz, B. C. & Heinitish, H. (1972). Effect of intravenous versus aspirated distilled water on serum electrolytes and blood gas tensions. *Journal of Applied Physiology*, **32**, 579–84.

Modell, J. H. & Moya, F. (1966). Effects of volume of aspirated fluid during chlorinated fresh water drowning. *Anesthesiology*, **27**, 662–72.

Montes, H. E. & Conn, A. W. (1980). Near-drowning: An unusual case. *Canadian Anaesthetists Society Journal*, **27**, 172–4.

Naylor, W. G., Poole-Wilson, P. A. & Williams, A. (1979). Hypoxia and calcium. *Journal of Molecular Cellular Cardiology*, **11**, 683–706.

Nichter, M. & Everett, P. B. (1989). Childhood near-drowning: is cardiopulmonary resuscitation always indicated? *Critical Care Medicine*, **17**, 993–5.

Nicodemus, H. F., Chancy, R. D. & Herold, R. (1981). Hemodynamic effects of inotropes during hypothermia and rapid rewarming. *Critical Care Medicine*, **9**, 325–8.

Nussbaum, E. (1985). Prognostic variables in nearly drowned, comatose children. *American Journal of Disease in Childhood*, **139**, 1058–9.

Nussbaum, E. & Maggi, J. C. (1988). Pentobarbital therapy does not improve neurological outcome in nearly-drowned, flaccid-comatose children. *Pediatrics*, **81**, 630–4.

Oakes, D. D., Sherek, J. P., Maloney, J. R. & Charters, A. C. (1982). Prognosis and management of victims of near-drowning. *Journal of Trauma*, **22**, 544–9.

O'Keefe, K. M. (1977). Accidental hypothermia: a review of 62 cases. *Journal of the American College of Emergency Physicians*, **6**, 491–6.

Orlowski, J. P. (1979). Prognostic factors in paediatric cases of drowning and near drowning. *Journal of the American College of Emergency Physicians*, **8**, 176–9.

O'Rourke, P. P., Stolar, C. J. H., Zwischenberger, J. B., Snedecor, S. M. & Bartlett, R. M. (1993). Extracorporeal membrane oxygenation: support for overwhelming pulmonary failure in the pediatric population. Collective experience from the Extracorporeal Life

Support Organization. *Journal of Pediatric Surgery*, **28**, 523–9.

Paulev, E.-P., Pokorski, H. Y., Ahn, B., Masuda, A., Kobayashi, T., Hishibayasiu, Y., Sakakibara, Y., Tanaka, M. & Nakamura, W. (1990). Facial cold receptors and the survival reflex diving bradycardia in man. *Japanese Journal of Physiology*, **40**, 701–12.

Pearn, J. H. (1980). Secondary drowning in children. *British Medical Journal*, **28**, 1103–5.

Pearn, J. H., Bart, R. D. & Yamaoka, R. (1979). Neurological sequelae after childhood near drowning: a total population study from Hawaii. *Pediatrics*, **64**, 187–91.

Peterson, B. (1977). Morbidity of childhood near-drowning. *Pediatrics*, **59**, 364–70.

Pfenninger, J. & Sutter, M. (1982). Intensive care after fresh water immersion in children. *Anesthesia*, **37**, 1157–62.

Pichard, J. D. (1981). Role of prostaglandins and arachidonic acid derivatives in the coupling of cerebral blood flow to metabolism. *Journal of Cerebral Blood Flow & Metabolism*, **1**, 361–84.

Pitt, W. R. & Balanda, K. P. (1991). Childhood drowning and near-drowning in Brisbane: the contribution of domestic pools. *Medical Journal of Australia*, **154**, 661–5.

Pratt, F. D. & Haynes, B. E. (1986). Incidence of 'secondary drowning' after salt water immersion. *Annals of Emergency Medicine*, **15**, 1084–7.

Quan, L. & Kinder, D. (1992). Pediatric submersions: prehospital predictors of outcome. *Pediatrics*, **90**, 909–13.

Quan, L., Wentz, K. R., Gore, E. J. & Copass, M. K. (1990). Outcome predictors in pediatric submersion victims receiving prehospital care in King County, Washington. *Pediatrics*, **86**, 586–93.

Ramey, C. A., Hayward, D. N. & Hayward, J. S. (1987). Dive response of children in relation to cold water drowning. *Journal of Applied Physiology*, **63**, 665–8.

Reuler, J. B. & Parker, R. A. (1978). Peritoneal dialysis in the management of hypothermia. *Journal of the American Medical Association*, **240**, 2289–90.

Rinaldo, J. E. & Rogers, R. M. (1982). Adult respiratory distress syndrome: changing concepts of lung injury and repair. *New England Journal of Medicine*, **306**, 900–9.

Rockoff, M. A., Marshall, L. F. & Shapiro, H. M. (1979). High dose barbiturate therapy in humans: a clinical review of 60 patients. *Annals of Neurology*, **6**, 194–9.

Rogers, M. C. (1985). Near-drowning: cold water on a hot topic? *Journal of Pediatrics*, **106**, 603–4.

Rowe, M. I., Arango, A. & Allington, G. (1977). Profile of paediatric head injuries in a water orientated society. *Journal of Trauma*, **17**, 587–99.

Sarnaik, A. P., Preston, G., Lieh-Lai, M. & Eisenbrey, A. B. (1985). Intracranial pressure and cerebral perfusion pressure in near drowning. *Critical Care Medicine*, **13**, 224–7.

Savard, G. K., Cooper, K. E., Veale, W. L. & Malkinson, T. J. (1985). Peripheral blood flow during rewarming from mild hypothermia in humans. *Journal of Applied Physiology*, **58**, 4–13.

Schissler, P., Parker, M. A. & Scott, S. J. (1981). Profound hypothermia: value of prolonged cardiopulmonary resuscitation. *South Medical Journal*, **74**, 474–7.

Sekar, T. S., MacDonnell, K. F., Namsirikul, P. & Herman, R. S. (1980). Survival after prolonged submersion in cold water without neurological sequelae; report of two cases. *Archives of Internal Medicine*, **140**, 775–9.

Shapiro, B. A. & Cane, R. D. (1981). Metabolic malfunction of the lung: noncardiogenic edema and adult respiratory distress syndrome. *Surgery Annual*, **13**, 271–98.

Shapiro, H. M., Wyte, S. R. & Loeser, J. (1974). Barbiturate augmented hypothermia for reduction of persistently elevated intracranial hypertension. *Journal of Neurosurgery*, **40**, 90–100.

Siebke, H., Rod, T., Breivik, H. & Lind, B. (1975). Survival after 40 minutes submersion without sequelae. *Lancet*, **1**, 1275–77.

Simcock, A. D. (1986). Treatment of near-drowning: a review of 130 cases. *Anaesthesia*, **41**, 643–8.

Smith, A. L., Hoff, J. T. & Nielson, S. L. (1974). Barbiturate protection in focal cerebral ischaemia. *Stroke*, **5**, 1–7.

Soung, L. S., Swank, L., Ing, T. S., Said, R. A., Goldman, J. W., Perez, J. & Geiss, W. P. (1977). The treatment of accidental hypothermia with peritoneal dialysis. *Canadian Medical Association Journal*, **117**, 1415–16.

Steward, D. J. (1976). A disposable condenser humidifier for use during anaesthesia. *Canadian Medical Association Journal*, **23**, 191–5.

Suter, P. M. & Fairley, H. B. (1975). Optimum end-expiratory airway pressure in patients with acute pulmonary failure. *New England Journal of Medicine*, **292**, 284–89.

Swann, H. G. & Spafford, N. R. (1951). Body salt and water changes during fresh and sea water drowning. *Texas Report of Biological Medicine*, **9**, 356.

Tate, R. M. & Repine, J. E. (1983). Neutrophils and the adult respiratory distress syndrome. *American Review of Respiratory Disease*, **128**, 552–9.

Towne, W. D., Geiss, W. P., Yanes, H. O. & Rahimtoola, S. H. (1972). Intractable ventricular fibrillation associated with profound accidental hypothermia: successful treatment with partial cardiopulmonary bypass. *New England Journal of Medicine*, **287**, 1135–7.

Truscott, D. G., Firor, W. B. & Clein, L. J. (1973). Accidental profound hypothermia. Successful resuscitation by core rewarming and assisted circulation. *Archives of Surgery*, **106**, 216–18.

Weinberger, L. M., Gibbon, M. H. & Gibbon, J. H. (1940). Temporary arrest of the circulation to the central nervous system. I. Physiological effects. *Archives of Neurological Psychology*, **43**, 615.

White, B. C., Winnegar, C. D., Wilson, R. F. & Krause, G. S. (1983). Calcium blockers in cerebral resuscitation. *Journal of Trauma*, **23**, 788–94.

Wickstrom, P., Ruiz, E., Lilja, G. P., Hinterkopf, J. P. & Haglin, J. J. (1976). Accidental hypothermia. Core rewarming with partial bypass. *American Journal of Surgery*, **131**, 622–5.

Winegar, C. D., Henderson, O., White, B. C. *et al.* (1983). Prolonged hypoperfusion in the cerebral cortex following cardiac arrest and resuscitation in dogs. *Annals of Emergency Medicine*, **12**, 471–7.

Wintemute, G. J. (1990). Childhood drowning in the United States. *American Journal of Disease in Childhood*, **144**, 663–9.

Wintemute, G. J., Drake, C. & Wright, M. (1991). Immersion events in residential swimming pools: evidence for an experience effect. *American Journal of Disease in Childhood*, **145**, 1200–3.

Wintemute, G. J., Kraus, J. F., Teret, S. P. & Wright, M. (1987). Drowning in childhood and adolescence: a population based study. *American Journal of Public Health*, **77**, 830–2.

Yatsu, F. M., Diamond, I., Graziano, C. & Lindquist, P. (1972). Experimental brain ischaemia: protection from irreversible brain damage with rapid acting barbiturate (methohexital). *Stroke*, **3**, 726–32.

Young, R. S. K., Zalneraitis, E. L. & Dooling, E. C. (1980). Neurological outcome in cold water drowning. *Journal of the American Medical Association*, **244**, 1233–5.

12

The acute response to burn injury in children

C. CHILDS

Introduction

Burns and scalds in infancy and childhood represent a significant proportion of all accidents (Lindblad & Terkelsen, 1990; Ryan et al., 1990; Smith & O'Neill, 1994; Enescu et al., 1994; Chapman et al., 1994). Before going to school one child in 130 will be admitted to hospital with a burn or scald (Lawrence & Wilkins, 1986).

Although the physical and emotional problems may be distressing, most children do survive their injuries. The number of children who die from burns and scalds each year is still very small. (Over a 14-year period to 1994 mortality at the Regional Paediatric Burns Unit for the North West of England, ranged from 0 to 1.8%, median 0.98%.) When burns are extensive the mortality rate rises. Complications after a burn can occur early from (for example) the inhalation of smoke and poisonous substances (Kinsella, 1988) and later on failure of one or more organs increases the mortality (Deitch, 1988). The probability of mortality can be predicted from the size and nature of the burn as well from the age of the patient (Bull, 1971). To audit the efficacy of treatment and clinical performance the predicted mortality can be compared with inpatient records of fatal cases; however this only tells us the final outcome: whether the patient recovered or died from his/her injuries. More useful would be the ability to measure illness. To do this, appropriate predictors which suggest worsening of the patient's condition need to be found. Adults can often give clinicians some idea of how they feel but babies and young children cannot say when they are starting to feel ill. This makes it even more important to try to find an objective measure of morbidity in children (Moir et al., 1991).

The nature of the burn provides a visual and relatively reliable estimation of the size and, in many cases, depth of the injury although the latter is more accurately assessed with specialised equipment (Bauer & Sauer, 1989; Cole et al., 1990; Shakespeare, 1992). For comparison of severity with other (non-burn) injuries the burn must be 'scored' formally (Baker et al., 1974). We know that there are occasions when children have a stormy illness (worse than one would have anticipated from the severity of the injury); it is also true that some children with extensive burns make a surprisingly uneventful recovery. Why does this happen and what markers are there, if any, which could be measured or recorded to alert us to the possibility of a change in the child's condition? The answer is that there are very few.

To correct this situation we need to know more about the pattern of the response to injury from admission to discharge within the context of a contemporary burns treatment protocol. We need to accept that disturbances to homeostasis are not just restricted to children with major burns as the mediators and mechanisms for severe illness probably have a common route (Anderson & Harken, 1990). It is possible, but by no means certain, that progressive clinical deterioration could have its origins during the acute phase of the burn. At the outset, inflammatory mediators of the immune system are undoubtedly supportive in maintaining homeostatic functions but continued release into the circulation may be counterproductive bringing a loss of control to homeostatic mechanisms as excessive production of inflammatory mediators exert their effects upon the host.

In this chapter the mediators of the acute response to injury and the mechanisms by which illness in burned children develops are discussed.

Acute inflammation

Within just a short time after an injury or infection there is a very well developed local and systemic response. In the burn patient the local response is directed towards inflammation of tissues at and around the wound (Zweifach, 1986). In the blood vessels, sticking of leucocytes and platelets to a progressively leaking endothelium of postcapillaries and venules is followed by migration of large molecules and leucocytes across the venule to tissue spaces. At the wound the immediate increase in permeability to macromolecules is mediated by histamine, bradykinin and serotonin (5-hydroxytryptamine, 5-HT) from mast cells as well as arachidonic acid derivatives (Zweifach, 1986). The combined, and overlapping, effects of these chemicals and molecules are responsible for chemotaxis of polymorphonuclear leucocytes (PMNs), the main mobile phagocytic cell. Leaking capillaries lead to local oedema and, if the burn is extensive, the escape of fluid from the circulation into the interstitium is also seen in the lung and brain and represents a 'vascular leak syndrome' (Schlag & Redl, 1990). Oedema after moderate to severe injury therefore occurs at the wound but also in distant tissues.

There are a vast number of mediators associated with the chemotactic, proinflammatory and inflammatory events after injury. Together they function to channel the inflammatory response towards activation of cells of the immune system; PMNs, activated monocytes, macrophages and lymphocytes (Clemens, 1991). From these cells a heterogeneous group of soluble polypeptide molecules, often referred to as cytokines (Dinarello, 1984), are produced and their biological effects become central to the development of our early reaction to trauma. Acting independently as 'cell hormones' or in conjunction with other mediators such as growth factors, acute phase proteins, autocoids, neurotransmitters and hormones of the endocrine system, these molecules exert their effects on a variety of tissues throughout the body. The injured host therefore has both a local and systemic component to the injury.

Cytokines and the acute phase response

The acute phase response or APR is the term used to describe both local and systemic changes to a variety of injuries: mechanical, thermal, infective or ischaemic. The initial damage to tissues causes disruption of cells as well as bleeding and the subsequent cascade of events involving clotting, activates platelets. These in turn produce a number of growth factors (Ross, 1989; Kiritsy & Lynch, 1993) including transforming growth factor-beta (TGF-β), platelet-derived growth factor (PDGF), epidermal growth factor (EGF), and proinflammatory cytokines such as interleukin 1 alpha and beta (IL-1α, IL-1β), tumour necrosis factor alpha (TNFα) and interleukin 8 (IL-8). The latter is chemotactic to neutrophils, monocytes, macrophages and T lymphocytes and once stimulated these cells also produce growth factors. IL-8 also stimulates proliferation of keratinocytes and fibroblasts. These, plus other immune cells, and peripheral cells such as endothelial cells, produce inflammatory mediators (Berczi & Nagy, 1994) such as IL-1, IL-6 and TNF. The clinical symptoms seen in patients are largely due to the biological effects of these mediators on the host.

Perhaps the best known of the symptoms of local inflammation are swelling and pain. Of the systemic changes, fever accompanied by sleepiness, loss of appetite and general malaise, are probably the most well appreciated clinical symptoms which can be attributed to the action of cytokines (Kent *et al.*, 1994). Of the biochemical disturbances, changes in liver export proteins characterise the systemic APR (Fleck *et al.*, 1985). Increases in some of the acute phase proteins (APP) (Shakespeare *et al.*, 1989); C-reactive protein (CRP), α-1 acid glycoprotein (A1AG or orosomucoid), α-1 antitrypsin (A1AT) and fibrinogen and a fall in albumin (Fleck *et al.*, 1985) are found after trauma and the mediator for this is IL-6 (Nijsten *et al.*, 1987).

Although difficult to detect in plasma during health, minute quantities of the interleukins, TNF, interferons and growth factors undoubtedly have a regulatory role in cellular growth and the maintenance of homeostasis (Clemens, 1991). After trauma, and indeed after burn injury, low levels of cytokines appear to have a beneficial effect upon the host, priming macrophages and triggering the immune system to the production of inflammatory mediators so that the person can respond effectively to the trauma or infection (Berczi & Nagy, 1994). The interleukins of importance in the development of the APR after injury are IL-1, IL-6 and TNF (Hopkins & Rothwell, 1995) but the major circulating cytokine is thought to be IL-1 and significant increases in plasma concentration after injury have been found in some (Baigrie *et al.*, 1991) but not all (Childs *et al.*, 1990a) studies.

There are reports of experimental difficulties with cytokine assays. Short half-lives (particularly IL-1) (Whicher & Ingham, 1990), endogenous inhibitors, circulating receptors and binding proteins will affect detection and measurement of these molecules in body fluids. This means that circulating levels of cytokines may not always give a precise indication of the biological activity and effects of these molecules on tissues and organs. Although originally isolated from immune cells (macrophages and monocytes for example) we now know that many more cells produce cytokines. Peripheral cells such as endothelial cells, keratinocytes, fibroblasts, T cells and B cells as well as cells of the central nervous system (neurons and glial cells) are an example (Rothwell & Hopkins, 1995). The production of cytokines released at local sites (of injury or infection for example) affect neighbouring cells as well as most other cells in the body. This undoubtedly requires a network of communication between the brain, the immune system and receptors on target tissues and organs (Deleplansque & Neveu, 1994). The changes in thermoregulatory and metabolic function after injury and the alterations to central nervous and neuroendocrine function are well documented (Delaplansque & Neveu, 1994; Rothwell & Hopkins, 1995; Salmon & Higgs, 1997) and while cytokines are involved in the genesis of these changes there is some evidence that secondary mediators like prostaglandins act as the final common pathway (Salmon & Higgs, 1987) in the local and systemic changes which follow injury.

The acute phase response to burn injury in children

Uncomplicated by pre-existing illness or co-morbid conditions, the physiological changes which occur in children reflect the response to injury per se, particularly during the first day or so after the accident. Differences in surgical and nursing treatment may modulate the response to injury so formulation of a treatment protocol which does not exacerbate the APR is important.

Children have a growing body mass (Johnson *et al.*, 1978) which is controlled by endocrine and metabolic mechanisms. The biological effects of anabolic hormones on normal physiology are different in the developing child compared with the adult who has achieved his/her final weight and stature. To what extent the response to injury in children differs from the adult has not been fully established; however some progress has been made in the study of children with moderate to severe burns. These patients provide a useful model to illustrate the acute response to burn injury in humans, albeit in the young of the species (Childs, 1994).

The first 24 hours after injury

Clinical evidence of the acute phase response

Thermoregulation

What happens to body temperature during the first hour or so after the burn, when patients are in transit to the admitting burn centre, is not really known because measurements are not usually made at this time. On arrival, and about 1–6 hours after the accident, deep body temperature, measured in the rectum (T_r) and skin surface temperature at the extremities, (acral regions, T_{ac}) is within the normal range (Childs, 1988) with a temperature gradient from core to skin of not more than 2.5 °C (Childs *et al.*, 1990b). If total body heat content (kJ/kg) is calculated during the first few hours after admission the evidence is that burned and healthy children have a similar heat content (Childs *et al.*, 1989) (Table 12.1). Similarities in the rate of heat storage between the two groups do not last long. By 5–8 hours, T_r starts to rise (Childs, 1988) and children move from a phase of relative thermal stability through a phase of rapid heat storage to a new and elevated plateau where the heat content of the body is as much as 7 kJ/kg higher than during the first few hours after admission (Childs *et al.*, 1989). The fifth to the eighth postburn hour marks the point at which thermoregulation becomes disrupted (Childs *et al.*, 1989). Twelve hours after the burn T_r peaks (Table 12.1), in excess of 40 °C (Childs & Little, 1989) in most cases and the temperature gradient between the inside and outside of the body increases. At this time the heat content of burn patients is significantly higher than in healthy children exposed to similar conditions (Childs *et al.*, 1989). There is now new evidence to show that the change in deep body temperature follows a similar pattern in most burned children and while a peak is reached in most cases between 10 to 12 hours after the accident, highest values are seen in children with more extensive injuries (C. Childs, unpublished results).

The rise in T_r is preceded by a fall in skin temperature at the extremities so T_{ac} can be used to predict the point at which thermoregulatory changes begin (Childs & Little, 1994). Rapid changes in peripheral skin temperature and perfusion occur (Wright *et al.*, 1995) and this can be shown within a short time after a burn (Table 12.1) in children and do not appear to be associated with the usual stimulus to changes in acral skin temperature and perfusion (Stoner *et al.*, 1991). In the burned children, despite the fall in skin temperature of the hands and feet, skin temperature in other areas remained elevated and this together with the rise in T_r, increased the heat content of the body

Table 12.1. *Deep body and skin surface temperature in children on admission and at approximately 10 hours after a burn*

Patient	Age (years)	Injury	On admission				At approximately 10 hours			
			T_r (°C)	T_{ac} (°C)	$\Delta T_r - T_{ac}$ (°C)	T_a (°C)	T_r (°C)	T_{ac} (°C)	$\Delta T_r - T_{ac}$ (°C)	T_a (°C)
1	1.83	25% scald	37.3	34.9	2.4	31.0	39.5	31.5	8.0	31.9
2	8.75	55% burn	37.2	35.3	1.9	32.6	40.4	30.1	10.3	31.1
3	1.08	12% scald	37.2	36.0	1.2	33.0	39.1	31.3	7.8	32.5
4	1.83	22% scald	37.8	36.3	1.5	34.7	38.9	32.2	6.7	30.0
5	0.92	10% scald	37.2	36.2	1.0	30.7	41.1	31.1	10.0	31.3
6	5.67	21% scald	37.2	35.5	1.7	31.0	40.1	30.0	10.1	31.9
7	1.42	23% scald	38.5	36.4	2.1	30.1	40.5	31.0	9.5	30.3
8	1.08	11% scald	37.1	35.0	2.1	30.0	39.3	31.0	8.3	30.3
9	1.58	12% scald	37.3	35.5	1.8	30.3	40.1	31.6	8.5	30.3
10	1.33	16% scald	37.5	35.6	1.9	29.0	39.6	30.1	10.8	28.8

Body temperature in young children with moderate to severe burns on admission to the Burns Unit and at approximately 10 hours after injury. In a constantly warm ambient temperature (T_a) there is an increase in rectal temperature (T_r) and fall in skin temperature measured at the hallux (T_{ac}), approximately 10 hours after the burn. The temperature gradient between deep body (rectal) and skin surface ($\Delta T_r - T_{ac}$) is given at the two time points.

(Childs *et al.*, 1989). The changes in body temperature are a characteristic of the APR. In burned children the rise in T_r and change in total body heat content has an identifiable starting point (Childs & Little, 1994).

Changing the ambient temperature does not alter the pattern of the thermoregulatory response. The increase in total body heat content appears to be independent of ambient conditions, occurring in cool as well as warm environments (Childs *et al.*, 1989).

With an increase in total body heat content a corresponding increase in heat loss might be expected to restore euthermia but this has not been shown. The rates of total heat loss in burned, compared with healthy children, are (somewhat inappropriately) much the same, but when the individual routes for heat loss by dry (radiant, convective and conductive) and wet (evaporative) routes were calculated, important differences emerged. Although dry heat loss was greater in the patients, wet heat loss, i.e. sweating, was low (Childs, 1989). This centrally mediated thermoregulatory mechanism was inhibited in these febrile children so although internally warm, the stimulus for activation of the sweating mechanism was inhibited (Childs *et al.*, 1990b, 1992a). Inhibition of thermoregulation after injury has been reported in response to nociceptive afferent stimulation and central control of heat loss can be influenced by incoming signals from neural afferents (Stoner, 1977). Burn injury in children appears to be associated with a central inhibition of at least one heat losing mechanism (sweating) which means that the threshold temperature for the onset of heat loss may increase, as shown under experimental conditions (Little & Stoner, 1968; Stoner, 1972). While there is only a very small transcutaneous loss of water from unburned skin in febrile burned children, sweating is marked in healthy children at the same ambient temperature (Childs *et al.*, 1992a). Over the exposed burn wound a high water (and heat) loss would be expected but when the wounds of burned children are covered (either with bandages or some sort of semi-permeable membrane) heat loss is reduced. As a consequence of bandaging, evaporative water loss is cut by about 50% (Childs *et al.*, 1992a).

In the past, excessive heat loss was shown to be an almost inevitable consequence of burn injury providing an important stimulus for thermoregulatory heat production (to offset a fall in body temperature) (Caldwell *et al.*, 1981). Limiting the rate of heat loss would seem an appropriate treatment to lower the metabolic demands for thermoregulation. This hypothesis was tested by Zawacki *et al.* (1970) but the postburn rise in metabolic rate was not lowered, suggesting that mechanisms other than those of a thermoregulatory nature played a more important role.

In acutely burned children heat loss is within the normal range despite a significant increase in the amount of heat stored in the body (Childs *et al.*, 1992a). Is this appropriate? One could argue that if the set-point for body temperature was normal (i.e. approximately 37°C) heat loss would have been higher; however, if the central thermoregulatory set-point was raised, as has been suggested after burn injury (Aulick *et al.*, 1979), by an endogenous pyrogen (Atkins & Bodel, 1972), then conservation of heat and/or endogenous heat production would be expected, and appropriate to raise body core temperature. In burned children there is a very characteristic pattern to the rise in deep body temperature and the mechanisms for this change are directed towards heat conservation. The inhibition of sweating is not the only mechanism for raising the temperature of the tissues of the body. A rise in metabolic heat production may be involved in the genesis of an increased T_r particularly in a cool environment (Morimoto *et al.*, 1988).

Metabolic activity

Until recently the early effect of a burn on thermoregulation and metabolism had been studied only in the experimental animal (Stoner, 1970). Why the acute metabolic response to burn injury in humans had been overlooked is unclear but difficulties in access to patients and the practical problems of indirect calorimetry in the first few hours after admission to hospital may be the explanation. In the last 5 years or so improvements in techniques for indirect calorimetry at the bedside have meant that measurements can be made without too much disruption to the nursing care of the patient (Figure 12.1). Recent studies show that the rise in T_r and heat content during the first 12 hours is associated with an increase in oxygen consumption ($\dot{V}O_2$) (Childs & Little, 1994) and this together with the fall in skin temperature at acral regions (Figure 12.2) and central inhibition in heat loss in certain areas of the body (Childs *et al.*, 1992a), supports the role for an upward readjustment in the thermoregulatory set-point temperature (Bligh, 1973).

Comparisons of burned children with controls

In most circumstances measurements of metabolic rate in patients need to be compared with an appropriate control group who have been studied under very similar conditions. For example, sleeping patients should be compared with sleeping controls and resting patients with resting controls. Separation of the results like this prevents the errors which can be made if factors which influence metabolic rate, like movement and activity, are not taken into account. The closest approximation to basal metabolic rate (BMR) (DuBois, 1924) which can reasonably be made in sick patients in bed is a sleeping metabolic rate (SMR) and burned children are indeed asleep (and sedated) for a large part of the resuscitation period. In sleeping burned children, $\dot{V}O_2$ is elevated above the control range (Figure 12.3) on about 50% of occasions (Childs & Little, 1994). In each child the pattern of T_r, $\dot{V}O_2$ and T_{ac} followed a remarkably similar pattern. The early rise in T_r involves an increase in oxygen consumption (and thus energy expenditure) (Childs & Little, 1994). In addition heat is conserved and the mechanisms for this appear to be an inhibition of sweating as well as a reduction in heat to the skin of the extremities (vasoconstriction). The characteristic fever of the APR is therefore brought about by both efferent routes of the thermoregulatory system, an increase in heat production as well as a central inhibition in the ability to lose heat by sweating.

All this information helps our understanding of the thermoregulatory and metabolic changes during the first day after a burn in patients treated by a specific treatment protocol (see Appendix) but how does this compare with the classic studies of the metabolic response to burns in the adult?

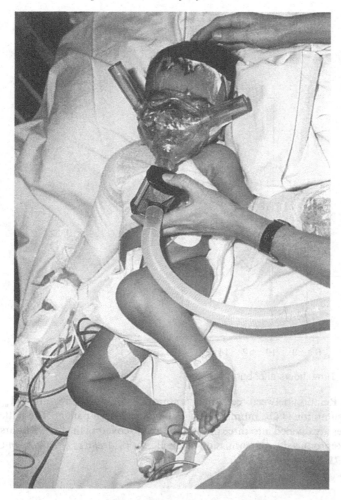

Figure 12.1. Method for collection of expired respiratory gas using a purpose built, flow-through system of indirect calorimetry. A close fitting mask is held over the nose and mouth. For a more detailed account of the design, construction and validation of the system see McGuinness and Childs (1991).

Early studies of the metabolic response to burn injury

In the past, most studies of the metabolic response to injury were undertaken during the later, 'flow' phase of injury (Cuthbertson, 1942), a time corresponding to the second or third week after injury. Patients with extensive wounds were at a stage when superficial wounds would have healed and granulation tissue formed from deeper

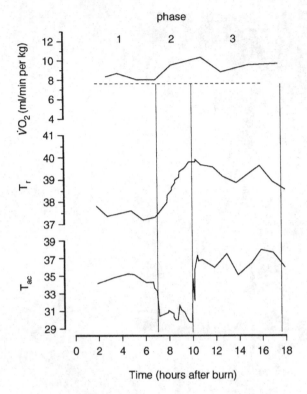

Figure 12.2. Relation between rectal temperature (T_r), toe skin temperature (T_{ac}) and oxygen consumption ($\dot{V}O_2$, ml/min per kg) in a typical burn patient. The pattern of these changes are divided into three phases (1, 2 and 3) covering the first 18 hours after the injury. Reproduced with permission of the Editor of *Archives of Disease in Childhood* (1994) **71**: 31–34.

wounds (if not infected) were ready to accept an autograft. Energy expenditure at this stage of the injury was reported to be as much as twice BMR (Wilmore *et al.*, 1974). Patients were referred to as 'hypermetabolic', requiring 'hyper' caloric diets to meet the patients' increased energy expenditure (Curreri *et al.*, 1974). Most children (and adults too) treated by contemporary burn protocols receive an autograft within the first few days and have a healed donor area within about 2 weeks. With supportive aftercare the child can be discharged from hospital at about this time. In contrast, the very nature of conservative treatment means that the wound is allowed to heal spontaneously and this takes time. A skin graft can be applied to areas which remain unhealed but compared with early closure at approximately 3 days, the wounds of conservatively treated patients will be open for much longer. If, as early studies show, the metabolic response is proportional to the severity of the burn (Wilmore *et al.*, 1975) (or the size of any unhealed wounds, including the donor area (Demling *et al.*, 1991)) it is not

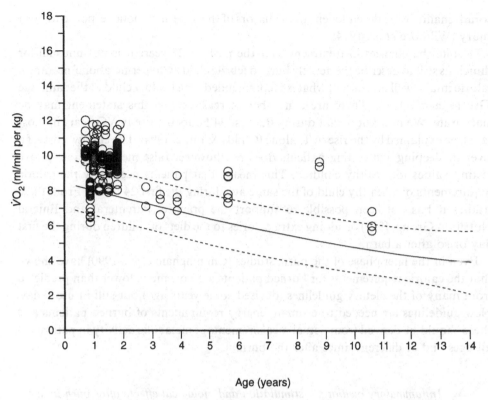

Figure 12.3. Oxygen consumption ($\dot{V}O_2$) in healthy sleeping children (mean $\pm$ 95% confidence interval). Superimposed on these control data are individual measurements of $\dot{V}O_2$ (O) in 17 sleeping burned children. Reproduced with permission of the Editor *Burns* (1994) **20**; 291–300.

surprising perhaps that energy requirements were once shown to be elevated for weeks or even months until complete closure of the burn.

The inevitable consequence of a large unhealed wound is uncontrolled loss of water and heat (Harrison *et al.*, 1964; Henane *et al.*, 1981) and if this is allowed to go unchecked deep body temperature falls if there is no compensatory increase in heat production and/or heat conservation (Morgan *et al.*, 1955). So great was the increase in cutaneous heat loss in exposed patients that compensatory thermoregulatory mechanisms were proposed as the real cause of the hypermetabolic response to burn injury (Caldwell *et al.*, 1981). While an obligatory heat loss certainly contributes to a disturbance in thermoregulation and metabolism this was not thought to provide a complete explanation for the changes seen during the 'flow' phase. Rather, it was argued that high levels of the circulating thermogenic hormones adrenaline and noradrenaline were the endogenous mediators of the hypermetabolic response to burn injury (Wilmore *et al.*, 1974).

Despite the changes in treatment over the past 20–25 years it is not unusual for clinicians still to describe the acutely burned febrile child as 'hypermetabolic' needing a calorie intake well in excess of what is recommended for a healthy child of the same age (Grotte *et al.*, 1982). There are a number of reasons why this statement may be inaccurate. We now know that during the first 24 hours the rise in $\dot{V}O_2$ can, in most cases, be explained by the rise in T_r alone (Childs & Little, 1994). The energy 'cost' of a fever in sleeping and resting patients does not however raise metabolic rate above resting values for healthy children. This means that patients need only the calorie requirements of a healthy child of the same age during the first 24 hours. From these studies it has not been possible to support the practice (Parenteral and Enteral Nutrition Group, 1989) of adding extra calories to the diets of children during the first day or so after a burn.

Even in the later phase of the burn, studies (Cunningham *et al.*, 1990) have shown that the calorie requirements for burned patients are now much lower than predicted from many of the dietary guidelines (devised some years ago) but still in use today. New guidelines are needed to estimate energy requirements of burned patients and these should be derived from actual measurements of metabolic activity in patients of all ages and at different times after the burn.

Inflammatory mediators: stimulation and biological effects after burn injury

There seems little doubt that the APR to burns in children is associated with a profound disturbances in thermoregulation and metabolism and cytokines do play a role in this. Traditionally burns have been associated with infection, initially by colonisation and invasion by Gram-positive organisms and later, typically by Gram-negative enterococci and anaerobes (Pruitt, 1984). Although fever is a classic symptom of infection it is seldom possible to identify a focus of infection which could account for the early fever in burned children. Wound swabs taken on admission are either free of microorganisms or have skin flora only. Pathogens, notably *Staphylococcus aureus* and *Streptococcus* species do not usually appear until the second day (Childs *et al.*, 1994).

On the other hand inflammatory mediators are present in the circulation within just a few hours and in much higher concentrations than in healthy subjects. In a series of 10 burned children, studied during the first 24 hours, there was a significant positive relationship in each patient between the pyrogenic cytokine, IL-6, and T_r (Figure 12.4). For the group, peak increases in T_r and plasma IL-6 occurred at 10–12 hours (Childs *et al.*, 1990a). Although it was not possible from these data to establish a cause and effect relationship between IL-6 and T_r, the early increases in plasma concentration at about 8 hours is in keeping with what has been shown in burned adults (Nijsten *et al.*, 1987).

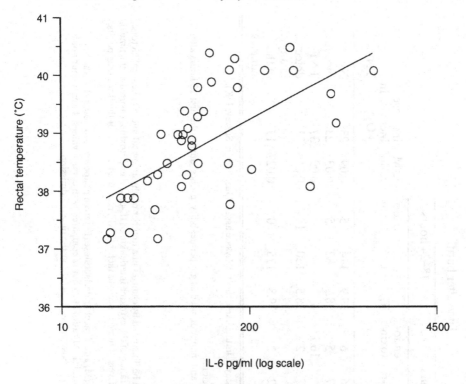

Figure 12.4. Relation between IL-6 (pg/ml, log scale) with rectal temperature in 10 patients, $r = 0.604757$, $P = 0.000017$ ($n = 43$ measurements).

The difficulties of detecting IL-1 in plasma are well recognised. There were few burned children in whom plasma levels were detectable (Childs *et al.*, 1990a) but this was not the case in tissue fluid. High levels of IL-1 probably produced from keratinocytes, were obtained from intact blisters. What influence local production of this cytokine would have on the overall sequence of events associated with the APR is unclear. There is now evidence however that the degree of inflammation and the hepatic acute phase response cannot be determined by plasma levels of either IL-1 or TNF and this is certainly the situation after a burn, for TNF was not detectable in plasma in any of the febrile children (Childs *et al.*, 1990c) (Table 12.2). TNF is probably more useful as an indicator for sepsis and mortality than for the changes associated with inflammation and the APR (Moldawer *et al.*, 1987). IL-1, IL-6 and TNF have all been identified as major mediators of the endocrine and metabolic changes characteristic of the APR but in the first 24 hours two of these cytokines avoid detection (Marano *et al.*, 1990) in clinical as well as experimental studies.

Table 12.2. *Acute responses to injury at three time points*

Name	Age	%burn	On admission			10–12 hours			18–24 hours			L/M ratio[d]	% increase in $\dot{V}O_2$[c]	TNF
			T_r	IL-6	endo-toxin[a]	T_r	IL-6	endo-toxin	T_r	IL-6	endo-toxin			
JA	13 m	11	37.2	21	5	39.0	66	6	39.9	114	5	0.09	23	No bioactive TNF detected in any of the samples
BD	16 m	16	37.3	30	5	39.1	77	5	38.9	82	5	0.03	23	
DM	17 m	23	38.3	16	2	38.6	—	16.1[b]	—	—	—	0.09	37	
AM	5.6 y	21	37.9	32	2	40.3	167	2	38.5	150	14	0.04	21	
SA	9 m	20	37.3	22	3.5	40.1	272	2	39.8	175	0	0.027	17	

[a] Lower limits of detection of endotoxin is 5–10 pg/ml using the LAL assay (Limulus Amoebocyte Lysate assay, Quadratech, Surrey, UK).
[b] Measured at 8.25 hours postburn.
[c] Change at 12 hours postburn from lowest value around time of admission.
[d] L/M ratio is the ratio of urinary excretion of the two sugars (lactulose and mannitol) used as gut permeability 'probes' during the first 12 hours after the burn.

Control values: range
IL-6,   20–34   (median 24.5 pg/ml)
L/M ratio, 0.008–0.044 (median 0.02)

The evidence for an acute phase response (APR) in burned children can be illustrated by changes in a number of physiological and biochemical factors. The table shows changes in rectal temperature (T_r) and plasma concentration of the cytokine interleukin 6 (IL-6) and endotoxin measured at the time of admission and at 10–12 hours and 18–24 hours after the burn. Plasma levels of tumour necrosis factor (TNF) measured at each of the three time points, was not detectable in any of the patients.

After an oral dose of two sugar 'probes', the monosaccharide, mannitol (M) and disaccharide, lactulose (L) (given at approx. 6–8 hours after the burn) there was a significant increase in the ratio of urinary lactulose to mannitol (L/M ratio) at 24 hours compared with control values. Twenty-four hours after the burn there was a 17–37% increase in oxygen consumption ($\dot{V}O_2$) above values measured at the time of admission.

The role of the gut in the inflammatory response to injury

The appearance of inflammatory molecules in plasma so soon after the injury leads us to question the source of the stimulus to their production. Some years ago, wound infection might have been an acceptable explanation but not now. Although the wound might appear to be the obvious site for pathogens and their toxins, few wounds are colonised during the acute period so a source of bacteria or their toxins distant from the wound could be involved.

In recent years the role of the gastrointestinal tract as a source of inflammatory material has been investigated (Gans & Matsumoto, 1974). Supported mainly by studies in animals (Alexander *et al.*, 1990) whole bacteria have been shown to cross the enterocyte to the circulation and gut-derived organisms have been identified in mesenteric lymph nodes (MLN), spleen and liver (Deitch, 1988). In healthy humans this would not normally be expected but after injury, infection or sepsis the gut becomes more permeable to microorganisms or their cell fragments like endotoxin (Braithwaite *et al.*, 1993) and the latter is known to be a potent stimulus to the production of inflammatory cells of the immune system. Penetration of bacteria through the enterocyte or passage of molecules via a disrupted tight junction (Alexander, 1990) may result in bacterial translocation (BT) alone or in conjunction with increased permeability of the enterocyte. BT and endotoxaemia stimulate production of biologically active inflammatory molecules like the interleukins and TNF. The clinical manifestation of increased gut permeability may be fever, discomfort and general malaise and at the extreme (and probably depending on the dose of the inflammatory molecules) septicaemia and multiple organ failure.

We know that the gut of young children with moderate to severe burns does become 'leaky' within the first 12 hours after the accident (Childs *et al.*, 1992b); however, the changes in gut permeability do not appear to be associated with an endotoxaemia because plasma endotoxins are not generally elevated (Table 12.2). There is a suggestion however that the increase in permeability, disturbances in thermoregulation and increased oxygen consumption may be related, but more research is needed to confirm this.

The inflammatory molecules of the immune system are also potent activators of the hypothalamo–pituitary axis and appear to be involved in the production of the 'classical' hormones of the endocrine system (Koenig, 1991).

The neuroendocrine response to acute burn injury

The neuroendocrine response to trauma is a feature of acute injury (Berkenbosch, 1994) and represents a coordinated response by the central nervous system to a variety of noxious signals: pain, fluid loss and tissue damage (Stoner, 1986). The initial changes in plasma hormone concentrations are produced as a result of stimulation of nociceptive afferents (Ganong, 1986; Stoner, 1986), the hypothalamo–pituitary–adrenal axis and the adrenal medulla.

Initiation of the neuroendocrine response must ultimately be traced to the nature of the injury and burned tissue is a very identifiable starting point. After burns and other injuries, high levels of plasma catecholamines have been reported (Hamberger et al., 1980; Davies et al., 1984; Frayn et al., 1985; Little et al., 1985). Increases in noradrenaline reflect 'spill over' from sympathetic nerve terminals, while plasma adrenaline is released from the adrenal medulla (Cryer, 1980) and this may be the most rapid and important response to injury (Wilmore, 1977).

In burned patients high levels of plasma catecholamines persist for many days (Chansouria et al., 1980) and this is exacerbated if patients are nursed in an environmental temperature below thermoneutrality (28–30°C) (Wilmore et al., 1974). Until recently little was known about the pattern of catecholamines during the first few hours after burn injury but it now seems that plasma catecholamines immediately after injury are elevated. In children plasma concentrations of adrenaline and noradrenaline are elevated but variable (Childs et al., 1990c). Whether catecholamines remain elevated (as shown in earlier studies) until (or even after) discharge from hospital is not clear at present.

Catecholamines are important in preparing the body to respond to sudden stress. Survival in extreme circumstances is dependent upon being able to mount a 'fight or flight' response (Cannon, 1929) and this involves redistribution of blood away from organs not directly involved in defending the person from danger to the heart, brain and muscle. Catecholamines also mobilise energy. This occurs by a direct action on the liver converting hepatic glycogen stores to glucose, by acting on skeletal muscle directly, converting muscle glycogen to lactate for resynthesis to new glucose in the liver via the Cori cycle. Catecholamines also suppress the normal release of insulin in response to an elevated blood glucose level (Heath, 1994) in adults and at the same time stimulate release of glucagon. The overall effect of these substrate changes soon after injury is a rise in plasma concentration of glucose.

In children hyperglycaemia seems to be more exaggerated than in the adult and is unrelated to the size of the injury (Childs et al., 1990c). Peak plasma glucose concentrations of 20 mmol/l are not uncommon during the first 12 hours whereas in the adult high values like this are less common (Taylor et al., 1944; Davies, 1982). Very high plasma glucose levels are not sustained but fall after about 8 hours and are maintained at a level well above normal (Childs et al., 1990c). Hyperglycaemia in injured children with, or without burns (e.g. head injury) (Parish & Webb, 1988) does not appear to predict outcome as it does in the adult (Pentelenyi et al., 1979). Why burned children have a high (but short) peak plasma glucose which fails to return to the normal range, is unclear but one possibility is that glycogenolysis is more readily stimulated by adrenaline. Like adults burned children develop insulin resistance but this is not immediate and not evident until about 8 hours postburn (the time at which other major physiological disturbances are noted).

Although the specific mechanisms by which injury affects the neuroendocrine system is unclear, it is known that corticotrophin releasing factor (CRF) is an important regulator of the hormones involved in the emotional and physical response to injury and stress (Berkenbosch, 1994). CRF is required to stimulate cells in the adenohypophysis to produce the pituitary hormone adrenocorticotrophin hormone (ACTH). In this way CRF, secreted from hypothalamic neurons, is transported via the portal hypophyseal vessels to the anterior pituitary, providing a neurosecretory link between the nervous system and the endocrine system (Rothwell, 1989). ACTH is released from the anterior pituitary into the circulation to the adrenal cortex where it stimulates cortisol release.

ACTH production is dependent upon release of CRF but recent evidence suggests that secretion of this hormone may be augmented by arginine vasopressin (AVP) from the neurohypophysis and also by adrenaline (Buckingham, 1985).

While ACTH is released in response to noxious, non-specific stimuli, AVP is released particularly in response to a change in blood volume such as haemorrhage or hypovolaemia (Buckingham, 1985). The nature of a brain injury represents a significant stimulus to release of the anterior pituitary hormone, ACTH, and the hormones of the adrenal cortex; cortisol and aldosterone as well as the posterior pituitary hormone, AVP. Cortisol increases after a burn (Sinha *et al.*, 1980) and in children, even those with moderate sized burns, there is a progressive and significant rise in plasma cortisol compared with values obtained at the time of admission (Childs *et al.*, 1990c). With time cortisol fluctuates widely and the normal, circadian pattern cannot be seen.

Cortisol promotes mobilisation of energy substrates (glycogen breakdown, regulation of glycerol and free fatty acid metabolism) (Barton, 1985) and the provision of energy from non-carbohydrate sources (in the form of amino acids from protein breakdown) is well documented after injury (Kirkpatrick, 1987). Mobilisation of protein, from skeletal muscle but also from visceral organs provides gluconeogenic precursors (such as lactate), respiratory fuel for rapidly dividing cells like enterocytes and immune cells as well as precursors for the synthesis of acute phase proteins (Kispert & Caldwell, 1990).

Loss of water, plasma and electrolytes from the burn surface as well as from the intravascular compartment (to the interstitium) represents the start of a disturbance in fluid balance which could if unchecked lead to hypovolaemia and electrolyte disturbances (Caldwell *et al.*, 1971). Compensatory mechanisms are activated via the renin–angiotensin–aldosterone system to conserve sodium, and with it water (Le Quesne *et al.*, 1985). Conservation of water alone is also aided by the pressor agent vasopressin (also known as antidiuretic hormone, ADH). In practice hypovolaemic patients are usually given some form of intravenous fluid therapy to correct the loss of circulating water volume (Le Quesne *et al.*, 1985) but it seems that vasopressin continues to be released, ensuring increased permeability to water in the distal tubules (Smith & MacIntosh, 1994). Thus even when fluid resuscitation has been started, sodium and water continues to be retained under the influence of vasopressin. In the event that fluid resuscitation is absent such protective mechanisms would support circulating blood volume for a limited period of time. When intravenous fluid therapy is started (the usual situation in severely burned patients admitted to hospital) some would argue that continued and elevated production of vasopressin is an inappropriate response leading to a clinical syndrome of fluid retention, dilutional hyponatraemia and the production of large urine volumes (Smith & MacIntosh, 1994). In the presence of fluid therapy the endocrine changes after burn injury should be borne in mind and care taken to avoid the problems which could follow, such as overtransfusion (Muir *et al.*, 1987). After all, from a teleological point of view the antidiuresis after burn injury is an adaptive biological response protecting the patient in the event that fluid support is delayed or possibly absent. In both adults and children a direct relation between plasma vasopressin and burn size has been shown and perhaps explains why patients with severe burns need careful management to balance the need for an adequate urine output with the danger of fluid overload.

Conclusions

In the past, study of the physiological changes associated with the early phase after the burn was often overlooked in favour of attention to the more profound clinical problems of the 'flow' phase (Cuthbertson, 1942) of injury. Providing the emergency treatment for immediate resuscitation, pain relief and wound treatment were dealt with and the patient's life was not in danger from the effects of the injury the clinical problems were probably very straightforward compared with those which would start to appear later. For after about 2 weeks profound muscle wasting and increased nitrogen loss became established as a consequence of a prolonged period of increased energy demands. The negative energy balance and gross debilitation of the patient were (and still are in some cases) extremely difficult to reverse and consequently this stimulated a variety of research interests. Problems like this were not considered to be a feature of the acute response for sufficient time had not elapsed for them to have developed.

In recent years, however, we have come to appreciate that the problems that appear later may have their roots in changes taking place much earlier; in fact within just hours (even minutes) after the accident. We know from the detailed studies which have been conducted in children that homeostasis is disturbed at an (almost) predictable time point and therefore must involve factors which are stimulated by a change in events, i.e. the injury itself. The mediators responsible have been shown to originate within the immune system but a network of communication between the nervous and endocrine systems are needed for the acute response to injury to become established. Measurement of the very many cytokines, growth factors and endocrine hormones make it clear that the first few hours and days is anything but an 'ebb phase' as described by Cuthbertson. Rather it is a volatile period during which the patients' homeostatic mechanisms are undergoing an adaptive response which ultimately must lead to healing. The problem is that these adaptive changes sometimes become exaggerated and the benefit may be outweighed by the effects of maladaptation and the chances of this happening may increase as the illness (injury) lingers (or the wound remains unhealed). An example of this is the development of SIRS (septic inflammatory response syndrome). At least we have come sufficiently far to recognise that, while an inflammatory response is essential and that cytokines for example, are fundamental to its development, there is a point at which adaptive changes become maladaptive and in some patients (and not always those with the most extensive injuries) this may ultimately lead to death. At the moment our ability to predict those patients who are at risk is limited but this may be explained by the fact that we still have an incomplete understanding of the basic biological processes associated with the response to an injury.

At least in the child we have made progress. It is now possible to characterise the typical response to a moderate to severe burn injury and therefore know what to expect from the time the child is admitted to hospital. Fever for example appears to be an inevitable consequence of the injury so one must question whether we really do need to make such a big effort to get rid of it. We have, as yet, to confirm the notion that it is beneficial, but we can at least state that it does not appear to be harmful. Perhaps it would be more expedient to monitor the pattern of body temperature, albeit elevated, which is expected until an unexpected event occurs and then consider the steps (treatment) which should be taken. As for the changes in the demand for oxygen we know now that this is not as great in the acute phase as shown previously in the 'flow' phase. Is this an inherent feature of the response itself or is it due to extraneous factors specific to the way in which patients are treated? If, for example, factors which raise the demand for oxygen, such as cold, pain, fear and activity, are eliminated then the rate of oxygen consumption may be reduced and the metabolic cost of the injury can be lowered with obvious savings on the need to mobilise endogenous energy stores.

The acute phase of injury can no longer be overlooked for it is within the first hours after the burn that the processes which ultimately lead to repair of injured tissues are established. In many cases the mechanisms by which this is brought about are successful but the potential for failure (morbidity and death) is inherent within the system. Finding a marker which could be used clinically to measure progress and/or predict outcome must be our greatest challenge.

References

Alexander, J. W. (1990). Nutrition and translocation. *Journal of Trauma*, 14 (Suppl.), 170S–174S.

Alexander, J. W., Boyce, S. T., Babcock, G. F., Gianotto, L., Peck, M. D., Dunn, D. L., Pyles, T., Childress, C. P. & Ash, S. K. (1990). The process of microbial translocation. *Annals of Surgery*, 212, 496–512.

Anderson, B. O. & Harken, A. H. (1990). Multiple organ failure: inflammatory priming and activation sequences promote autologous tissue injury. *Journal of Trauma*, 30 (Suppl.), S44–S49.

Aulick, L. H., Hander, E. H., Wilmore, D. W., Mason, A. D. & Pruitt, B. A. (1979). The relative significance of thermal and metabolic demands on burn hypermetabolism. *Journal of Trauma*, 19, 559–66.

Atkins, E. & Bodel, P. (1972). Fever. *New England Journal of Medicine*, 286, 27–34.

Baigrie, R. J., Lamont, P. M., Dallman, M. & Morris, P. J. (1991). The release of interleukin 1β (IL-1) precedes that of interleukin 6 (IL-6) in patients undergoing major surgery. *Lymphokine Cytokine Research*, 10, 253–6.

Baker, S. P., O'Neill, B., Haddon, W. Jr. & Long, W. B. (1974). The injury severity score: a method for describing patients with multiple injuries and evaluating emergency care. *Journal of Trauma*, 14, 87–196.

Barton, R. N. (1985). Neuroendocrine mobilisation of body fuels after injury. *British Medical Bulletin*, 41, 218–25.

Bauer, J. A. & Sauer, Th. (1989). Cutaneous 10 mhz ultrasound B scan allows the quantitative assessment of burn depth. *Burns*, 1, 49–51.

Berczi, I. & Nagy, E. (1994). Neurohormonal control of cytokines during injury. In *Brain Control of Responses to Trauma*, ed. N. J. Rothwell & F. Berkenbosch, pp. 32–107. Cambridge, Cambridge University Press.

Berkenbosch, F. (1994). Neuroendocrine responses to physical trauma. In *Brain Control of Responses to Trauma*, ed. N. J. Rothwell & F. Berkenbosch, pp. 239–59. Cambridge, Cambridge University Press.

Bull, J. P. (1971). Revised analysis of mortality due to burns. *Lancet*, 2, 1133–4.

Bligh, J. (1973). *Temperature Regulation in Mammals and Other Vertebrates*. London, North Holland, pp. 153–247.

Brathwaite, C. E. M., Ross, S. E., Nagele, R., Mure, A. J., O'Malley, K. F. & Garcia-Perez, F. A. (1993). Bacterial translocation occurs in humans after traumatic injury: evidence using immunofluorescence. *Journal of Trauma*, 34, 586–90.

Buckingham, J. C. (1985). Hypothalamo–pituitary responses to trauma. *British Medical Bulletin*, 41, 203–11.

Caldwell, F. T., Bowser, B. H. & Crabtree, J. H. (1981). The effect of occlusive dressings on the energy metabolism of severely burned children. *Annals of Surgery*, 193, 579–90.

Caldwell, F. T., Casali, R. E., Flanigan, W. J. & Bowser, B. (1971). What constitutes the proper solution for resuscitation of the severely burned patient? *American Journal of Surgery*, 122, 655–61.

Cannon, W. B. (1929). *Bodily Changes in Pain, Hunger, Fear and Rage*, 2nd edn. New York, Appleton.

Chansouria, J. P. N., Sinha, K., Mathur, A. K., Patel, V., Tripathi, F. M. & Udupa, K. N. (1980). Hormonal and associated metabolic alterations following burn injury: Part 1. Relationship to degree of burn. *Burns*, 7, 10–15.

Chapman, J. C., Sarhadi, N. S. & Watson, A. C. H. (1994). Declining incidence of paediatric burns in Scotland: a review of 1114 children with burns treated as inpatients and outpatients in a regional centre. *Burns,* **20**, 106–10.

Childs, C. (1988). Fever in burned children. *Burns,* **14**, 1–6.

Childs, C. (1989). *Changes in heat content and heat loss during the acute phase of burn injury.* PhD thesis, University of Manchester.

Childs, C. (1994). Studies in children provide a model to re-examine the metabolic response to burn injury in patients treated by contemporary burn protocols. *Burn,* **20**, 291–300.

Childs, C. & Little, R. A. (1989). Paracetamol (acetaminophen) in the management of burned children with fever. *Burns,* **14**, 343–8.

Childs, C. & Little, R. A. (1994). Acute changes in oxygen consumption and body temperature after burn injury. *Archives of Disease in Childhood,* **71**, 31–4.

Childs, C., Edwards-Jones, V., Heathcote, D. N., Dawson, M. & Davenport, P. J. (1994). Patterns of *S. aureus* colonisation, toxin production, immunity and illness in burned children. *Burns,* **20**, 514–21.

Childs, C., Heath, D. F., Little, R. A. & Brotherston, M. (1990c). Glucose metabolism in children during the first day after burn injury. *Archives of Emergency Medicine,* **7**, 135–47.

Childs, C., Ratcliffe, R. J., Holt, I., Hopkins, S. J. & Little, R. A. (1990a). The relationship between interleukin-1, interleukin-6 and pyrexia in burned children. In *Physiological and Pathophysiological Effects of Cytokines. Progress in Leucocyte Biology,* ed. C. A. Dinarello, M. Kluger, M. Powanda & J. Oppenheim, vol. 10b, pp. 295–300. New York, Wiley Liss.

Childs, C., Stoner, H. B. & Little, R. A. (1990b). Evidence of a central inhibition of heat loss during the acute phase of burn injury in children. *Archives of Emergency Medicine,* **7**, 303–4.

Childs, C., Stoner, H. B., Little, R. A. & Davenport, P. J. (1989). A comparison of some thermoregulatory responses in healthy children and in children with burn injury. *Clinical Science,* **77**, 425–9.

Childs, C., Stoner, H. B., Little, R. A. & Davenport, P. J. (1992a). Cutaneous heat loss shortly after burn injury in children. *Clinical Science,* **83**, 117–26.

Childs, C., Watson, S. B., Fisher, M. I., Ward, I. D., Davenport, P. J. & Little, R. A. (1992b). Gut permeability in the acutely burned child. *Proceedings of the Association of Clinical Biochemists,* June. 52.

Clemens, M. J. (1991). *Cytokines,* pp. 57–73. Oxford, Bios Scientific Publishers.

Cole, R. P., Jones, S. G. & Shakespeare, P. G. (1990). Thermographic assessment of hand burns. *Burns,* **16**, 60–6.

Cryer, P. E. (1980). Physiology and pathology of the human sympathoadrenal neuroendocrine system. *New England Journal of Medicine,* **303**, 436–44.

Cunningham, J. J., Lydon, M. K. & Russell, W. E. (1990). Calorie and protein provision for recovery from severe burns in infants and young children. *American Journal of Nutrion,* **51**, 553–7.

Curreri, P. W., Richmond, D., Marvin, J. & Baxter, C. R. (1974). Dietary requirements of patients with major burns. *Journal of the American Dietetic Association,* **65**, 415–17.

Cuthbertson, D. P. (1942). Post shock metabolic response. *Lancet,* **1**, 433–7.

Davies, J. W. L. (1982). *Physiological Responses to Burning Injury,* pp. 424–529. London, Academic Press.

Davies, C. L., Newman, R. J., Molyneux, S. G. & Grahame-Smith, D. G. (1984). The relationship between plasma catecholamines and severity of injury in man. *Journal of Trauma,* **24**, 99–105.

Deitch, E. A. (1990). Intestinal permeability is increased in burn patients shortly after injury. *Surgery*, **107**, 411–16.

Deleplansque, B. & Neveu, P. J. (1994). Brain regions involved in modulation of immune responses. In *Brain Control of Responses to Trauma*, ed. N. J. Rothwell & F. Berkenbosch, pp. 108–22. Cambridge, Cambridge University Press.

Demling, R. H., Frye, E. & Read, T. (1991). Effect of sequential early burn wound excision and closure on postburn oxygen consumption. *Critical Care Medicine*, **19**, 861–6.

Dinarello, C. A. (1984). Interleukin-1. *Reviews of Infectious Disease*, **6**, 51–95.

Du Bois, E. (1924). *Basal Metabolism in Health and Disease*. New York, Lea and Febiger.

Enescu, D., Davidescu, I. & Enescu, M. (1994). Paediatric burns in Bucharest, Romania; 4327 cases over a 5-year period. *Burns*, **20**, 154–1565.

Fleck, A., Colley, C. M. & Myers, M. A. (1985). Liver export proteins and trauma. *British Medical Bulletin*, **41**, 265–73.

Frayn, K. N., Little, R. A., Maycock, P. & Stoner, H. B. (1985). The relationship of plasma catecholamines to acute metabolic and hormonal responses to injury in man. *Circulatory Shock*, **16**, 229–40.

Ganong, W. F. (1986). Neuroendocrine responses to injury. In *The Scientific Basis for the Care of the Critically Ill*, ed. R. A. Little & K. N. Frayn, pp. 61–73. Manchester University Press.

Gans, H. & Matsumoto, K. (1974). The escape of endotoxin from the intestine. *Surgery, Gynecology and Obstetrics*, **139**, 395–402.

Grotte, G., Meurling, S. & Retland, A. (1982). Parenteral nutrition. In *Textbook of Paediatric Nutrition*, vol. 2, 2nd edn, ed. D. McLaren & D. Burman, pp. 228–58. Edinburgh, Churchill Livingstone.

Hamberger, B., Farnebo, L.-O. & Liljedahl, S.-O. (1980). Plasma noradrenaline and dopamine in burn patients. *Burns*, **7**, 20–4.

Harrison, H. N., Moncrief, J. A., Duckett, J. W. & Mason, A. D. (1964). The relationship between energy metabolism and water loss from vaporization in severely burned patients. *Surgery*, **56**, 203–11.

Heath, D. F. (1994). Glucose, insulin and other plasma metabolites shortly after injury. *Journal of Accident and Emergency Medicine*, **11**, 67–77.

Henane, R., Bittel, J. & Bansillon, V. (1981). Partitional calorimetry measurements of energy exchange in severely burned patients. *Burns*, **7**, 180–9.

Hopkins, S. J. & Rothwell, N. J. (1995). Cytokines and the nervous system. 1. Expression and recognition. *Trends in Neuroscience*, **18**, 83–8.

Johnson, T. R., Moore, W. M. & Jeffries, J. E. (eds) (1978). *Children are Different: Developmental Physiology*, 2nd edn. Ohio, Ross Laboratories.

Kent, S., Bluthe, R.-M., Goodall, G., Kelley, K. W. & Dantzer, R. (1994). Central nervous system control of sickness behavior. In *Brain Control of Responses to Trauma*, ed. N. J. Rothwell & F. Berkenbosch, pp. 152–82. Cambridge, Cambridge University Press.

Kinsella, J. (1988). Smoke inhalation. *Burns*, **14**, 269–79.

Kiritsy, C. P. & Lynch, S. E. (1993). Role of growth factors in cutaneous wound healing. *Critical Reviews in Oral Biology and Medicine*, **4**, 729–60.

Kirkpatrick, J. R. (1987). The neuroendocrine response to injury and infection. *Nutrition*, **3**, 221–7.

Kispert, P. & Caldwell, M. D. (1990). Metabolic changes in sepsis and multiple organ failure. In *Multiple Organ Failure. Pathophysiology and Basic Concepts of Therapy*, ed. E. A. Deitch, pp. 104–25. New York, Thieme Medical Publishers.

Koenig, J. L. (1991). Presence of cytokines in the hypothalamic–pituitary axis. *Progress in NeuroEndocrinImmunology*, **4**, 143–53.

Lawrence, J. C. & Wilkins, M. D. (1986). The epidemiology of burns. In *Burncare – Proceedings of a teaching symposium arranged by the British Burn Association*, pp. 13–17. Hull, published by Smith and Nephew.

Le Quesne, L. P., Cochrane, J. P. S. & Fieldman, N. R. (1985). Fluid and electrolyte disturbance after trauma: the role adrenocortical and pituitary hormones. *British Medical Bulletin*, **41**, 212–17.

Lindblad, B. E. & Terkelsen, C. J. (1990). Domestic burns among children. *Burns*, **16**, 254–6.

Little, R. A. & Stoner, H. B. (1968). The measurement of heat loss from the rats' tail. *Quarterly Journal of Experimental Physiology*, **53**, 76–83.

Little, R. A., Frayn, K. N., Randall, P., Stoner, H. B. & Maycock, P. (1985). Plasma catecholamine concentrations in acute states of stress and trauma. *Archives of Emergency Medicine*, **2**, 46–52.

Marano, M. A., Fong, Y., Moldawer, L. L., Wei, H., Calvano, S. E., Tracy, K. J., Barie, P. S., Manogue, K., Cerami, A., Shires, G. T. & Lowry, S. F. (1990). Serum cachectin/tumor necrosis factor in critically ill patients with burns correlates with infection and mortality. *Surgery, Gynecology and Obstetrics*, **170**, 32–8.

Marcuson, R. W. (1991). Relationships between skin temperature and perfusion in the arm and leg. *Clinical Physiology*, **11**, 27–40.

McGuinness, K. & Childs, C. (1991). Development of an indirect calorimeter for use in infants and children. *Clinical Physics and Physiological Measurement*, **12**, 343–51.

Moir, G. C., Shakespeare, V. & Shakespeare, P. G. (1991). Audit of thermally injured children under 4 years of age. *Burns*, **17**, 406–10.

Moldawer, L. L., Gelin, J., Schersten, T. & Lundholm, K. G. (1987). Circulating interleukin-1 and tumor necrosis factor during inflammation. *American Journal of Physiology*, **253**, R922–R928.

Morgan, H. C., Andrews, R. P. & Jurkiewicz, M. J. (1955). The effect of thermal injury on insensible weight loss in the rat. *Surgical Forum*, **6**, 78–84.

Morimoto, A., Murakami, N., Nakorami, T. & Watanabe, T. (1988). Multiple control of fever production in the central nervous system of rabbits. *Journal of Physiology*, **397**, 269–80.

Muir, I. F. K., Barclay, T. L. & Settle, J. A. D. (1987). *Burns and Their Treatment*, pp. 14–54. London, Butterworth & Co (publishers) Ltd.

Nijsten, M. W. N., De Groot, E. R., Ten Duis, H. J., Klasen, H. J., Hack, C. E. & Aarden, L. A. (1987). Serum levels of Interleukin-6 and acute phase responses. *Lancet*, **2**, 921.

Parenteral and enteral nutrition group (PENG) of the British Dietetic Association (BDA). (1989). *Guide to Clinical Nutrition*. Abbot Laboratories.

Parish, R. N. & Webb, K. S. (1988). Hyperglycaemia is not a poor prognostic sign in head-injured children. *Journal of Trauma*, **28**, 517–19.

Pentelenyi, T., Kammerer, L., Peter, F. *et al.* (1979). Prognostic significance of the changes in carbohydrate metabolism in severe head injury. *Acta Neurochirurg.* Suppl. **28**, 103–7.

Pruitt, B. A. (1984). The diagnosis and treatment of infection in the burn patient. *Burns*, **11**, 79–91.

Ross, R. (1989). Platelet-derived growth factor. *Lancet*, **1**, 1179–82.

Rothwell, N. J. (1989). CRF is involved in the pyrogenic and thermogenic effects of interleukin 1β in the rat. *American Journal of Physiology*, **256** (*Endocrinol. Metab.* **19**): E111–E115.

Rothwell, N. J. & Hopkins, S. J. (1995). Cytokines and the nervous system. II. Actions and mechanisms of action. *Trends in Neurscience*, **18**, 130–6.

Ryan, C. A., Shankowsky, H. A. & Tredget, E. E. (1990). Profile of the paediatric burn patient in a Canadian burn centre. *Burns*, **18**, 267–2,

Salmon, J. A. & Higgs, G. A. (1987). Prostaglandins and leukotrienes as inflammatory mediators. *British Medical Bulletin*, **43**, 285–96.

Schlag, G. & Redl, H. (1990). Endothelium as the interface between blood and organ in the evolution of organ failure. In *Shock, Sepsis, and Organ Failure*, ed. G. Schlag, H. Redl & J. H. Siegel, pp. 210–77. Berlin, Springer-Verlag.

Shakespeare, P. G. (1992). Looking at burn wounds. The A. B. Wallace Memorial Lecture. *Burns*, **18**, 287–95.

Shakespeare, P. G., Ball, A. & Spurr, E. D. (1989). Serum protein changes after abdominal surgery. *Annals of Clinical Biochemistry*, **26**, 49–57.

Sinha, J. K., Mathur, A. K., Chansouria, J. P. N., Patel, V., Tripathi, F. M. & Udupa, K. (1980). Hormonal and associated metabolic alterations following burn injury: Part II. A comparative evaluation in surviving and non surviving patients. *Burns*, **7**, 16–19.

Smith, A. & McIntosh, N. (1994). Regulation of fluid and metabolic balance following thermal injury. *British Journal of Intensive Care*, **4**, 271–81.

Smith, R. W. & O'Neill, T. J. (1994). An analysis into childhood burns. *Burns*, **11**, 117–24.

Stoner, H. B. (1970). The acute effects of trauma on heat production. In *Energy Metabolism in Trauma*, ed. R. Porter & J. Knight, pp. 1–22. London, Churchill.

Stoner, H. B. (1972). Effect of injury on the responses to thermal stimulation of the hypothalamus. *Journal of Applied Physiology*, **33**, 665–71.

Stoner, H. B. (1973). The acute effects of trauma on heat production. In *Energy Metabolism in Trauma*, ed. R. Porter & J. Knight, pp. 1–22. London, Churchill.

Stoner, H. B. (1977). The role of catecholamines in the effects of trauma on thermoregulation, studies in rats treated with 6-hydroxydopamine. *British Journal of Experimental Pathology*, **58**, 42–9.

Stoner, H. B. (1986). A role for the central nervous system in the responses to trauma. In *The Scientific Basis for the Care of the Critically Ill*, ed. R. A. Little & K. N. Frayn, pp. 215–29. Manchester University Press.

Stoner, H. B., Barker, P., Riding, G. S. G., Hazelhurst, D. E., Taylor, L. & Marcuson, R. W. (1991). Relationships between skin temperature and perfusion in the arm and leg. *Clinical Physiology*, **11**, 27–40.

Taylor, F. H. L., Levenson, S. M. & Adams, M. A. (1944). Abnormal carbohydrate metabolism in human thermal burns. *New England Journal of Medicine*, **231**, 437–46.

Whicher, J. & Ingham, E. (1990). Cytokine measurement of body fluids. *European Cytokine Network*, **1**, 239–43.

Wilmore, D. W., Long, J. M., Mason, A. D., Skreen, R. W. & Pruitt, B. A. (1974). Catecholamines: mediator of the hypermetabolic response to thermal injury. *Annals of Surgery*, **180**, 653–69.

Wilmore, D. W., Mason, A. D., Johnson, D. W. & Pruitt, B. A. (1975). Effect of ambient temperature on heat production and heat loss in burn patients. *Journal of Applied Physiology*, **38**, 593–7.

Wilmore, D. W. (1977). *The Metabolic Management of the Critically Ill*, pp. 91–128. New York, Plenum Medical Book Co.

Wright, I. P., Griffiths, M. & Childs, C. (1995). A microprocessor based photoplethysmograph for use in clinical practice. *Anaesthesia*, **50**, 875–8.

Zawacki, B. E., Spitzer, K. W., Mason, A. D. & Johns, L. A. (1970). Does increased evaporative water loss cause hypermetabolism in burned patients? *Annals of Surgery*, **171**, 235–40.

Zweifach, B. W. (1986). Dynamic sequelae of the acute inflammatory process: a state-of-the-art review. In *The Scientific Basis for the Care of the Critically Ill*, ed. R. A. Little & K. N. Frayn, pp. 15–32. Manchester University Press.

Appendix

Brief outline of the treatment protocol for patients admitted to the Regional Paediatric Burns Unit, Manchester, UK.

Admissions: mainly urgent (with some late) referrals of patients up to age 16 years. Intensive nursing care for patients with burns equal to or more than 10% total body surface area (+ bsa).

Fluid resuscitation: initial colloid resuscitation with human albumin solution (HAS), replaced by fresh frozen plasma (FFP) when blood typed. Maintenance requirement given as 0.45% NaCl, 5% Dextrose. Fluid volume guided by Mount Vernon Formula*.

Analgesia and sedation: intravenous or oral analgesia initially with morphine sulphate IV, 0.2 mg/kg (oral 0.2 mg/kg for patients less than 12 months of age. For patients over the age of 12 months, IV morphine 0.3 mg/kg and Oromorph 0.2–0.5 mg/kg. Sedation with trimeprazine tartrate (Vallergan) 2 mg/kg.

Postoperatively, and with the exception of those patients with very small autografts, Patient Controlled Analgesia (PCA) with morphine sulphate.

Initial wound management: initial debridement of blisters followed by cleansing with 0.9% NaCl. For small burns (less than 10% tbsa) wounds treated with Mupiricin (Bactroban) and for those with more extensive burns, Betadine (Seton Health Care Group plc, Oldham, U.K.). Dressed with dry gauze and crepe bandages to give a semi-occlusive dressing.

Surgery: usually at about day three. Tangential excision for deep, partial thickness burns or radical excision for full thickness burns.

Ambient temperature: air temperature (dry bulb) maintained at approximately 30°C.

Nutrition: early enteral feeding with proprietary feed, starting within the first 12 hours after the accident. Calorie requirements during the first 2 days based on formula of actual measurements of oxygen consumption (an energy expenditure) in burned children.

13

Nutritional support of the severely burned child

M. J. MULLER and D. N. HERNDON

Introduction

Children and adolescents have gained the most from improvements in burn care. Modern techniques have made it unlikely that any child will succumb to burn injury even if it is associated with a significant smoke inhalation injury. Table 13.1 shows an increase in the size of burn associated with a 50% mortality from 49% body surface area (BSA) to 98% BSA. (Muller & Herndon, 1994). This remarkable achievement has been accomplished by the development of specialised burn centres, which in turn have fostered basic and clinical research. Appropriate fluid resuscitation has decreased early deaths from acute renal failure to a negligible level. Control of sepsis with early, total excision of full-thickness burn wounds combined with topical antimicrobial therapy and rapid wound closure has promoted survival. Prolonged survival unmasked a hypermetabolic, protein catabolic state that can be attenuated by appropriate nutritional support. This chapter describes the hypermetabolic response which follows injury; discusses the metabolic, wound healing and immunomodulating aspects of nutritional support of a severely injured child; and expands on pharmacological manipulations of the hypermetabolic response which allows better use to be made of provided nutrients.

Response to injury

The response to any injury is similar and varies only in its extent and duration. In this respect, burn is a good model of injury as the extent of injury is quantifiable and recovery is often delayed for many weeks, allowing investigation (Vaughan, et al., 1990). This prolonged state of critical illness leads to marked weight loss with accompanying reduction in wound healing and increased mortality (Newsome et al., 1973).

Table 13.1. *Burn size and associated mortality*

Age (years)	Burn size of expected 50% mortality	
	1942–52 (%BSA)	1983–93 (%BSA)
0–15	49	98
15–44	46	70

BSA: body surface area.
Source: Muller & Herndon (1994), Bull & Fisher (1954).

Weight loss of 30% was common among survivors of 40% BSA burns only 20 years ago. This was in spite of 'force-feeding' from hospital trays.

The site of injury stimulates an inflammatory response which, in the case of a burn, becomes generalised with greater than a 20% BSA burn. (Demling & Lalond, 1990b). Activated leucocytes produce and release histamine, thromboxanes and cytokines in sufficient quantity that serum levels become measurable and are elevated in direct proportion to the increasing burn size (Herndon, 1984; Kupper *et al.*, 1986; Drost, *et al.*, 1993a).

Cutaneous burn wounds have an increased xanthine oxidase activity which produce damaging oxygen radicals and hydrogen peroxide. In turn, hydroxyl ion release leads to distant organ lipid peroxidation and systemic inflammation. Malondialdehyde levels, an indicator of lipid peroxidation, are increased in the wound, serum and lung (Demling, 1990). Levels of naturally occurring antioxidants such as vitamin E are decreased because of consumption by both regional and systemic inflammation (Nguyen *et al.*, 1993).

The result of this tremendous outpouring of inflammatory mediators is to alter the thermoregulatory set-point in the hypothalamus and to drive a series of alterations in the hormonal and metabolic milieu (Hume & Egdahl 1959; Volenec, 1979; Herndon *et al.*, 1987b). The nervous system plays an important role in the stress response. The limbic system is activated by fear, emotion and thalamic relay of peripheral nociceptive stimuli and inflammatory mediators such as bacterial endotoxin, and various cytokines, such as interleukin 1 and tumor necrosis factor-alpha, stimulate the hypothalamus directly (Wilmore *et al.*, 1975; Dinarello *et al.*, 1986, 1988; Bentler & Cerami, 1987; Morimoto *et al.*, 1988; Michie & Wilmore, 1990). The central reset mechanism producing hyperthermia and the hormonal metabolic response results in elevation of the metabolic rate which can approach 200% of normal in severely burned subjects and has been verified experimentally in a rat burn model with manipulation of the preoptic anterior hypothalamus (Caldwell *et al.*, 1994). Increased substrate cycling contributes to increased thermogenesis and metabolic rate and is under beta-adrenergic control (Wolfe et al., 1990). Greatly increased adrenergic activity is a feature of the stress response.

Hormonal activity

While inflammatory mediators initiate and maintain the stress response, altered hormonal activity drives the thermogenic metabolic response and is certainly responsible for maintenance of a hyperdynamic circulatory response which is, of itself, thermogenic. Catecholamines, along with cortisol and glucagon, are characterised as the stress hormones. They are all elevated following injury and all have synergistic effects (Herndon et al., 1977; Shamoon et al., 1981). Catecholamine levels are raised two to tenfold, directly proportional to burn size (Wimore, 1980; Ziegler et al., 1990). A close correlation exists between the increase in plasma catecholamines and metabolic rate (Wilmore et al., 1974a). Catecholamine levels remain elevated until wound repair is complete. Catecholamines, via alpha, beta-1 and beta-2 adrenoreceptors, accelerate hepatic gluconeogenesis, hepatic glycogenolysis, adipocyte lipolysis, (beta-2) and muscle proteolysis (Herndon et al., 1994). The power of this effect is sufficient to maintain blood glucose levels at or above normal values, even if a patient is fasting. Substrate availability for gluconeogenesis (glycerol, pyruvate, lactate, alanine) is also increased. This increase in sympathomimetic activity is accompanied by a proportional decrease in thyroid hormone levels. Control of metabolic rate shifts from the thyroid axis to the sympathoadrenal axis (Herndon et al., 1977). Free thyronine (T_4) and free 3, 5, 3' tri-iodothyronine (T_3) serum levels decrease while levels of reverse T_3, an inactive metabolite, increase (Becker et al., 1983). Plasma norepinephrine (noradrenaline) and epinephrine (adrenaline) are correlated negatively with T_3 while plasma catecholamine levels are correlated positively with T_3 levels. This syndrome of hypermetabolic, low T_3 of burn injury is similar to other states of critical illness and is also known as the sick euthyroid syndrome (Becker et al., 1980, 1982; Aun et al., 1983). The thyroid remains responsive to thyroid stimulating hormone (TSH), whose levels are also diminished. Glucagon production is elevated in burned patients subsequent to adrenergic stimulation of pancreatic alpha cells. Levels are raised to two to four times normal values. Glucagon promotes gluconeogenesis, glycogenolysis, lipolysis and ketogenesis in the liver. Continued adrenergic stimulation of glucagon prevents suppression of its release during subsequent hyperglycemia (Vaughan et al., 1985). Glucagon and catecholamines synergise to promote gluconeogenesis. If they are infused together into normal subjects, gluconeogenesis is more prolonged than if they are infused alone (Shamoon et al., 1981).

Cortisol facilitates the action of catecholamines and helps maintain cardiovascular stability during stress. It synergises with catecholamines and glucagon so as to divert glucose utilisation from skeletal muscle to central organs such as the brain. Cortisol stimulates gluconeogenesis, increases proteolysis and alanine synthesis, sensitises adipocytes to the action of lipolytic hormones (catecholamines), and has an anti-inflammatory action. It also causes insulin resistance. The net result is to increase glucose production and promote proteolysis and lipolysis. Post-injury hyperglycaemia is usually proportional to the degree of insult (Wolfe *et al.*, 1970; Long *et al.*, 1971).

Substrate metabolism: substrate cycling

A substrate cycle exists when opposing, non-equilibrium reactions catalysed by different enzymes are active simultaneously (Newsholme & Crabtree, 1976). Substrate cycling involves the use of high-energy phosphate bonds in ATP, with the net result being the production of heat. There is no change in the amount of either the substrate or the product, but energy expenditure is increased in order to re-synthesise ATP. This process is therefore known as futile or wasteful substrate cycling. One such example is a glucose-lactate-glucose metabolic sequence known as the Cori cycle. Burned extremities metabolise a large amount of glucose to lactate and pyruvate (Wilmore *et al.*, 1977). The inflammatory cells in burn wounds (leucocytes and fibroblasts) primarily metabolise glucose in an anaerobic fashion for energy generation (Im & Hoops, 1979). The anaerobic metabolites of glucose (lactate and pyruvate) are then returned to the liver along with gluconeogenic amino acids which are released from muscle tissue for the synthesis of additional glucose. Burned patients have a significant rate of hepatic uptake of lactate and pyruvate, which have been generated from anaerobic metabolism of glucose peripherally. From these substrates, the liver synthesises glucose which is then reutilised as an energy source by the leucocytes and fibroblasts in the burn wound (Falcone & Caldwell, 1990). Thus, burned patients have an accelerated Cori cycle in which glucose is synthesised by the liver and metabolised through anaerobic metabolism by the various cells present in a burn wound.

Burned patients require large amounts of glucose to avoid excessive protein catabolism; however, burned patients begin to develop difficulties in metabolising glucose when the rate of infusion exceeds 4 mg/kg per minute (Wolfe *et al.*, 1987b). Lipid and protein are then utilised to meet the remaining metabolic requirements (Jahoor *et al.*, 1989). The stress response causes increased lipolytic activity and results in elevated serum levels of free fatty acids and glycerol and a decreased rate of ketogenesis (Harris *et al.*, 1982; Abbot *et al.*, 1985; Wolfe *et al.*, 1987a). As ketone bodies are one of the primary energy sources utilised to decrease protein catabolism, it follows that burned patients may require increased amounts of carbohydrate and protein in their diet to prevent protein catabolism and achieve a positive nitrogen balance (Shaw & Wolfe, 1989). The metabolism of fatty acids by the cyclooxygenase enzyme system is significantly increased in burned patients.

Protein breakdown and synthesis rates are both elevated following burn injury, but the rate of protein breakdown is elevated in excess of protein synthesis and results in net protein/nitrogen loss (Jahoor *et al.*, 1988). There is increased efflux of amino acids, especially alanine, glutamine and phenylalanine, from muscle following a burn injury (Herndon *et al.*, 1978; Aulick & Wilmore, 1979; Stinnett *et al.*, 1982). Alanine efflux occurs from muscle tissue distant from the site of a burn injury (an unburned limb) indicating a generalised response (Herndon *et al.*, 1978). The branched-chain amino acids, valine, leucine and isoleucine, supply nitrogen for transamination of pyruvate in order to produce alanine which is subsequently utilised for glucose production. Glutamate is converted to glutamine by the action of glutamine synthetase before conversion to alanine and ammonia in the gut mucosa. Alanine is transported to the liver for gluconeogenesis and ammonia is converted to urea and subsequently excreted in the urine (Stinnett *et al.*, 1982; Birkhahn *et al.*, 1987; Jahoor *et al.*, 1990).

Nutritional requirements

Caloric intake can be estimated and provided with formulae based on retrospective analysis of maintenance of body weight or by measurement of metabolic rate using indirect calorimetry. Accurate provision of calories is important. Overfeeding leads to respiratory failure from excess CO_2 production, hepatic steatosis, increased blood urea nitrogen which worsens renal failure, and promotion of hypermetabolism. Underfeeding causes increased loss of lean body mass, muscle wasting, poor wound healing and susceptibility to infection.

Total energy expenditure (TEE) is made up of basal metabolism, resting energy expenditure, diet-induced thermogenesis and energy consumed by muscular activity. In burned patients, anxiety, futile substrate cycling, shivering and pain all increase total energy expenditure. Direct calorimetry measures actual heat elaborated when a subject is placed in a sealed, insulated chamber. Indirect calorimetry uses the stoichiometric relation between oxygen consumption and carbon dioxide production during respiratory gas exchange analysis. Indirect calorimetry can be performed as a bedside procedure with a mobile metabolic cart which measures the volume of gas expired and the concentration of oxygen and carbon dioxide of inspired and expired gas (Westenskow *et al.*, 1984). Oxygen consumption and carbon dioxide production are estimated and equations calculated to give measured resting energy expenditure (Turner *et al.*, 1985). Obviously, measurements should be performed in the resting state (at least 1 hour following activity) and in the same absorptive state. If performed in a postabsorptive state, basal metabolic rate or basal energy expenditure is measured. As many burned patients undergo continuous feeding, a measurement taken during this process also accounts for the thermic effect of food and is known as measured resting energy expenditure (MREE). The metbolism of different substrates gives known ratios of carbon dioxide production to oxygen consumption. This ratio is known as the respiratory quotient (RQ). Fat oxidation produces an RQ of 0.7 while glucose oxidation gives an RQ of 1.0. A respiratory quotient of greater than 1.0 indicates net fat synthesis. This can occur with overnutrition and leads to hepatic steatosis (Wolfe *et al.*, 1980). Alternatively, low RQ readings indicate inadequate nutrition (Saffle *et al.*, 1985).

Extrapolation of measured resting energy expenditure to total energy expenditure over 24 hours requires multiplication by an activity factor. Total energy expenditure can be quantified with the doubly-labelled water technique which involves the infusion of two stable isotopes of water: $H_2^{18}O$ and ^2H_2O. ^2H_2O is lost from the body at a rate proportional to water flux alone while $H_2^{18}O$ is lost in water and in CO_2 during rapid equilibration through carbonic anhydrase. The difference in turnover rates gives total CO_2 production and total energy expenditure can be calculated if dietary intake is known. Application of this technique in severely burned children during convalescence revealed that total energy expenditure exceeded measured resting energy expenditure by a factor of $1.18 + 0.17$ ($r^2 = 0.92$) (Goran *et al.*, 1990). Analysis of the determinants of measured resting energy expenditure has shown that for predicted basal energy expenditure (PBEE) derived from the Harris–Benedict equation, total body surface area and weight are the most important predictors (Harris & Benedict, 1919). Burn size and time after burn accounted for smaller increments, 24% and 21%, respectively, of the measured over predicted energy expenditure (Goran *et al.*, 1991). The following equation will predict the energy required to ensure that 95% of burned children will receive sufficient calories to reach a state of energy balance:

$$TEE = (1.55 \times PBEE) + (2.39 \times OBEE \ 0.75).$$

In most cases, this is close to: $TEE = 2 \times PBEE$.

As this formula will provide excess calories to half the patients, indirect calorimetry is needed to evaluate individual requirements. Indirect calorimetry represents the most reliable method of estimating energy requirements, if performed often and in a similar state. Measured resting energy expenditure multiplied by an activity factor of 1.2 to 1.3 will provide appropriately for the majority of patients (Gore *et al.*, 1990). Although mobile metabolic carts are the ideal, they require a sizable financial outlay initially and a trained technician to use and maintain them. Also, when using indirect calorimetry, two factors should be considered: energy expenditure may be less than energy requirement if malabsorption or diarrhoea is present and indirect calorimetry loses accuracy at $FiO_2 > 0.6$ or if gas leak occurs.

Many burn units will depend on feeding formulae to calculate requirements. These formulae have been derived from retrospective analyses of dietary intake which was associated with the maintenance of body weight averaged over hospital stay. The Curreri formula, long used for adult patients, is based on only nine patients receiving parenteral nutrition over the first 20 days of recovery. In fact, the only patient in the group who lost weight received only 20% of requirements while weight was maintained in the other patients whose energy intake was significantly less than that prescribed by the formula. Therefore, it too commonly overestimates energy requirements. The formulae depicted in Table 13.2 are based on body surface area and have been shown to maintain body weight to within 5% of pre-burn values (Curreri *et al.*, 1974; Hildreth & Carvajal, 1982; Hildreth *et al.*, 1980, 1982, 1988, 1990, 1993).

It has been shown that resting energy expenditure rarely exceeds predicted basal metabolic rate (Harris–Benedict) by more than 50% in patients with burns of more than 45% if treated with occlusive dressings and modern techniques (Rutan, 1986). This indicates that an injury factor less than that previously used in some predictive formulae is more appropriate (Table 13.3).

Enteral nutrition

Ischaemic mucosal erosions are seen in the stomach and duodenum within hours of significant burn injury and are most likely present throughout the gut (Czaja *et al.*, 1974). An ileus results but is limited by reperfusion with adequate fluid resuscitation and early enteral feeding. A transgastric jejunal tube, per nasal or percutaneous, advanced past the ligament of Trietz under fluoroscopy, allows enteral feeding to commence well before gastroduodenal function is restored and seems to diminish the extent and duration of ileus (Mass, 1981).

Experimental models have shown attenuation of catecholamine elaboration and maintenance of gut mucosal integrity with immediate enteral, but not parenteral, nutrition. Other studies have shown that when continuous enteral tube feedings were started immediately following burn injury, the postburn hypermetabolic response was prevented and elevations of serum of glucagon, cortisol and catecholamines failed to develop (Mochizuki *et al.*, 1985; Saito *et al.*, 1987b). Intestinal permeability, as assessed by lactulose-mannitol absorption and polyethylene glycol (Ryan *et al.*, 1992), is increased in a burn size dependent fashion early after injury. Thereafter, supervening infection will again induce increased intestinal permeability (Ziegler *et al.*, 1988; Levoyer *et al.*, 1992). Passage of these macromolecules implies that bacterial translocation or leak of endotoxin can occur (Demling, 1992; Munster *et al.*, 1993).

Certainly, burn size-dependent increases in levels of circulating endotoxin and cytokines, such as IL-1, TBF, and IL-6, occur postburn, and these may originate from

Table 13.2. *Predictive formulae for caloric requirement of burned children*

Age (years)	Maintenance TBSA (Kcal/m²/day)	Plus	Burn requirement BSA burned (Kcal/m²/day)
12–18	1500	+	1500
1–12	1800	+	1300
< 1	2100	+	1000

TBSA: body surface area (m²); BSA burned; body surface area burned.
N.B. Caloric requirement may plateau at 50–60% BSA burned hence the importance of indirect calorimetry.

Table 13.3. *Estimating caloric requirements*

- Formulae based on body surface area are appropriate for children
- Injury factor is approximately 1.5
- Indirect calorimetry vital for infants and those with massive injuries
- TEE = MREE × 1.25 (MREE includes thermic energy of food)

the gut (Winchurch *et al.*, 1987; Drost, 1993a,b). Animals which received immediate enteral feeding did not develop gut mucosal atrophy, while it did develop in a comparative group whose enteral feeding was delayed. Gut mucosal atrophy allows translocation of bacteria and endotoxin into the portal circulation. Endotoxin transport across the gut has been shown to be enhanced in parenterally fed animals compared with chow-fed controls (Gonella *et al.*, 1992; Herndon & Zeigler, 1993). Postburn ileus affects the stomach and colon, sparing the small bowel (Tinckler, 1965). Therefore, duodenal or jejunal tube feeding can be commenced early in the postburn period. Immediate intragastric feeding in a clinical trial was associated with only a 3% daily incidence of vomiting, no aspiration pneumonia and delivery of calculated needs by the third postburn day; it is therefore suitable for those with burns of moderate size (McDonald *et al.*, 1991).

Enteral feeding is far preferable to total parenteral nutrition in the critically ill, burned patient (Moore *et al.*, 1992). Parenteral supplementation in severely burned children increased mortality *three-fold* and decreased the amount of enteral calories tolerated (Herndon *et al.*, 1987b, 1989).

Nutritional modulation of postburn response

Lipids

Cyclooxygenase activity leads to an increased rate of production of the physiologically active prostaglandins which have immunosuppressive activity. One means of limiting this effect is to supply dietary lipids as omega-3 fatty acids which are metabolised by the cyclooxygenase enzyme system to yield PGE-3. The more common dietary fatty acids are of the omega-6 group and are metabolised to yield PGE-1 and PGE-2. PGE-1 and PGE-2 have been reported to have significant immunosuppressive properties, while PGE-3 has been reported to be immunologically inert. It has therefore been hypothesised that by replacing the omega-6 fatty acids obtained from standard vegetable and animal oils with the omega-3 fatty acids from fish oil, postburn immunosuppression might be avoided or reversed (Alexander & Gottschlich, 1990).

Protein

Protein availability is essential for adequate wound healing. Protein malnutrition is associated with a decreased rate in gain of strength of skin, incisions, abdominal wounds and intestinal anastomoses. More specifically, a shortage of protein blunts fibroblastic proliferation, neoangiogenesis, collagen synthesis and wound remodelling (Ruberg, 1984; Zaizen *et al.*, 1990). It is therefore essential that negative nitrogen balance be avoided. The ideal amount of protein which should be provided in the diet of burned patients has not yet been determined. Increasing protein intake in burned patients from 1.4 g protein/kg per day to 2.2 g protein/kg per day did not alter the nitrogen balance (Wolfe *et al.*, 1983). Another study showed that increasing the percentage of protein in the diet of burned patients resulted in a number of immunological benefits. They compared patients receiving 16.5% of their calories as protein to those receiving 23% of their calories as protein. Although neither group was able to achieve the desired caloric intake, the group receiving the higher protein content was found to have significantly higher serum levels of IgG, transferrin and complement factor 3. More important, they experienced fewer bacteraemic days and had a significantly lower mortality rate (Alexander *et al.*, 1980).

Amino acids

Arginine is an integral substrate of the urea cycle and is not considered an essential amino acid; however, under periods of severe stress it is thought to become an essential dietary nutrient. An experimental deficiency of arginine in the traumatised rat produced decreased collagen deposition and decreased wound breaking strength (Nirgiotis *et al.*, 1991). Arginine is not only important to wound healing when deficient, it also appears to promote wound healing when given as a supplement. High arginine levels were shown to improve wound healing in rats as demonstrated by increased collagen deposition and increased wound breaking strength. In healthy humans, it was shown to increase the deposition of total protein and hydroxyproline (an indicator of collagen content) into wound cylinders. Supplemental arginine has also been shown to decrease skin weight loss under stress, therefore retaining more dermal protein for wound healing. It also promotes retention of nitrogenous calories and decreased protein catabolism. Arginine appears to achieve most of its stimulatory action second-arily via the hypothalamic–pituitary axis as a secretagogue of insulin, glucagon, prolactin and growth hormone as these effects are absent in hypophysectomised rats. In support of these mechanisms, arginine supplementation appears to be most effective in the first 3 days of wound healing, the period of inflammation and fibroblast migration and activation. On the cellular level, there has been demonstrated an altered metabolism of arginine in wounded tissues. Although arginase is present in fibroblasts only in very low levels, its presence is significant in macrophages and in extracellular wound fluid, presumably released from dying macrophages.

Arginase catalyses the conversion of arginine to ornithine which is a precursor to proline, a collagen precursor. Arginine supplementation in an experimental burn model and in postsurgical cancer patients improved the indices of immune function (Saito *et al.*, 1987b; Daly *et al.*, 1988). In this fashion, supplemental arginine may directly enhance collagen production in the wound (Barbul & Regan, 1993; Barbul *et al.*, 1985, 1990; Albina *et al.*, 1988; Saito *et al.*,1987b; Kirk, 1990).

Glutamine is an amino acid thought to play an integral role in wound healing. It is known to be utilised in substantial amounts by macrophage metabolism (Caldwell, 1989). Glutamine is considered to be a major fuel of rapidly dividing cells, such as fibroblasts, enterocytes and stimulated lymphocytes (Donnelly & Scheffer, 1976; Dud-rick *et al.*, 1993). Cultures of fibroblasts require more glutamine to survive than any other amino acid and the glutamine metabolised is primarily oxidised to carbon dioxide to provide a source of energy (Griffiths, 1970). Fibroblasts may even derive more energy from glutamine metabolism than from glucose (Reitzer *et al.*, 1979).

Glutamine is also important in the production of collagen because glutamate, a primary metabolite of glutamine, is the primary precursor to proline in pure fibro-blasts cultures. Glutamine is the preferred fuel of the small bowel enterocyte (Souba *et al.*, 1985). Sepsis has been shown to decrease glutamine uptake by the small bowel enterocyte which may result in barrier failure (Souba *et al.*, 1990) and the addition of glutamine to the nutritional regimen has been theorised to improve barrier function. Methionine and cysteine have important roles in antioxidant production. Sulphydryl groups produced directly from cysteine, or indirectly from methionine, act as oxygen radical scavengers. Cysteine and glutamine form glutathione, which is a strong sulphydryl reducing substance and is required in the synthesis of the leukotriene. Their presence is therefore required to limit lipid peroxidation (Linder *et al.*, 1993a).

Vitamins

Vitamins and trace elements play key roles in wound healing, which is the ultimate goal in the management of severely injured children.

Scurvy is characterised by weakening and dehiscence of previously healed wounds. Supplemental ascorbic acid delivery has been demonstrated to have two complementary effects on healing. Within the first 24 hours, there is a reduction in the degradation of intracellular collagen; and after 24 hours, supplementation increases the synthesis of collagen protein and favours its release into the extracellular medium (Anderson, 1977; Sengupta & Deb, 1978; Lacroix *et al.*, 1988).

Vitamin A has been shown to affect cell morphology and epithelial cell differentiation. Vitamin A binds to specific intracellular receptor proteins which carry the vitamin to the nucleus where it affects the gene expression of glycosyltransferases, fibronectin, and perhaps even transglutaminases (Goodson & Hunt, 1988). It also appears necessary as a cofactor in collagen synthesis and crosslinking. T lymphocyte function is enhanced by vitamin A (Barbul & Regan, 1993). Supplemental vitamin A also increases fibroplasia and collagen accumulation in wounds and increases the differentiation rate of fibroblasts (Demetriou *et al.*, 1985).

Vitamin E is an antioxidant and free radical scavenger which appears to act in preventing the oxidation of cell membrane polyunsaturated phospholipids (Maderazo *et al.*, 1990; Hinder & Stein, 1991). It is a promising means of counteracting the oxidative changes induced by systemic inflammation. As vitamin E levels are decreased in burned children, supplementation is most appealing.

The B vitamin group is central to the metabolism of all cells because they are coenzymes in reactions which are necessary for energy metabolism. Riboflavin is a coenzyme in oxidation–reduction reactions involved in fatty acids synthesis and oxidation, amino acid oxidation, electron transport, xanthine oxidase function and glutathione reductase function (Lakshmi *et al.*, 1989). Pantothenic acid functions as part of coenzyme-A and phosphopantheine involved in the Krebs cycle and in β-oxidation of fatty acids. It also appears to play an important role in collagen production by the wound. Alone, it has been shown to increase skin strength and the fibroblastic content of scar tissue (Grenier *et al.*, 1982).

Zinc oxide has been used in surgical dressings for a long time. Zinc deficiency impairs the rate of epithelialisation and lessens the gain in wound strength through impaired amino acid utilisation (Prasad, 1986). A hypercatabolic state induces hyperzincuria which can progress to zinc depletion (Larson *et al.*, 1970). In addition to substantial urinary loss, a redistribution of zinc occurs after tissue injury and surgical stress. Zinc uptake is increaseed in the wound, liver, spleen and lung while zinc levels decrease in plasma and skin (Okada *et al.*, 1990; Linder, 1991). Zinc supplementation has not been shown to accelerate wound healing in non-burned, normozinc subjects (Barcia, 1970). Injured children have substantial sequestration of zinc into the wound as well as high urinary losses and should benefit from zinc supplementation.

Selenium has an influence on wound healing through its presence in selenium-dependent glutathione peroxidase (Linder, 1991). This enzyme protects the cell from oxidative damage by catalysing the reduction of hydrogen peroxide. Selenium deficiency may also affect wound healing by altering macrophage and polymorphonuclear cell function. A state of selenium deficiency often occurs in burned patients and is thought to be secondary to silver therapy (Boosalis *et al.*, 1986).

Too little is known of the appropriate degree of vitamin supplementation; however, children and adolescents who have suffered major burns should receive a B group multivitamin, ascorbic acid 500 mg, vitamin A 10 000 IU, and vitamin E 10 mg daily. Infants should receive half these amounts. It is preferable to deliver these supplements as part of the enteral feed in suspension in order to decrease gastrointestinal upset (Gottschlich & Warden, 1990).

Nutrient utilisation

Recombinant growth factors

Transmembrane amino acid transport has been shown to be decreased in burned patients (Biolo *et al.*, 1993). This may explain, in part, the relative inability of increased amino acid availability to completely reverse net protein catabolism in trauma patients whereas, in normal subjects, hyperaminoacidaemia is a potent stimulus to net protein synthesis (Wolfe *et al.*, 1983; Tessari *et al.*, 1987). It may be that increased cytokine levels, especially tumor necrosis factor and interleukin 1 or endotoxemia, may have a direct effect upon amino acid transport at the cell membrane. Certainly, intrinsic anabolic growth factor levels are decreased and this may have a direct permissive role (Jeffries & Vance, 1992). Both recombinant growth hormone and insulin-like growth factor-1 (IGF-1) increase transmembrane amino acid transport *in vitro* (Kostyo, 1968; Shorwell *et al.*, 1983; Goldstain *et al.*, 1989). Growth hormone (GH) enhanced wound healing in protein malnourished, glucocorticoid-induced protein catabolic rats (Jorgensen & Andreassen, 1988; Atkinson *et al.*, 1992).

GH promotes protein synthesis by increasing the cellular uptake of amino acids and accelerating nucleic acid translation and transcription, thereby enhancing cell proliferation. Fatty acids are released from the hydrolysis of fat for conversion to acetyl Co-A, an essential energy producing molecule for the tricarboxylic acid cycle. Through the

Table 13.4. *Donor site healing times (days)*

	First	Second	Third
Placebo	9.0 ± 0.4	9.0 ± 0.7	8.0 ± 1.0
GH	7.0 ± 0.5*	6.0 ± 0.4	6.0 ± 1.0

Data presented as mean ± SEM.
Source: Herndon *et al.* (1990).

Table 13.5. *Donor site healing times in infants and children presenting late for treatment*

	n	Age (years)	TBSA (% burns)	Healing times (days)
rhGH < 2 years	9	9.4 ± 0.2	56 ± 5	6.0 ± 0.4
rhGH: late	6	5.2 ± 1.2	57 ± 7	6.0 ± 0.7
Control	26	8.4 ± 0.9	67 ± 3	8.5 ± 0.5

Data presented at mean ± SEM.
Source: Gilpin *et al.* (1994).

preferential use of adipose tissue for energy production, there is a decrease in body fat with the result that protein is spared from catabolism (Van Vlient *et al.*, 1987). GH treatment of obese dieters allowed lean body mass conservation at the expense of adipose stores (Clemmons *et al.*, 1987).

GH seems to have a more marked anabolic action in those whose protein balance is catabolic. No improvement in muscle mass or strength was detected in young adults undergoing exercise training while non-trained subjects showed improved net protein balance through an increased rate of whole-body protein synthesis with no change in protein degradation (Yarasheski, 1993). Furthermore, the protein catabolic effect of prednisone, a glucocorticoid, was prevented by the concomitant administration of GH (Horber & Haymond, 1990).

Injury, especially burn injury, is well known to induce an accelerated rate of protein breakdown with a concomitant failure to increase synthesis sufficiently to compensate (Wolfe *et al.*, 1989). GH anabolic action appears to be primarily mediated by an increase of protein synthesis. Brachial artery infusion of GH in both normal and postoperative patients revealed a direct effect of GH on skeletal muscle (Fryburg *et al.*, 1991; Mjaaland *et al.*, 1993). GH also acts in a stimulation of insulin-like growth factor synthesis. GH administration increases IGF-1 blood concentration via increased IGF-1 production by the liver (Daughaday *et al.*, 1987). GH also increases IGF-1 production in other tissues, such as skeletal muscle and cartilage, where IGF-1 may exert an autocrine/paracrine action.

Clinical trials of recombinant growth hormone have revealed potent, protein anabolic effects. Amino acid efflux was decreased from the forearms of patients after having undergone abdominal surgery (Mjaaland *et al.*, 1993). The beneficial metabolic effects of growth hormone in adult burned patients have been known for some time (Soroff *et al.*, 1960, 1967; Liljadahl *et al.*, 1961; Wilmore *et al.*, 1974b). Increased availability of the recombinant product has allowed its remarkable metabolic and wound healing properties in children to be fully explored.

A group of severely burned adolescents, mean burn size of 70% BSA, underwent isolated limb and whole body stable isotope assessment with N^{15}lysine and indocyanine green (Gore *et al.*, 1991b). GH treatment (0.2 mg/kg) raised leg blood flow significantly from 1.7 ± 0.1 l/min per 100 ml leg volume/mean $\pm$ SEM to 2.7 ± 0.3. This increase in peripheral blood flow did not cause an increase in cardiac index which was raised equally in both groups to twice the normal range. Urinary nitrogen excretion was also decreased. A hyperinsulinaemic, euglycaemic, eukalaemic clamp showed a decrease in net protein breakdown in control groups but no further benefit in the GH group. Furthermore, a 30-fold increase in GH and a threefold increase in IGF-1 serum levels were noted with no change in insulin, glucagon or cortisol levels. Overall, GH treatment resulted in a 50% reduction in protein loss.

Carbohydrate metabolism in burned children is significantly affected by GH treatment. Severely burned adolescents were given GH (0.2 mg/kg per day) or placebo in blinded fashion (Gore *et al.*, 1991a). All were hypermetabolic at 140% predicted resting energy expenditure. A euglycaemic hyperinsulinaemic clamp showed a significant reduction in glucose uptake and inhibition of glucose oxidation in the GH group. Glucose utilisation (percentage glucose uptake oxidised) in both patient groups remained similar. This implies that GH induces an insulin resistance by inhibiting glucose transport. As counter-regulation, plasma levels of insulin then increase to maintain euglycaemia. Clinically, about one-third of patients treated with GH require therapeutic insulin for 2–3 days, after which time borderline hyperglycaemia persists but not at a level requiring insulin.

These profound metabolic effects result in greatly enhanced wound healing in massively burned children. The rate limiting step in closing a burn wound in children whose injury is extensive is donor-site wound healing. Skin is a target tissue for GH, either indirectly via circulating insulin-like growth factor-1 (IGF-1) or directly by GH interaction with specific receptors on the surface of epidermal and dermal cells (Tavakkol *et al.*, 1992). GH treatment of the severely burned improves wound healing dramatically if the dose is sufficient. A dose of 0.2 mg/kg per day, but not 0.1 mg/kg per day, accelerated skin graft donor site wound healing by 25% in children with a mean burn size of 60% BSA. The significance of these results was that these massively burned children could be taken to the operating room for further skin grafting about 2 days earlier if treated with GH. The overall time to totally close the burn wound was reduced from 46 to 32 days for those with the mean burn size for the group of 60% BSA. Alternatively, the treated group took 0.54 ± 0.04 D/% TBSA (mean $\pm$ SD) and the placebo group to 0.80 ± 0.09 days/% BSA to achieve total wound closure (Herndon *et al.*, 1990).

Infants less than 2 years of age showed the same beneficial effects of rhGH as those who were older, without adverse effect. Also, patients presenting 2 or 3 weeks after injury, who were all in poor condition and looked cachectic from sepsis, hypermetbolism, and inadequate nutrition were noted to have donor site healing times of about 7 days. This is remarkable in patients so nutritionally and metabolically disadvantaged (Gilpin *et al.*, 1994).

The effect of GH on burned children is profound and beneficial. Protein anabolism is induced in the most ill patients. Wound healing is accelerated by about 25% and has sped wound closure by weeks in those with massive burns. An overall cost saving of 18% is achieved in this group due to the large decrease in intensive care days and overall length of stay (Rutan & Herndon, 1994).

Insulin-like growth factor-1

Growth hormone acts both directly and indirectly via IGF-1 production in the liver and elsewhere (Chwans & Bistrian, 1991; Boulivare *et al.*, 1992). IGF-1 serum levels are decreased in burned patients (Moller *et al.*, 1991). This is consistent with the observation that hepatic IGF-1 secretion is directly impaired despite normal pituitary GH secretion in many disease states and that simultaneous use of GH and IGF-1 gives enhanced anabolic effects in normal humans (Dahn *et al.*, 1988; Kupfer *et al.*, 1993).

The IGF-1 response to GH treatment is attenuated with increasing severity of injury (Kimbrough *et al.*, 1991). These facts have led to speculation that IGF-1 alone, or in combination with GH, may achieve better results, particularly in malnourished, septic, burned patients. Early animal work has been most encouraging. Fifty per cent scald-burned rats were given 1 mg/day of IGF-1 or placebo via osmotic pumps implanted subcutaneously (Strock *et al.*, 1990). The pump capacities allowed for evaluation of IGF-1 effects over a 14-day study period. It was noted that circulating IGF-1 levels were significantly decreased in untreated animals following thermal injury compared with unburned controls. IGF-1 treated animals showed IGF-1 levels which had been restored to levels similar to unburned controls. The metabolic rates (estimated by oxygen consumption) of burned animals treated with IGF-1 were comparable to those of the unburned (sham) control group, while placebo treated burned rats had significantly elevated metabolic rates, i.e. postburn hypermetabolism was completely obviated with this treatment. Using the same model, small intestinal mucosal DNA and protein content, gut mucosal weight, splenic weight and body weight were increased with 3 mg/kg per day IGF-1. Additionally, the IGF-1 treated rats had a decrease in the usual postburn hyperglycaemia, a positive nitrogen balance, and increased weight gain for 5 days. The incidence of bacterial translocation to the mesenteric lymph nodes was reduced from 90% to 30% as gut mucosal function was improved (Huang *et al.*, 1993).

Beta-adrenergic-receptor agents

Tachycardia of 120–150 beats per minute is often sustained for many weeks in massively burned patients, and cardiac dysfunction commonly contributes to mortality with myocarditis, cardiomyopathy and focal myocardial infarcts often found at autopsy (Joshi, 1970; Linares, 1988). These findings are similar to those found in patients who succumb to other hypercatecholamine states such as phaeochromocytoma. The hyperdynamic circulatory response to burn injury is stimulated by 10-fold increases in catecholamines which play a significant role in increasing energy expenditure. Adrenergic blockade had been used with success in pathological hypercatecholamine states and thyrotoxicosis by decreasing myocardial work load, whole-body irritability and tremulousness (Gelfland *et al.*, 1987).

Catecholamines also stimulate lipolysis in burned patients (Wolfe *et al.*, 1982, 1987a). Acute administration of beta-blocking agents precipitously decreases the rate of release or appearance of free fatty acids (FFA) in plasma, indicating the important role that pre-existing sympathetic activity plays in the mobilization of FFA. Chronic catecholamine blockade could, therefore, indirectly increase protein catabolism, as FFA are a primary endogenous energy substrate. The concern that adrenergic blockade could have a detrimental metabolic effect has been amplified by the notion that catecholamines may have a direct protein anabolic effect (Garder *et al.*, 1976; Miles *et al.*, 1984; Keller *et al.*, 1987).

Wilmore examined adrenergic blockade in exposed patients with alpha, beta, and combined alpha and beta blockade (Wilmore *et al.*, 1974a). Alpha blockade alone did not change metabolic rate; however, significant decreases were seen with combined alpha and beta blockade and with beta blockade alone. The decrease in metabolic rate was associated with a decrease in pulse rate, blood pressure, minute ventilation and free fatty acids. Larger than normal doses were required to obtain adequate blockade. In the same study, a significant correlation between increasing urinary catecholamine excretion and an increasing metabolic rate was induced by cold stress.

Four non-responders to cold stress who showed a paradoxical decrease in metabolic rate later succumbed. Consequently, adrenergic blockade which interferes with cold stress response (catecholamine-induced calorigenic response), would seem to be best avoided.

A number of more recent and extensive studies have shown that limited beta blockade can be safely used in severely burned patients. Propranolol, 2 mg/kg per day, was given intravenously to 18 patients for 5 days with burns of $70 \pm 30\%$ TBSA (Herndon *et al.*, 1988). Heart rate was decreased 20%, left ventricular work index by 22%, and rate pressure product by 36%. Plasma glucose, free fatty acids, triglyceride and insulin levels remained unchanged; however, blood urea nitrogen was elevated in the treated group. Stable isotope infusions of urea were then performed in both the fed and fasted state with rate of urea production (Ra) increased one to fivefold in the treated group. This led to speculation that blockade of the skeletal muscle cell beta-2 adrenoreceptor was preventing normal agonist activity of elevated catecholamines with alteration in net protein balance to further catabolism. Burned patients have an increase in both protein synthesis and protein breakdown, both possibly as a result of catecholamine activity.

A group of six, septic, severely burned adolescents, aged 17 ± 3 years, with burns $82 \pm 11\%$ TBSA, were given propranolol with continuous hemodynamic monitoring with a swan-ganz catheter (Minifee *et al.*, 1989). Pressure-work index and rate pressure product were significantly decreased with both 0.5 and 1.0 mg/kg. Cardiac index, oxygen delivery index and oxygen consumption were improved without adversely affecting overall oxygen delivery or total body oxygen consumption. Further propranolol, 1–2 mg/kg per day, achieved a 25% decrease in heart rate, in adolescents who were still able to appropriately respond to cold stress and isoproteronol challenge (Honeycutt *et al.*, 1992).

Beta-1 selective blockade has been compared with beta-1, beta-2 non-selective blockade. Stable isotope infusions of leucine, urea, and glycerol were used to assess protein and lipid metabolism during treatment with either propranolol, 2.1 ± 0.3 mg/ kg per day, or metoprolol, 1.8 ± 0.4 mg/kg per day for 5 days. Both drugs caused a significant, 20% decrease in heart rate. Unlike the previous study, rate of urea appearance, urea production rate, and rate of appearance of leucine were not significantly altered by either agent. Propranolol did, however, significantly decrease the rate of appearance of glycerol. This means that whole body protein catabolism was not altered but that propranolol diminished lipolytic activity by blockade of the beta-2 adrenoreceptor (Herndon *et al.*, 1994).

Selective beta-adrenergic receptor agonists have long been used in animals to increase lean meat production. Clenbuterol, a totally selective beta-2 agonist, has structural similarities to epinephrine (adrenaline) and is well known to promote protein anabolism in normal animals via beta-2 adrenergic receptor activation (Choo *et al.*, 1992). Postsurgical rats and burned rats showed increased muscle mass and body weight with Clenbuterol with evidence that hypermetabolism was also increased (Carter *et al.*, 1991; Chance *et al.*, 1991). In 30% BSA burned rats given a dorsal incision and Clenbuterol, 2 mg/kg per day, by continuous infusion, muscle and body mass were increased. Increased wound breaking strength was induced by Clenbuterol in a free-feeding group but not in pair-fed animals, indicating a need for substrate availability to allow Clenbuterol to act (Hollyoak *et al.*, 1994).

Summary

Proper provision of calories for severely injured children has decreased mortality, improved wound healing and increased resistance to infection. Indirect calorimetry improves estimation of energy requirements and decreases over and under feeding. Increased protein, omega-3 fatty acids, and amino acids such as arginine and glutamine, together with antioxidant vitamin supplementation, should further speed recovery. Stimulation of protein anabolism with recombinant growth factors and beta-2 adrenoreceptor agonists improves substrate utilisation and has remarkable wound healing effects.

References

Abbott, W. C., Schiller, W. R., Long, C. L., Birkhahn, R. H. & Blakemore, W. S. (1985). The effect of major thermal injury on plasma ketone body levels. *JPEN.* **9**, 153–8.

Albina, J. E., Mills, C. D., Barbul, A., Thirkill, C. E., Henry, W. I. Jr, Mastrofrancesco, B. & Caldwell, M. D. (1988). Arginine metabolism in wounds. *American Journal of Physiology*, **254**, E459–E467.

Alexander, J. W. & Gottschlich, M. M. (1990). Nutritional immunomodulation in burn patients. *Critical Care Medicine*, **18**(Suppl.), S149–S153.

Alexander, J. W., Macmillan, B. G., Stinnett, J. D., Ogle, C. K., Bozian, R. C., Rischer, J. E., Oakes, J. B., Morris, M. J. & Krummel, R. (1980). Beneficial effects of aggressive protein feeding in severely burned children. *Annals of Surgery*, **192**, 505–17.

Anderson, T. W. (1977). Vitamin C. *Nutrition Today*, **12**, 6–13.

Atkinson, J. B., Kosi, M. & Srikanth, M. S. (1992). Growth hormone reverses impaired wound healing in protein-malnourished rats treated with corticosteroids. *Journal of Pediatric Surgery*, **27**, 1026–8.

Aulick, L. H. & Wilmore, D. W. (1979). Increased peripheral amino acid following burn injury. *Surgery*, **85**, 560–5.

Aun, F., Medeiros-Neto, G. A., Younes, R. N., Birogini, D. & Ramos de Oliveira, M. (1983). The effect of major trauma on the pathways of thyroid hormone metabolism. *Journal of Trauma*, **23**, 1048–50.

Barbul, A. & Regan, M. C. (1993). Biology of wound healing. In *Surgical Basic Science*, ed. Fischer, J. E., pp. 67–89. St Louis, Mosby.

Barbul, A., Fishel, R. S., Shimazu, S. & Efron, G. (1985). Intravenous hyperalimentation with high arginine levels improves wound healing and immune function. *Journal of Surgical Research*, **38**, 328–34.

Barbul, A., Laazarou, S. A., Efron, D. T., Efron, D. T., Wakkerdrug, H. L. & Efron, G. (1990) Arginine enhances wound healing and lymphocyte immune responses in humans. *Surgery*, **108**, 331–7.

Barbul, A., Rettura, G., Levenson, S. & Seifter, E. (1983). Wound healing and thymotrophic effects of arginine: a pituitary mechanism of action. *American Journal of Clinical Nutrition*, **37**, 786–94.

Barcia, P. J. (1970). Lack of acceleration of healing with zinc sulphate. *Annals of Surgery*, **172**, 1048–50.

Becker, R. A., Vaughan, G. M., Goodwin, C. W., Ziegler, G., Harrison, T. S., Mason, A. D. Jr & Pruitt, B. A. Jr (1980). Plasma nor-epinephrine and thyroid hormone interactions in severely burned patients. *Archives of Surgery*, **115**, 439–43.

Becker, R. A., Vaughan, G. M., Goodwin, C. W., Ziegler, M. G., Zitska, C. A., Mason, A. D. Jr & Pruitt, B. A. Jr (1983). Interactions of thyroid hormones and catecholamines in severely burned patients. *Reviews of Infectious Diseases*, **5**, S908–S913.

Becker, R. A., Vaughan, G. M., Zeigler, M. G., Seraile, L. G., Goldfarb, W., McManus, W. F., Pruitt, B. A. Jr & Mason, A. D. Jr (1982). Hypermetabolic low triiodothyronine syndrome of burn injury. **10**, 870–5.

Bentler, B. & Cerami, A. (1987) Cachectin: more than a tumour necrosis factor. *New England Journal of Medicine*, **316**, 379–85.

Biolo, G., Maggi, S. P., Fleming, R. Y. D., Herndon, D. N. & Wolfe, R. R. (1993). Relationship between amino acid transport and protein kinetics in muscle tissue of severely burned patients. *Clinical Nutrition*, **12**, 4–7.

Birkhahn, R. H., Long, C. L., Fitikin, D., Jeevanandam, B. & Blakemore, W. S. (1987) Whole-body protein metabolism due to trauma in man as estimated by L-(^{15}N)-alanine. *American Journal of Physiology*, *(Endocrinology/Metabolism)*, **241**, E64–E71.

Boosalis, M. G., Solem, L. D., Ahrenholz, D. H., McCall, J. T. & McClain, C. J. (1986). Serum and urinary selenium levels in thermal injury. *Burns*, **12**, 236–40.

Boulivare, S. D., Tamborlane, W. V., Matthews, L. S. & Sherwin, R. S. (1992). Diverse effects of insulin-like growth factor 1 on glucose lipid and amino acid metabolism. *American Journal of Physiology (Endocrinology Metabolism*, **25**) **262**, E130–E133.

Bull, J. P. & Fisher, A. J. (1954). A study of mortality in a burns unit: a revised estimate. *Annals of Surgery*, **139**, 269–74.

Caldwell, F. T., Graves, D. B. & Wallace, B. H. (1994). The response in heat production, plasma catecholamines, and body temperature of burned rats to hypothalamine temperature displacement. *Journal of Burn Care Rehabilitation*, **15**, 315–22.

Caldwell, M. D. (1989). Local glutamine metabolism in wounds and inflammation. *Metabolism* (Suppl. 1), **38**, 34–9.

Carter, W. J., Dang, A. S. Q., Faas, F. G. & Lynch, M. E. (1991). Effects of clenbuterol on skeletal mass, body composition and recovery from surgical stress in senescent rats. *Metabolism*, **40**, 855–60.

Chance, W. T., Von Allman, D., Benson, D., Zhang, F. S. & Fisher, J. E. (1991). Clenbuterol decreases catabolism and increases hypermetabolism in burned rats. *Journal of Trauma*, **31**, 365–70.

Choo, J. J., Horan, M. A., Little, R. A. & Rothwell, N. J. (1992). Anabolic effects of clenbuterol on skeletal muscle are mediated by beta-2 adrenoreceptor activation. *American Journal of Physiology* (Endocrinology and Metabolism 26) 263, E50–E56.

Chwans, W. J. & Bistrian, B. R. (1991). Role of exogenous growth hormone and insulin-like growth factor 1 in malnutrition and acute metabolic stress: A hypothesis. *Critical Care Med.* 19(10), 1317–22.

Clemmons, D. R., Snyder, D. K., Williams, R. & Underwood, L. E. (1987). Growth hormone administration conserves lean body mass during dietary restriction in obese subjects. *Journal of Clinical Endocrinology and Metabolism,* **64,** 878–83.

Curreri, P. W., Richmond, D., Marvin, J. & Bacter, C. R. (1974). Dietary requirements of patients with major burns. *Journal of the Diatetic Association,* **65,** 415–19.

Czaja, A. J., McAltraney, J. C. & Pruitt, B. A. Jr (1974). Acute gastroduodenal disease after thermal injury. *New England Journal of Medicine,* **291,** 925–9.

Dahn, M. S., Lange, M. P. & Jacobs, L. A. (1988). Insulin-like growth factor-1 production is inhibited in human sepsis. *Archives of Surgery,* **123,** 1409–14.

Daly, J. M., Reynolds, J., Thorm, A., Kinsley, L., Dietrick-Gallagher, M., Shou, J. & Ruggieri, B. (1988). Immune and metabolic effects of arginine in the surgical patient. *Annals of Surgery,* **208,** 512–23.

Daughaday, W. H., Hall, K. & Salmon, W. D. Jr (1987). Letter to the editor: On the nomenclature of the somatomedins and insulin-like growth factors. *Journal of Clinical Endocrinology and Metabolism,* **65,** 1075–6.

Demetriou, A. A., Levenson, S. M., Retture, G. & Seifter, E. (1985). Vitamin A and retinoic acid: induced fibroblast differentiation in vitro. *Surgery,* **98,** 931–4.

Demling, R. H. (1992). Early increased gut permeability after burns. *Critical Care Medicine,* **20,** 1503–12.

Demling, R. H. & Lalond, C. (1990a). Early postburn lipid peroxidation: effect of ibuprofen and allopurinol. *Surgery,* **107,** 85–93.

Demling, R. H. & Lalond, C. (1990b). Identification and modification of the pulmonary and systemic inflammatory and biochemical changes caused by a skin burn. *Journal of Trauma,* **30,** 557–62.

Dinarello, C. A., Cannon, J. G., Wolff, S. M., Bernheim, H. A., Beutler, B., Cerami, A., Figari, I. S., Palladino, M. A. Jr & O'Connor, J. V. (1986). Tumor necrosis factor (cachectin) is an endogenous pyrogen and induces production of interleukin-1. *Journal of Experimental Medicine,* **163,** 1433–50.

Dinarello, C. A., Conno, J. G. & Wolff, S. M. (1988). New concepts on pathogenesis of fever. *Reviews of Infectious Diseases,* **10,** 168–9.

Donnelly, M. & Scheffer, I. E. (1976). Energy metabolism in respiration-deficient and wild-type Chinese hamster fibroblasts in culture. *Journal of Cell Physiology,* **89,** 39–51.

Drost, A. C., Burleson, D. G., Cioffi, W. G., Jordan, B. S., Mason, A. D. Jr & Pruitt, B. A. Jr (1993a). Plasma cytokines following thermal injury and their relationship with patient mortality, burn size and time postburn. *Journal of Trauma,* **35,** 335–9.

Drost, A. C., Burleson, D. G., Cioffi, W. G., Mason, A. D. Jr & Pruitt, B. A. Jr (1993b). Plasma cytokines after thermal injury and their relationship to infection. *Annals of Surgery,* **218,** 74–8.

Dudrick, P. S., Copeland, E. M., Bland, K. I. & Souba, W. W. (1993). Divergent regulation of fuel utilization in human fibroblasts by epidermal growth factor. *Journal of Surgical Research,* **54,** 305–10.

Falcone, P. A. & Caldwell, M. D. (1990). Wound metabolism. *Clinics in Plastic Surgery,* **17,** 443–56.

Fryburg, D. A., Gelfand, R. A. & Barrett, E. J. (1991). Growth hormone acutely stimulates forearm muscle protein synthesis in normal humans. *America Journal of Physiology (Endocrinology and Metabolism* 23) **260**, E499–E504.

Garder, A. J., Karl, I. E. & Kipnis, D. M. (1976). Alanine and glutamine synthesis and release from skeletal muscle. IV. B-adrenergic inhibition of amino acid release. *Journal of Biological Chemistry*, **251**, 851–7.

Gelfand, R. A., Hutchinson-Williams, K. A., Bonde, A. A., Castellino, P. & Sherman, R. S. (1987). Catabolic effects of thyroid hormone excess: the contribution of adrenergic activity to hypermetabolism and protein breakdown. *Metabolism*, **36**, 562–9.

Gilpin, D. A., Barrow, R. E., Rutan, R. L., Broemeling, L. D. & Herndon, D. N. (1994). Recombinant human growth hormone accelerates wound healing in children with large cutaneous burns. *Annals of Surgery*, **220**, 19–24.

Goldstain, R. H., Poliks, C. F. & Pilch, B. D. (1989). Stimulation of collagen formation by insulin and insulin-like growth factor in cultures of human lung fibroblasts. *Endocrinology*, **124**, 964–70.

Gonnella, P. A., Helton, W. S., Robinson, M. & Wilmore, D. (1992). O-side chain of Escherichia coli endotoxin O111: B4 is transported across the intestinal epithelium in the rat: evidence for increased transport during total parenteral nutrition. *European Journal of Cell Biology*, **59**, 224–7.

Goodson, W. H. & Hunt, T. K. (1988). Wound healing. In *Nutrition and Metabolism in Patient Care*, ed. Kinney, J. M., Jeejeebhoy, N. N., Hill, G. L. & Owen, O. E., pp. 635–42. Philadelphia, W. B. Saunders.

Goran, M. I., Broemeling, L. D., Herndon, D. N., Peters, E. J. & Wolfe, R. R. (1991). Estimating energy requirements in burned children: a new approach derived from measurements in resting energy expenditure. *American Journal of Clinical Nutrition*, **54**, 35–40.

Goran, M. I., Peters, E. J., Herndon, D. N. & Wolfe, R. R. (1990). Total energy expenditure in burned children using the doubly labelled water technique. *American Journal of Physiology (Endocrinology/Metabolism)* **259**, E576–E585.

Gore, D. C., Honeycutt, D., Jahoor, F., Rutan, T., Wolfe, R. R. & Herndon, D. N. (1991a). Effect of exogenous growth hormone on glucose utilization in burn patients. *Journal of Surgical Research*, **51**, 518–23.

Gore, D. C., Honeycutt, D., Jahoor, F., Wolfe, R. & Herndon, D. N. (1991b). Effect of exogenous growth hormone on whole-body and isolated limb protein kinetics in burned patients. *Archives of Surgery*, **126**, 38–43.

Gore, D. C., Rutan, R. L., Hildreth, M., Desai, M. H. & Herndon, D. N. (1990). Comparison of resting energy expenditures and caloric intake in children with severe burns. *Journal of Burn Care and Rehabilitation*, **11**, 400–4.

Gottschlich, M. M. & Warden, G. D. (1990). Vitamin supplementation in the patient with burns. *Journal of Burn Care and Rahabilitation*, **11**, 275–9.

Grenier, J. F., Aprahamian, N., Genot, C. & Dentinger, A. (1982). Pantothenic acid (vitamin B) efficiency on wound healing. *Acta Vitaminology and Enzymology*, **4**, 81–5.

Griffiths, J. B. (1970). The quantitative utilization of amino acids and glucose and contact inhibition of growth in cultures of the human diploid cell. *Journal of Cell Science*, **6**, 739–49.

Harris, J. A. & Benedict, F. G. (1919). *Biometric studies of basal metablism in man.* Carnegie Institution of Washington, Publication 270.

Harris, R. L., Frenkel, R. A., Cottam, G. L. & Baxter, C. R. (1982). Lipid mobilization and metabolism after thermal injury. *Journal of Trauma*, **22**, 194.

Herndon, D. N. & Ziegler, S. T. (1993). Bacterial translocation after thermal injury. *Critical Care Medicine*, **21**, 550–4.

Herndon, D. N., Abston, S. & Stein, M. D. (1984). Increased thromboxane B₂ levels in the plasma of burned and septic burned patients. *Surgery, Gynaecology and Obstetrics*, **159**, 210–13.

Herndon, D. N., Barrow, R. E., Kunkel, K. R., Browemeling, L. & Rutan, R. L. (1990). Effects of recombinant human growth hormone on donor-site healing in severely burned children. *Annals of Surgery*, **212**, 424–31.

Herndon, D. N., Barrow, R. E., Rutan, T. C., Minifee, P., Jahoor, F. & Wolfe, R. R. (1988). Effect of propranolol administration on hemodynamic and metabolic responses of burned pediatric patients. *Annals of Surgery*, **208**, 484–92.

Herndon, D. N., Barrow, R. E., Stein, M., Linares, H., Rutan, T. C. & Rutan, R. (1989). Increased mortality with intravenous supplemental feeding in severely burned patients. *Journal of Burn Care and Rehabilitation*, **27**, 195–204.

Herndon, D. N., Curreri, P. W., Abston, S., Rutan, T. & Barrow, R. E. (1987a). Treatment of burns. *Current Problems in Surgery*, **2**, 347–97.

Herndon, D. N., Nguyen, T. T., Wolfe, R. R., Maggi, S. P., Biolo, G., Muller, M. & Barrow, R. E. (1994). Lipolysis in burned patients is stimulated by the Beta-2 receptor for catecholamines. *Archives of Surgery*, **129**, 1301–5.

Herndon, D. N., Stein, M. D., Rutan, T. C., Abston, S. & Linares, H. (1987b). Failure of TPN supplementation to improve liver function, immunity, and mortality in thermally injured patients. *Journals of Trauma*, **27**, 195–204.

Herndon, D. N., Wilmore, D. W., Mason, A. D. Jr & Pruitt, B. A. Jr (1977). Humoral mediators of nontemperature dependent hypermetabolism in 50% burned rats. *Surgery Forum*, **28**, 37–9.

Herndon, D. N., Wilmore, D. W., Mason, A. D. Jr & Pruitt, B. A. Jr (1978). Abnormalities of phenylalanine and tyrosine kinetics: significance in septic and nonseptic patients. *Archives of Surgery*, **113**, 133–5.

Hildreth, M. & Carvajal, H. F. (1982). Calorie requirements in burned children: a simple formula to estimate daily caloric requirements. *Journal of Burn Care and Rehabilitation*, **3**, 78–80.

Hildreth, M. A., Herndon, D. N., Desai, M. H. & Broemeling, L. D. (1993). Caloric requirement of burn patients under 1 year of age. *Journal of Burn Care and Rehabilitation*, **14**, 108–12.

Hildreth, M. A., Herndon, D. N., Desai, M. H. & Broemeling, L. D. (1990). Current treatment reduces calories required to maintain weight in pediatric patients with burns. *Journal of Burn Care and Rehabilitation* **11**, 405–9.

Hildreth, M. A., Herndon, D. N., Desai, M. H. & Duke, M. A. (1980). Caloric needs of adolescent patients with burns. *Journal of Burn Care and Rehabilitation*, **10**, 523–6.

Hildreth, M. A., Herndon, D. N., Desai, M. H. & Duke, M. A. (1988). Re-assessing caloric requirements in pediatric burn patients. *Journal of Burn Care and Rehabilitation*, **9**, 916–18.

Hildreth, M. A., Herndon, D. N., Parks, D., Desai, M. & Rutan, T. (1982). Evaluation of a caloric requirements formula in burned children treated with early excision. *Journal of Trauma*, **27**, 188–9.

Hinder, R. A. & Stein, H. J. (1991). Oxygen-derived free radicals. *Archives of Surgery*, **126**, 104–5.

Hollyoak, M. A., Muller, M. J., Meyers, N. A., Williams, W. G., Barrow, R. E. & Herndon, D. N. (1995). Beneficial wound healing at metabolic effects of clenbuterol in burned and non-burned rats. *Journal of Burn Care and Rehabilitation* 16, 233–240.

Honeycutt, D., Barrow, R. & Herndon, D. N. (1992). Cold stress response in patients with severe burns after beta-blockade. *Journal of Burn Care and Rehabilitation*, 13, 181–6.

Horber, F. F. & Haymond, M. W. (1990). Human growth hormone prevents the protein catabolic side effects of prednisone in humans. *Journal of Clinical Investigation*, 86, 265–72.

Huang, K. F., Chung, D. H. & Herndon, D. N. (1993). Insulin-like growth factor-1 (IGF-1) reduces gut atrophy and bacterial translocation after severe burn injury. *Archives of Surgery*, 128, 47–54.

Hume, D. M. & Egdahl, R. H. (1959). The importance of the brain in the endocrine response to injury. *Annals of Surgery*, 150, 697–712.

Im, M. J. C. & Hoops, J. E. (1979). Energy metabolism in healing skin wounds. *Journal of Surgical Research*, 10, 459.

Jahoor, F., Desai, M., Herndon, D. N. & Wolfe, R. R. (1988). Dynamics of the protein metabolic response to burn injury. *Metabolism*, 37, 330–7.

Jahoor, F., Peters, E. J. & Wolfe, R. R. (1990). The relationship between gluconeogenic substrate supply and glucose production in humans. *American Journal of Physiology (Endocrinology/Metabolism)*, 258, E288–E296.

Jahoor, F., Shangraw, R. E., Mihoshi, H., Wallfish, H., Herndon, D. N. & Wolfe, R. R. (1989). Role of insulin and glucose oxidation in mediating the protein catabolism of burns and sepsis. *American Journal of Physiology* (Endocrinology/Metabolism), 257, E323–E331.

Jeffries, M. K. & Vance, M. L. (1992). Growth hormone and cortisol secretion in patients with burn injury. *Journal of Burn Care and Rehabilitation*, 13, 391–5.

Jorgensen, P. H. & Andreassen, T. T. (1988). The influence of biosynthetic human growth hormone on biomechanical properties of rat skin incisional wounds. *Acta Chirurgia Scandinavica*, 154, 623–6.

Joshi, V. V. (1970). Effects of burns on the heart. *Journal of the American Medical Association*, 211, 2130–4.

Keller, U., Kraenzlin, W., Stauffacher, W. & Arnaud, M. (1987). B-adrenergic stimulation results in diminished protein breakdown, decreased amino acid oxidation and increased protein synthesis in man. *JPEN*, 11(Suppl.), 7S (abstract).

Kimbrough, T. D., Shernan, S., Ziegler, T. R., Scheltinga, M. & Wilmore, D. W. (1991). Insulin-growth factor-1 response is comparable following intravenous and subcutaneous administration of growth hormone. *Journal of Surgical Research*, 51, 472–6.

Kirk, S. J., Hurson, M., Regan, M. C., Holt, D. R., Wasserkrug, H. L. & Barbul, A. (1990). Arginine stimulates wound healing and immune responses in humans. *Surgery*, 108, 331–7.

Kostyo, J. L. (1968). Rapid effects of growth hormone on amino acid transport and protein synthesis. *Annals of the New York Academy of Sciences*, 148, 389–407.

Kupfer, S. R., Underwood, L. E., Baxter, R. C. & Clemmons, D. R. (1993). Enhancement of the anabolic effects of growth hormone and insulin-like growth factor 1 by use of both agents simultaneously. *Journal of Clinical Investigation*, 91, 391–6.

Kupper, T. S., Deitch, E. A., Baker, C. C. & Wong, W. C. (1986). The human burn wound as a primary source of interleukin-1 activity. *Surgery*, 100, 409–15.

Lacroix, B., Didier, E. & Grenier, J. F. (1988). Role of pantothenic and ascorbic acid in wound healing processes: in vitro study on fibroblasts. *International Journal of Vitamin and Nutritional Research*, 58, 407–13.

Lakshmi, R., Lakshi, A. V. & Bamji, M. S. (1989). Skin wound healing riboflavin deficiency. *Biochemical Medicine and Metabolic Biology,* **42**, 185–91.

Larson, D. L., Mawell, R., Abston, S. & Dobrovsky, M. (1970). Zinc deficiency in burned children. *Plastic Reconstructive Surgery,* **46**, 13–21.

LeVoyer, T., Cioffi, W. G., Pratt, L., Shippee, R., McManus, W. F., Mason, A. D. Jr & Pruitt, B. A. Jr (1992). Alterations in intestinal permeability after thermal injury. *Archives of Surgery,* **127**, 26–30.

Liljadahl, S. O., Gemzell, C. A. & Plantin, L. O. (1961). Effect of human growth hormone in patients with severe burns. *Acta Chirurgia Scandinavica,* **122**, 1–4.

Linares, H. A. (1988). Autopsy findings in burned children. In *Pediatric Burn Management,* ed. Carvajal, H. F. & Parks, D. H., pp. 298–9. Chicago, IL, Yearbook Medical Publishers.

Linder, M. C. (1993a). Nutrition and metabolism of proteins. In *Nutritional Biochemistry and Metabolism,* 2nd edn, ed. Linder, M. C., pp. 87–109. New York, Elsevier.

Linder, M. C. (1993b). Nutrition and metabolism of vitamins. In *Nutritional Biochemistry and Metabolism,* 2nd edn, ed. Linder, M. C., pp. 111–89. New York, Elsevier.

Linder, M. C. (1991). Nutritional and metabolism of the trace elements. In *Nutritional Biochemistry and Metabolism,* 2nd edn, ed. Linder, M. C., pp. 215–76. New York, Elsevier.

Long, C. L., Spencer, J. L., Kinney, J. M. & Geiger, J. W. (1971). Carbohydrate metabolism in man: effect of elective operation and major injury. *Journal of Applied Physiology,* **31**, 110–16.

Maderazo, E. G., Woronick, C. L., Hickingbotham, N., Mercier, E., Jacobs, L. & Bhagavan, H. (1990). Additional evidence of autooxidation as a possible mechanism of neutrophil locomotory dysfunction in blunt trauma. *Critical Care Medicine,* **18**, 141–7.

McDonald, W. S., Sharp, C. W. & Deitch, E. A. (1991). Immediate enteral feeding in burn patients is safe and effective. *Annals of Surgery,* **213**, 177–83.

Mass, G. (1981). Maintenance of gastrointestinal function after bowel surgery and immediate enteral feeding nutrition: clinical experience with objective demonstration of intestinal absorption and motility. *JPEN,* **5**, 215–20.

Michie, H. R. & Wilmore, D. W. (1990). Sepsis, signals, and surgical sequelae: a hypothesis. *Archives of Surgery,* **125**, 531–6.

Miles, J. M., Nissen, S. L., Gerich, J. E. & Haymond, M. W. (1984). Effects of epinephrine infusion on leucine and alanine kinetics in humans. *American Journal of Physiology,* **247**, E166–E172.

Minifee, P. K., Barrow, R. E., Abston, S., Desai, M. & Herndon, D. N. (1989). Improved myocardial oxygen utilization following propranolol infusion in adolescents with postburn hypermetabolism. *Journal of Pediatric Surgery,* **24**, 806–11.

Mjaaland, M., Unneberg, K., Larsson, J., Nilson, L. & Reuhang, A. (1993). Growth hormone after abdominal surgery attenuated forearm glutanine, alanine, 3-methylhislidine and total amino acid efflux in patients receiving total parenteral nutrition. *Annals of Surgery,* **217**, 413–22.

Mochizuki, H., Trocki, O., Dominioni, L. & Alexander, J. W. (1985). Reduction of postburn hypermetabolism by early enteral feedings. *Current Surgery,* **42**, 121–5.

Moller, S., Jensen, M., Svensson, P. & Skakkebaek, N. E. (1991). Insulin-like growth-factor-1 (IGF-1) in burn patients. *Burns,* **17**, 279–81.

Moore, F. A., Feliciano, D. V., Andrassy, R. J., McCardle, A. H., Booth, F. V. & Morgenstein-Wagner, XX (1992). Early enteral feeding, compared with parenteral, reduces postoperative septic complications: the results of a meta-analysis. *Annals of Surgery,* **216**, 172–83.

Morimoto, A., Murakami, N., Nakamori, T. & Watanabe, T. (1988). Multiple control of fever production in the central nervous system of rabbits. *Journal of Physiology*, **397**, 269–80.

Muller, M. J. & Herndon, D. N. (1994). The challenge of burns. *Lancet*, **343**, 216–20.

Munster, A. M., Smith Meek, M., Dickerson, C. & Winchurch, R. A. (1993). Translocation; Incidental phenomenon or true pathology? *Annals of Surgery*, **218**, 321–7.

Newsholme, E. A. & Crabtree, B. (1976). Substrate cycles in metabolic regulation and in heat generation. *Biochemical Society Symposium*, **41**, 61–109.

Newsome, T. W., Mason, A. D. & Pruitt, B. A. (1973). Weight loss following thermal injury. *Annals of Surgery*, **178**, 215–17.

Nguyen, T. T., Cox, C. S., Traber, D. L., Gasser, H., Redl, H., Schlag, G. & Herndon, D. N. (1993). Free radical activity and loss of plasma antioxidants, vitamin E and sulfhydryl groups in burned patients. *Journal of Burn Care and Rehabilitation*, **14**, 602–9.

Nirgiotis, J. G., Hennessey, P. J., Black, C. T. & Andrassy, R. J. (1991). The effects of an arginine-free enteral diet on wound healing and immune function in the postsurgical rat. *Journal of Pediatric Surgery*, **26**, 936–41.

Okada, A., Takagi, Y., Nezu, R. & Lee, S. (1990). Zinc in clinical surgery: a research review. *Journal of Pediatric Surgery*, **20**, 635–44.

Prasad, A. S. (1986). Clinical, endocrinological and biochemical effects of zinc deficiency. *Clinical Endocrinology and Metabolism*, **3**, 567–89.

Reitzer, L. J., Wice, B. M. & Kennell, D. (1979). Evidence that glutamine, not sugar, is the major energy source for culture HeLa cells. *Journal of Biological Chemistry*, **254**, 269–76.

Ruberg, R. L. (1984). Role of nutrition in wound healing. *Surgical Clinics of North America*, **64**, 705–14.

Rutan, R. & Herndon, D. N. (1994). Justification for the use of growth hormone in a pediatric burn center. *Proceedings of the American Burn Association*, Orlando, Fl.

Rutan, T. C., Herndon, D. N., Van Osten, T. & Abston, S. (1986). Metabolic rate alteration in early excision and grafting versus conservative treatment. *Journal of Trauma*, **26**, 140–2.

Ryan, C. N., Yarmush, M. I., Burk, J. F. & Tompkins, R. G. (1992). Increased gut permeability after burns correlate with the extent of burn injury. *Critical Care Medicine*, **20**, 1508–12.

Saffle, J. R., Medina, E., Raymond, J., Westenskow, D., Kravitz, M. & Warden, G. D. (1985). Use of indirect calorimetry in the nutritional management of burned patients. *Journal of Trauma*, **25**, 32–9.

Saito, H., Trocki, O., Alexander, J. W., Kopcha, R., Heyd, T. & Joffe, S. N. (1987a). The effect of route of nutrient administration on the nutritional state, catabolic hormone secretion and gut mucosal integrity after burn injury. *JPEN*, **11**, 1–7.

Saito, H., Trocki, O., Wang, S. L., Gonce, S. J. & Alexander, J. W. (1987b). Metabolic and immune effects of dietary arginine supplementation after burn. *Archives of Surgery*, **122**, 784–9.

Santos, A. A., Rodrick, M. L., Jacobs, D. O., Dinarello, C. A., Wolff, S. M. & Mannick, J. A. (1994). Does the route of feeding modify the inflammatory response? *Annals of Surgery*, **220**, 155–63.

Sengupta, K. P. & Deb, S. K. (1978). Role of vitamin C in collagen synthesis. *Journal of Experimental Biology*, **16**, 1061–3.

Shamoom, H., Hendler, R. & Sherwin, R. S. (1981). Synergistic interactions among anti-insulin hormones in the pathogenesis of stress hyperglycemia in humans. *Journal of Clinical Endocrinology and Metabolism*, **52**, 1235–41.

Shaw, J. H. F. & Wolfe, R. R. (1989). An integrated analysis of glucose, fat, and protein metabolism in severely burned traumatized patients. Studies in the basal state and the response to total parenteral nutrition. *Annals of Surgery*, **209**, 63–72.

Shorwell, M. A., Kilberg, M. S. & Oxender, D. L. (1983). The regulation of neutral amino acid transport in mammalian cells. *Biochemica Biophysica Acta*, **737**, 267–84.

Soroff, H. S., Pearson, E., Green, N. L. & Artz, C. P. (1960). The effect of growth hormone on nitrogen balance at various levels of intake in burned patients. *Surgery Gynecology and Obstetrics*, **111**, 259–73.

Soroff, H. S., Rozin, R. R., Mooty, J., Lister, J. & Raben, M. S. (1967). Role of human growth hormone in the response to trauma: metabolic effects following burns. *Annals of Surgery*, **166**, 739–52.

Souba, W. W., Herskowitz, K., Klimberg, V. S., Salloum, R. M., Plumley, D. A., Flynn, T. C. & Copeland, E. M. (1990). The effects of sepsis and endotoxemia on gut glutamine metabolism. *Annals of Surgery*, **211**, 543–9.

Souba, W. W., Smith, R. J. & Wilmore, D. W. (1985). Glutamine metabolism by intestinal tract. *JPEN*, **9**, 608–17.

Stinnett, J. D., Alexanader, J. W., Watanabe, C., MacMillan, B. G., Fischer, J. E., Morris, M. J., Trocki, O., Miskell, P., Edwards, L. & James, H. (1982). Plasma and skeletal muscle amino acids following severe burn injury in patients and experimental animals. *Annals of Surgery*, **195**, 75.

Strock, L. L., Singh, H. Abdullah, A., Miller, J. A. & Herndon, D. N. (1990). The effect of insulin-like growth factor-1 on postburn hypermetabolism. *Surgery*, **108**, 161–4.

Tavakkol, A., Edler, J. T. & Griffiths, C. E. M. (1992). Expression of growth hormone receptor, insulin-like growth factor 1 (IGF-1) and IGF-1 receptor mRNA and proteins in human skin. *Journal of Investigative Dermatology*, **99**, 343–9.

Tessari, P., Inchiostro, S., Biolo, G., Trevisan, R., Fantin, G., Marescotti, M. C., Iori, E., Tiengo, A. & Crepaldi, G. (1987). Differential effects of hyperinsulinemia and hyperaminoacidemia on leucine-carbon metabolism in vivo. *Journal of Clinical Investigation*, **79**, 1062–9.

Tinckler, L. F. (1965). Surgery and intestinal mortality. *British Journal of Surgery*, **52**, 140–50.

Turner, W. W., Ireton, C. S., Hunt, J. L. & Baxter, C. R. (1985). Predicting energy expenditures in burned patients. *Journal of Trauma*, **259**, 11–16.

Van Vliet, G., Bosson, D. & Craen, M. (1987). Comparative study of the lipolytic potencies of pituitary-derived and biosynthetic human growth hormone in hypopituitary children. *Journal of Clinical Endocrinology and Metabolism*, **65**, 876.

Vaughan, G. M., Becker, R. A., Unger, R. H., Ziegler, M. G., Siler-Khodr, T. M., Pruitt, B. A. & Mason, A. D. Jr (1985). Non-thyroidal control of metabolism after burn injury: possible role of glucagon. *Metabolism*, **34**, 637–41.

Vaughan, G. M., Pruitt, B. A. Jr & Mason, A. D. Jr (1990). Burn trauma as a model of severe illness. In *Endocrinology of Thermal Trauma*, ed. Dolecek, R., Brizio-Molteni, L., Molteni, A. & Traber, D., pp. 307–49. Philadelphia, Lea and Febiger.

Vaughan, G. M., Becker, R. A., Allen, J. P., Goodwin, C. W. Jr, Pruitt, B. A. Jr & Mason, A. D. Jr (1982). Cortisol and corticotropin in burned patients. *Journal of Trauma*, **22**, 263–73.

Volence, F. J. (1979). Metabolic profiles of thermal trauma. *Annals of Surgery*, **190**, 694–8.

Westenskow, D. R., Cutler, C. A. & Wallace, W. D. (1984). Instrumentation for monitoring gas exchange and metabolic rate in critically ill patients. *Critical Care Medicine*, **12**, 183–7.

Wilmore, D. W., Aulick, L. H. & Mason, A. D. Jr (1977). Influence of burn wound on local and systemic responses to injury. *Annals of Surgery*, **186**, 44.

Wilmore, D. W., Lang, J. M., Mason, A. D., Skreen, R. W. & Pruitt, B. A. Jr (1974a). Catecholamines: mediator of the hypermetabolic response to thermal injury. *Annals of Surgery*, **180**, 653–69.

Wilmore, D. W., Moyland, J. A. Jr, Bristow, B. F., Mason, A. D. & Pruitt, B. A. (1974b). Anabolic effects of growth hormone and high caloric feedings following thermal injury. *Surgery Gynecology and Obstetrics*, **138**, 875–84.

Wilmore, D. W., Orcutt, T. W., Mason, A. D. Jr & Pruitt, B. A. Jr (1975). Alterations in hypo-thalamic function following thermal injury. *Journal of Trauma*, **15**, 697–703.

Winchurch, R. A., Thupari, J. N. & Munster, A. M. (1987). Endotoxemia in burn patients: levels of circulating endotoxins are related to burn size. *Surgery*, **102**, 808–12.

Wolfe, R. R., O'Donnell, T. F. Jr, Stone, M. D., Richmand, D. A. & Burke, J. F. (1980). Investigation of factors determining the optimal glucose infusion rate in total parenteral nutrition. *Metabolism*, **29**, 892–900.

Wolfe, R. R. & Durkot, M. J. (1982). Evaluation of the role of the sympathetic nervous system in the response of substrate kinetics and oxidation to burn injury. *Circulatory Shock*, **9**, 395–406.

Wolfe, R. R., Durkot, M. J., Alison, J. R. & Burke, J. F. (1970). Glucose metabolism in severely burned patients. *Metabolism*, **28**, 1031–9.

Wolfe, R. R., Goodenough, R. D., Burke, J. F. & Wolfe, M. H. (1983). Response of protein and urea kinetics in burn patients to different levels of protein intake. *Annals of Surgery*, **197**, 163–71.

Wolfe, R. R., Herndon, D. N., Peters, E. J., Jahoor, F., Desai, M. H. & Holland, O. B. (1987a). Regulation of lipolysis in severely burned children. *Annals of Surgery*, **206**, 214–21.

Wolfe, R. R., Herndon, D. W., Jahor, F., Mihoshi, H. & Wolfe, M. H. (1987b). Effect of severe burn injury on substrate cycling by glucose and fatty acids. *New England Journal of Medicine*, **317**, 403–8.

Wolfe, R. R., Jahoor, F. & Hartl, W. H. (1989). Protein and amino acid metabolism after injury. *Diabetes/Metabolism Reviews*, **5**, 149–64.

Wolfe, R. R., Klein, S., Herndon, D. N. & Jahoor, F. (1990). Substrate cycling in thermogenesis and amplification of net substrate flux in human volunteers and burned patients. *Journal of Trauma*, **30** (12 Suppl.), 56–59.

Yarasheski, K. E., Zachwieja, J. J., Angelopoulos, T. J. & Bier, D. M. (1993). Short-term growth hormone treatment does not increase muscle protein synthesis in experienced weight lifters. *Journal of Applied Physiology*, **74**, 3073–6.

Zaizen, Y., Ford, E. G., Costin, G. & Atkinson, J. B. (1990). The effect of perioperative exogenous growth hormone on wound bursting strength in normal and malnourished rats. *Journal of Surgery*, **25**, 70–4.

Ziegler, M. G., Morrisey, E. C. & Marshal, L. F. (1990). Catecholamine and thyroid hormones in traumatic injury. *Critical Care Medicine*, **18**, 253–8.

Ziegler, T. R., Smith, R. J., O'Dwyer, S. T., Demling, R. H. & Wilmore, D. W. (1988). Increased intestinal permeability associated with infection in burn patients. *Archives of Surgery*, **123**, 1313–19.

14

Recovery, rehabilitation and the neuropsychological sequelae of head injury

M. CROUCHMAN

Introduction

Trauma in children is more likely to involve the head than in adults, and head injury is the commonest cause of acquired disability in childhood, with an estimated prevalence in the UK of at least 75 per 100 000.

In spite of this, our understanding of head injury outcome in children has been limited by a relative lack of information. In the past most studies were carried out by epidemiologists or by surgeons who did not separate children from adults, or if they did, saw childhood as ending at 14, even 12, years of age. Clinical follow-up of children was often brief, with no clearly defined hand-over to a paediatrician for longer term management. There were (and still are) considerable problems with case definition: not all the children who suffer a significant blow to the head are brought to medical attention (Rune, 1970), and the traditional measures of severity (Glasgow Coma Scale, duration of unconsciousness, duration of postraumatic amnesia) are less easily applied and interpreted in the very young child; very large data sets may mask significant findings in small subgroups (Klonoff et al., 1977); and local variations and changing practice in retrieval and acute management may be affecting outcome. These factors must be taken into account when interpreting head injury information in children, and in particular when attempting to compare results between studies.

Problems with definition of severity

Field (1976) enigmatically defined head injury as 'trauma which carries some risk of damage to the brain'. Assessment of severity is usually made on the basis of length of coma, concussion, post-traumatic amnesia (PTA) [the time interval between injury and the reinstatement of continuous day-to-day memory, as assessed clinically], and/or demonstrable damage to brain tissue. There is no uniformity in the way that studies have used these parameters, and most contain a mixture of cases of different degrees of severity (Ruijs *et al.*, 1992). For example, Fay *et al.* (1993) in their study of 129 children with minor head injury [an injury causing unconsciousness for 15 minutes or less], included 13 with abnormal CT scans. Coma scales and PTA do not always reflect extensive localised damage. They may be useful for predicting overall outcome in this type of injury, but may not truly reflect disability.

Studies based on Accident and Emergency Department attendances, such as the one carried out by Hawthorne (1978), inevitably include many more cases of mild head injury. Most research has looked at hospital admissions, and although these studies will certainly include the severe cases [defined as an injury causing unconsciousness for 6 hours or more, or a PTA of 24 hours or more], guidelines for admission of head injuries have changed over the years, may vary between hospitals, and are not always followed. Concussion [brief loss of consciousness with prompt recovery, and no localising neurological signs], often used in case definition as an indication of significant injury, might be thought to be a universal admission criterion. In a Swedish community study (Rune, 1970), however, only one-third of children with a history of concussion or unconsciousness had been admitted and Kraus *et al.* (1986) estimated that 44% of children presenting at hospital with head injury had not been unconscious. Some of the large studies have used clinical terms such as 'pressurised brain involvement' for case definition (Annegers *et al.*, 1980), while many others have resorted to International Classification of Diseases (ICD) codings. This may include 'all types of facial injuries, including lacerations or head injury resulting in at least 1 day of restricted activity and/or prompting the patient to seek medical attention' (Field, 1976). Such definitions have not improved uniformity.

Finally, studies using computed tomography (CT) scans in head injured patients (Zimmermann *et al.*, 1978; Sekino *et al.*, 1981) have confirmed Oppenheimer's finding in 1968 that 'permanent damage, in the form of microscopic destructive foci, can be inflicted in the brain by what are regarded as trivial head injuries' and, more recently, advances in magnetic resonance imaging (MRI) and spectroscopy show that reciprocal circulatory metabolic and functional depressions may occur in undamaged areas remote from the localised injury (diaschisis) (Stirling-Mayer *et al.*, 1987). Zimmermann found that generalised brain swelling was more common in children. More than one-quarter of consecutive closed head injury admissions showed this within 24 hours, and regional blood flow studies confirmed transitory hyperaemia. Brain scans are not routinely repeated the day after admission, and the severity of injury may thus be underestimated in some children.

Factors that may affect outcome

Age

There is a general perception that children have greater powers of recovery from illness and injury. This has been shown not to be the case in relation to head injury, where the outcome is poorest in infancy (Mahoney *et al.*, 1983; Raimondi & Hirscauer, 1984; Gennarelli & Thibault, 1985). Ewing-Cobbs *et al.* (1989) found that very young toddlers showed more problems on intellectual, motor and expressive language testing from 6 months after injury than older children in this study. A number of other researchers have shown that age effect becomes less marked when the injured child is of school age or an adolescent.

There are three possible reasons for this age effect. First, the cause, and therefore the mechanisms, of brain injury vary with age. Second, there may be an age-specific physiological response to brain trauma (Zimmerman *et al.*, 1978). Third, there is evidence that the earlier theories of 'plasticity' (see below) have been overoptimistic, and it is becoming increasingly apparent that damage to the very young brain results in severe disruption of the normal developmental pathways for a number of cortical functions.

Mechanisms of injury

Brain injury has been described as the brain's way of managing the forces delivered to it. Different types of injury are associated with different outcomes, and a detailed account of the accident is important. Localised injury may initially produce dramatic focal neurological signs (e.g. weakness of the arm and aphasia after a blow to the left parietal region) but has a very good prognosis for recovery. Injuries which result from high acceleration and deceleration forces within the brain substance, such as con-tracoup contusions, subdural haemorrhage and diffuse cerebral oedema are more likely to be associated with axonal damage, and therefore a poorer prognosis. The degree of damage depends on both the acceleration of the brain tissue and the duration of that acceleration. The greater the acceleration, and the longer it lasts, the greater the risk of brain injury (Gennarelli, 1992).

When the element of rotation is added to these forces the risk to the brain increases. Laboratory studies using a deformable mesh imbedded in a gel with similar properties to brain tissue have been used to measure these shearing forces. The major sites of rotation are the deep areas of the frontal and temporal poles. This concords with clinical findings of predominantly frontal and temporal lobe contusions in children who have been subjected to non-accidental impacted shaking (McClelland *et al.*, 1980). Such injury results in permanent neurological and intellectual impairment in 50% of cases, and head injury is the cause of death in 30% of child abuse fatalities (Caffey, 1972). Rotation, and more commonly, angulation injury may also be a feature of road traffic accidents, particularly when a pedestrian child is flung into the air on impact. The resultant severe cerebral oedema and scattered haemorrhages are associated with a high incidence of residual disability.

The infant skull is soft (it can be cut with scissors) and only partially fused. This ability to change shape confers a degree of protection but also results in more shearing injuries (Cummins & Potter, 1970). The smooth surface of the baby's brain compared with that of the adult is thought to contribute to the problem (Gurdjian & Webster, 1958). The effects of this movement of the infant brain's shallow convolutions against the skull produces splits in the grey–white matter junction, which may then calcify. These have been described as being cranial ultrasound evidence of shaking injury. Considerable damage can therefore be caused to the child's brain without fracturing the skull or causing scalp injury (Duhaime et al., 1987) and this adds to the difficulties of making a confident diagnosis of child abuse. Undiagnosed abuse may be one of the reasons why the outcome in babies has been described as worse than in older children, i.e. the history is one of a minor head injury, the child does not have a protracted period of unconsciousness (but see below), and yet the injury to the brain and the subsequent outcome is that of a severe injury. On the other hand, the presence of multiple 'egg-shell' skull fractures in babies, although usually associated with shock from subgaleal haemorrhage, is compatible with a complete absence of brain injury. The energy delivered to the head appears to be dissipated by fracturing of the skull.

As well as the injury itself, and any secondary brain insult, a period of primary anoxia before or during retrieval profoundly influences the prognosis and long-term outcome.

Predisposing factors (Chapter 9)

These suggest a combination of risk-taking behaviour and adverse environment in the aetiology of injury. They are important in that they may confound outcome data. They also give a picture of the social and educational background to which the injured child will return, and which has been shown to influence outcome (Greenspan & MacKenzie, 1996). For example, Brown et al. (1981) showed that while half of 31 children with severe head injuries had developed psychiatric problems within a year, all of the study population with mild premorbid problems demonstrated psychiatric problems within this time. Additionally, repeat head injuries which occur in 15% of accident prone individuals are likely to be cumulative (Klonoff et al., 1993).

Plasticity (the capacity of the brain to reorganise after injury)

In 1898 Cotard pointed out that damage to the left hemisphere in early life did not result in aphasia. The increased capacity for recovery was confirmed in the infant monkey by Kennard in 1938, and further evidence has accumulated from experience with elective hemispherectomy (Wilson, 1970; Teuber, 1975; Vargha-Khadem & Polkey, 1992). This operation is usually carried out as a treatment for intractable epilepsy, in children with a pre-existing hemiplegia. The fact that only a minor degree of additional neurological deficit results from surgery in younger children is taken as evidence that transfer of function has already occurred as a result of the original condition. Undoubtedly plasticity forms an important part of recovery from brain injury in the very young child, but as more in-depth assessments are carried out it is unfortunately becoming apparent that the optimism expressed by Bruce *et al.* (1979) is not entirely justified. On the contrary, there is growing evidence to confirm the earlier view that injury to the rapidly developing brain results in failure to acquire new learning, leading to developmental stagnation (Hebb, 1942). Thus some specific deficits are more commonly observed in younger children, e.g. written language and visual recognition memory. Wo *et al.* (1970) compared children under 8 and over 10 years, and found that although the younger group had shorter comas they had more severe cognitive deficits as a result of their injuries.

Transfer of function takes place both within and between hemispheres. Although commitment of the left hemisphere to language development may begin during the second year of life (Woods & Carey, 1979) the ability to transfer this function continues until about the age of 10 years, but with evidence of a cost to the right hemisphere (Teuber, 1975). Language appears to be preferentially relocated, whereas damage to the right hemisphere may result in permanent visuospatial problems, i.e. the theory of hemispheric equipotentiality has not been substantiated by clinical observations (Aram, 1988). When both hemispheres are damaged the prognosis for recovery is poor, and this is a particular problem in shaking and other diffuse axonal injuries.

Normal brain development is based on additive and subtractive processes; the latter probably continue throughout childhood (Cowan *et al.*, 1984; Finger *et al.*, 1986). Head injuries in childhood generally occur in the midst of these subtractive processes but at a time when the additive processes are complete or nearly complete (Goodman, 1989). When axons are transected by injury, the distal portion dies, but the proximal regenerates by sprouting. Over longer distances regeneration may be hampered by problems with tissue alignment, vasculisation and scar tissue barriers. If the brain is injured at a very early stage while developing axons have still not reached their destination there is an increased risk of misconnections. Recovery can also occur in function in the absence of structural change by reactivation of latent synapses (Wall, 1977). The degree of recovery is also related to whether injury occurs suddenly or gradually.

In summary, cerebral plasticity will be most evident when brain injury has occurred gradually, very early in life and has affected just one hemisphere. For this reason, head injury produces greater disability than, for example, a slow-growing tumour (Finger & Stein, 1982).

Predictors of outcome

Clinicians involved in the early care of head injured children are often pressed for answers about long-term outcome. Unfortunately, there are only two long-term follow-ups (Gaidolfi, & Vignolo, 1980; Klonoff *et al.*, 1993) and as yet there are no certain predictors. Extrapolation down the age scale of experience with adults is inappropriate. A reliable multimodal prognostic index of predictive factors for disability remains to be separately identified for children, but in the meantime a number of methods have been used.

Duration of loss of consciousness

There is evidence for differences in the pattern of loss of consciousness, between adults and children. Todorow & Heiss (1978) described a delayed reduction in consciousness ('fall asleep syndrome') in 24 of 300 consecutive admissions, and a similar clinical picture was described by Takahashi & Nakazawa (1980) in a group of young children who had fits following minor head injury. The author has observed that impairment of consciousness in very young babies may be poorly recognised by medical and nursing staff (but less so by mothers), perhaps because they continue to cry and feed. This may contribute to the commonly held belief that very young children are less likely to suffer impaired consciousness, but also has important implications for the assessment of the severity of injury. On the other hand, a Glasgow Coma Scale (GCS) of 4 or less appears to carry a less gloomy prognosis in children, who have a lower threshold for displaying extensor rigidity (Frowein *et al.*, 1992).

Nonetheless, measures of loss of consciousness have been found to be useful for outcome prediction, even though the most commonly used (the GCS) contains verbal items inappropriate to small children. Levin & Isenberg (1979) found admission GCS verbal and motor scores more predictive of subsequent neuropsychological deficit than GCS eye scores. Sequential GCS assessments, particularly the motor component, were shown to provide better prediction of the level of disability in children (Michaud *et al.*, 1992); however, with the increased use of paralysis and ventilation, such information is not readily obtained.

Alteration in the level of consciousness does not always reflect localised damage so that assessment of coma and PTA can underestimate disability outcome in this type of injury.

Post-traumatic amnesia

PTA [the time interval between injury and the reinstatement of continuous day-to-day memory, as assessed clinically] was described by Russell in 1932, and proposed as a way of classifying injury severity by Jennett in 1976. It may be a more useful guide to outcome (Gronwall & Wrightson, 1980; Chadwick *et al.*, 1981) but is difficult to assess in small children. Where it has been used for case definition care must be taken to distinguish between objective serial documentation using, for example, the Childrens Orientation and Amnesia Test (COAT) (Ewing-Cobbs *et al.*, 1984) rather than subjective accounts. Ruijs *et al.* (1992) described retrospective testing of 54 head injured children aged 2–15 years which they claimed to be as good prognostically as the duration of coma. McDonald *et al.* (1994) in their study of 98 children aged 6–15 years showed a high association between days to COAT 75% and a range of initial and 1 year outcome measurements of neurobehaviour and cognitive function, and this was significantly better than other traditional methods, e.g. coma scales, duration of coma, Abbreviated Injury Score, both initially and at 1 year.

They also found that days to GCS 15 was an easier and more objective measurement than duration of impaired consciousness, and recommend this as an alternative. Although Michaud *et al.* (1992) concluded that the GCS at 72 hours is a better predictor of the severity of early disability, it was not a better predictor of longer term neurobehavioural and functional outcome. Ewing-Cobbs *et al.* (1990) found no relation between duration of PTA and early non-verbal memory, but a significant relationship between PTA duration and non-verbal memory at 6 months and 1 year. Children who had PTA for at least 2 weeks showed less recovery in non-verbal memory performances over the first 12 months than those with a shorter period of PTA.

Scans

CT scans have been said to add little to short-term outcome prediction in children (Levin *et al.*, 1992), but those showing evidence of damage after 2 months have been demonstrated to be associated with poor outcome. On the other hand, motor and neuropsychological deficits can persist in spite of normal MRI appearances.

As children recover from severe head injury the secondary evidence of brain damage may appear. Ventricular dilatation can be the manifestation of communicating hydrocephalus which occurs in 1–2% of cases (Granholm & Srendgaard, 1972). More commonly it is evidence of loss of cerebral tissue, particularly when there is focal dilatation of the temporal horn of a lateral ventricle. Thirty-two young adults showed a relation between ventricular enlargement and both duration of coma and persistence of cognitive deficits including problems with memory (Levin *et al.*, 1981).

Functional MRI and single photon emission computed tomography (SPECT) will undoubtedly revolutionise knowledge in the field of head injury outcome, but are not practicable investigations in children as yet.

Electroencephalograms

EEG changes on stimulation may be regarded as signs of cortical and autonomic reactions and lack of change on EEG after stimulation may be associated with poor outcome (Pfurtscheller *et al.*, 1986). Signals from frontal scalp leads are the most significant predictors, and phase and coherence, which are less affected by oedema or medication, exhibit the highest discriminant accuracy (Thatcher *et al.*, 1991).

Evoked responses

The long pathways of somatosensory, hearing and particularly vision, through the brain may be disrupted by diffuse injuries. Measurements of latencies of these evoked responses may be useful in monitoring acute recovery, but may also prove important in the prediction of long-term disability (Rappaport *et al.*, 1977, 1978).

Vestibular function

Oculovestibular responses may be abnormal in the acute stage and have been related to poor neuropsychological outcome in severely head injured adults (Levin *et al.*, 1979). They are also thought to play an important role in sensory integration during normal child development and vestibular stimulation is advocated as a rehabilitation technique (Johnson, 1989).

Multivariant factors

Intracranial pressure (ICP), presence of severe potentially hypoxic injuries, hypoxia and hypotension are known to be predictors of survival (Michaud *et al.*, 1992) but it is not known how they relate to longer term outcomes. The Abbreviated Injury Scale (AIS) head region score, which is based on initial clinical assessment and CT findings, is said to be predictive of outcome, but is too crude to be of value in children.

Thatcher *et al.* (1991), in 162 adults, found that the most predictive of both early and 1 year outcome across all neurobehavioral and functional measures were, in order, days to an age adjusted 75% performance on the COAT, days to a GCS score of 15, initial GCS, and coma duration. In the only long-term follow-up (23 years), however, Klonoff *et al.* (1993) showed that unconsciousness was of limited predictive value, and

EEG alone of no predictive value. The combination of length of unconsciousness, skull fractures, EEG, post-traumatic seizures, and neurological status was the most discriminating of long-term subjective sequelae. This confirms the complexity of outcome prediction, and the need for multicentre standardised collection and multivariant analysis of data. Currently, the Systematic Review Unit at the Institute of Child Health in London is carrying out work which will hopefully clarify which measurements are of predictive value.

Sequelae of head injury

Motor disability

Recovery from motor deficits produced by head injury in children is more rapid and complete than in adults (see Plasticity). Mahoney *et al.* (1983) and Raimondi & Hirschauer (1984) found that severe persistent motor impairment is common in very young children, probably for the reasons outlined above. Brink *et al.* (1980) followed 344 children under 18 years who had been in coma for a mean of 5 weeks. After 1–7 years they found increased reflexes in 93%, but most were functionally normal; 73% were independent in walking and self-care skills at 1 year and only three of those who regained consciousness were unable to walk by the end of follow-up. Klonoff *et al.* (1977) found neurological abnormalities were the least likely to change over 5-year follow-up and 38% of under 9 year olds and 31% of over 9 year olds showed persistent neurological deficits. Many of these were permanent, as physical problems at long-term follow-up were reported by 36 out of 159 patients (Klonoff *et al.*, 1993).

The severest motor sequelae are seen when the brainstem is involved. Pyramidal damage results in weakness and spasticity, while cerebellar damage results in scanning speech, ataxia and incoordination. Injury to the extrapyramidal nuclei produces rigidity, slowness, delayed initiation and involuntary movements.

Swallowing and feeding difficulties

These are common after severe head injury, and may be due to coma, bulbar palsy, or mechanical problems arising from injuries to the face, neck or chest. Assessment by a Speech and Language Therapist trained in dysphagia is essential to look at head positioning, oral reflexes, phonation, facial muscle control, swallowing sequence and saliva control (Lees, 1989). Videofluoroscopy is used when there is any doubt about the child's ability to protect the airway during oral feeding. This provides the only really good objective measure but obviously cannot be repeated frequently. Many children pass through a phase of hyperphagia following head injury even in the absence of detectable thalamic damage, and this may be encountered as a side-effect of drugs such as haloperidol and chlorpromazine when these are used to reduce severe agitation. Agitation is most commonly a feature of frontal contusion which in itself may be associated with eating disinhibitions.

Post-traumatic epilepsy (PTE)

PTE (epilepsy appearing for the first time following a head injury) occurs in one-third of patients with intracranial contusions, haemorrhages, or prolonged coma (Brink *et al.*, 1980), and in 15% of those with depressed fractures.

Early PTE (i.e. within the first week of injury) occurs in 5% of all cases of concussion, and predisposes to the development of later PTE, particularly when one or both of the above two conditions also apply. Thus one-quarter of all patients fitting within the first week of injury proceed to late PTE. A patient who does not fit in the first few days after injury is unlikely to proceed to late PTE (only 3% of the latter did not fit within the first week). Late PTE usually starts within 1 year of injury (one-half of cases) and 80% have an onset within 4 years. Caveness *et al.* (1979) postulated multifactorial factors which determine the likelihood, frequency and persistence of PTE. The overall prevalence of epilepsy in the population is 0.6%, which raises the question as to whether, in any one individual, the onset of fits after 4 years can truly be attributed to head injury.

The above statements apply to head injured patients of all ages. Children under the age of 5 years at time of injury are more susceptible to fits in the early phase, and infants in particular (perhaps because of the severity of injury and a lower fit threshold) are likely to present with early convulsions. Recovery of the EEG also appears age-related. Klonoff *et al.* (1977) recorded annual EEGs in their prospective 5-year follow-up of 131 children under, and 100 over, 9 years of age. In older children the EEG stabilised by 3 years, whereas improvements were still evident in the younger group 5 years after injury. By the fifth year 15% of EEGs were still abnormal.

In Klonoff's original study post-traumatic seizures occurred in ten out of 231 children, of whom 90% had a mild head injury. In their 23-year follow-up study (Klonoff *et al.*, 1993) only two of these ten said that they had had fits at any time following the head injury! Of the two who reported continuing seizures one had had a second head injury, and the other was in the severe injury group. This suggests a relatively low risk of PTE as a result of childhood head injury.

For the individual child these statistics are of only limited prognostic value. In all age groups it is apparent on follow-up that social functioning and psychological adjustment is significantly worse in those patients who develop PTE, but the use of anticonvulsants to prevent early and late PTE has not been shown to be effective.

When fits occur, carbamazepine is probably the drug of first choice, but intravenous anticonvulsants (usually phenytoin) are used in the acute period. All anticonvulsants have side-effects, and the decision to start them should not be taken lightly. Even more important, the basis on which they are to be discontinued should be clearly stated from the outset in each child to prevent unnecessary prolongation of therapy. PTE is currently undergoing Systematic Review (see above) the results of which will hopefully lead to a more logical approach to use of anticonvulsants in head injured children.

Post-traumatic stress disorder (PTSD)

The psychological trauma experienced by children involved in accidents and disasters has only recently been acknowledged. PTSD has been defined, somewhat unhelpfully, as resulting from experience of a traumatic event outside the range of normal experience. It is manifested in distressing recollections of the event; avoidance of stimuli associated with the trauma; and a range of signs of increased physiological arousal (Horowitz, 1976). Foa *et al.* (1989) suggest that trauma resulting in PTSD violates more of the victim's assumptions about safety than other forms of trauma. Natural disasters appear to be less traumatic than deliberate violence. There is no information about the child's perception of being hit by a person driving a vehicle but certainly anger and recrimination feature prominently in parents and in some injured adolescents.

The overwhelming symptoms of PTSD are anxiety and the generalisation of fear. Children frequently complain of terrifying recurrent nightmares in which their injuries may be horrifically exaggerated, are frightened to be left alone, or to go out to play. Children may somatise their feelings, refuse to talk about them, or may perseverate vivid descriptions. A teenage girl with a tibial fracture and frontal contusions after a road traffic accident spent the first week singing an account of this experience and her anger against the driver in 'rap'. At the time this was attributed to frontal damage, but in retrospect was probably evidence of PTSD. Distinguishing between the effects on behaviour produced by acute brain injury and those resulting from PTSD may require the skills of a child psychologist. The latter condition has an excellent prognosis if treated, and help should be sought when a child shows more than the expected confusional response during the early stage of recovery.

There may be changes in the child's attitude to life. A 9-year-old girl, who had made a full recovery from evacuation of an extradural haematoma resulting from tripping on the ground and banging her head against a wall, was tearful and generally anxious 6 weeks later. She was obviously aware that she could have died. She said that she felt the accident had been a good thing in that it made her realise the lack of importance of her previous worries about how she looked and how her friends behaved. This reaction has also been described by Yule (1994) in child survivors of ship sinkings, but it is difficult to know how much children's verbalisations are influenced by family responses and conversations.

'Survivor guilt', recognised in adult victims, probably occurs not only in the child, but also in parents and siblings. PTSD is less severe in children who know the victim but were not directly involved in the incident (Lonigan *et al.*, 1991). Many road traffic accidents take place on the way to or from school, and are witnessed by siblings and friends. These also need to be monitored for evidence of distress. Many do not confide in parents or teachers, and keep their repetitive, intrusive thoughts to themselves (Yule & Williams, 1990).

Children suffering from PTSD have symptoms which overlap with those resulting from brain injury: poor concentration, irritability, problems with memory, low mood (Yule, 1994), and a drop in academic performance which likewise may persist (Tsui, 1990).

Children who are the victims of accidents (as opposed to disasters) are a selected group and may be particularly vulnerable. Pre-existing problems in the family, and the ways in which the family react to the child's injury, may affect the course of PTSD. Black *et al.* (1971) in their 5-year study of 105 children up to the age of 14 years, concluded that premorbid personality may influence the nature, rather than the incidence, of post-traumatic behaviour problems. The overriding factor, however, in the genesis of PTSD is the severity of the trauma, and loss of consciousness may not be protective (McMillan, 1991). A recent study in 70 adults (Sbordone & Liter, 1995) strongly suggests that mild traumatic brain injury does not produce PTSD, but more studies are needed in children.

Speech and language

Speech and language appear to have preferental relocation after brain injury in the young child (see Plasticity). If language development is normal before injury, and the child has made a good cognitive recovery, the prognosis for reasonable recovery of speech and language is good (Klonoff *et al.*, 1977; Winogron *et al.*, 1984).

Abnormalities of speech production are one of the most dramatic consequences of brain injury, and it is hardly surprising that a large proportion of head injury research has been carried out in this area. Temporary disruption of speech and language is commonly encountered in children with a focal contusion following a blow to the left parietal region. There may be a brief period of total aphasia, often associated with transitory weakness of the right upper limb. The prognosis is excellent, with only occasional isolated defects, usually anomia or word retrieval problems (Levin *et al.*, 1979; Chadwick *et al.*, 1981; Ewing-Cobbs *et al.*, 1985), but the experience can be very frightening for the child and family. Showing them the scan with an explanation based on their understanding of the normal evolution of bruises, albeit with a caveat about epilepsy (see above), is usually reassuring. Rapid recovery of aphasia occurs during the first 3 months, but may continue during the first year, after which progress tails off.

In the presence of bilateral or severe damage, disruption of language may be more serious or long lasting. Hecaen (1976) found that anomia was frequent, and complete aphasia persisted for up to 3 months; however, aphasia carries a better prognosis in children than in adults. Ewing-Cobbs *et al.* (1987) investigated 23 children aged 5–10 years old and 33 children aged 11–15 years old, 6 months after injury, and found similar language deficits to those described in adults, but with a disproportionate affect on written language. This appears to be age-related, and children have greater difficulty with written language than adolescents, regardless of severity of the injury.

Perseveration is common in the first 6 months after head injury but carries a poor prognosis if it persists after 1 year, suggesting that the child is making self-monitoring errors.

Although damage to the basal ganglia has a better prognosis than diffuse cortical injury, the effects on speech are more frequently seen in children (Levin *et al.*, 1983). Severe persistent motor impairment is likely to be associated with dysarthric speech problems, including monotonous slow speech, hypernasality, and less commonly, rapid or cluttered speech (Ylvisaker, 1993). Such children may understand speech, and communicate non-verbally.

Problems with language comprehension are unusual beyond the acute recovery phase (Ewing-Cobbs *et al.*, 1985), when they begin to carry a more guarded prognosis (van Dongen & Loonen, 1977). In Levin *et al.*'s study (1979) of 64 children and adolescents, only one in ten of those with language problems during the first 6 months had comprehension difficulties, but speech and language deficits were more likely to persist in those injured in late adolescence. Gaidolfi & Vignolo (1980) found a reduction in spontaneous speech in four of 21 young adults 10 years after closed head injury.

Residual language deficits may not become apparent until the child is older. This may be because expectations increase with age, or because current testing methods do not detect 'real life' difficulties in communication. Ylvisaker (1993) showed that in 90% of cases teachers reported severe deterioration in the reading of long passages, compared with 25% who had difficulties in reading individual words. The same problems were encountered with the ability to express simple versus complex ideas. Additionally, there may be a problem with children failing to acquire new language over time (Cooper & Flowers, 1987).

Reading and writing

Children with persisting spelling problems frequently have problems with high level auditory comprehension, discrimination and word finding. The premorbid characteristics of many head injured children make it important to assess for pre-existing specific learning difficulties in the family history and school work (Lees, 1989). Dyslexia or unexpectedly poor school achievement may be found in up to 40% of cases. Children have greater difficulty with written language than adolescents, regardless of the severity of injury (Ewing-Cobbs *et al.*, 1987), underlining the vulnerability of newly acquired developmental skills. Such findings have important implications for language rehabilitation.

Perceptual deficits

Damage to sensory modalities is common, but tends to be given lower priority during the acute stage. This is less likely to happen if there is involvement of the rehabilitation team from the outset.

Vision and visuomotor function

Decompression of the orbit may be required as an emergency procedure after severe impact injury, but trauma or haemorrhage around the base of the brain may result in III or VI nerve palsies. If these persist and interfere with binocular vision for prolonged periods amblyopia may develop. Ophthalmic advice within the first 2 weeks is essential, and patching or glasses which lift a ptosic eyelid may be prescribed. Alternate eye patching is sometimes useful to alleviate the common symptom of diplopia.

Di Scala *et al.* (1992) found an instance of visual problems of 7.1% in a group with predominantly mild head injuries, rising to 42% in a group with predominantly severe injuries, but the type of problem was not specified and reference was not made to background prevalence (up to 20% of 12-year-olds have visual problems (Crouchman, 1987)). In Klonoff's long-term follow-up (1993) of 159 patients, perceptive problems or field defects were present in two, diplopia in two and retinal damage in one.

Visuomotor performance has been shown to be impaired 1 year after injury in nearly one-third of head injured children after resolution of PTA. This was related to coma duration and initial GCS, and associated with a slowed reaction time and somatosensory problems (Levin & Eisenberg, 1979).

Visual field defects are a common association with hemiplegia, but in some instances may be due to unilateral neglect (see below).

Hearing

Disruption of hearing is particularly associated with temporal or base of skull fractures and may be caused by blows to a static head, as well as the shearing forces in angular acceleration. The VIII nerve may be damaged directly in its path from the brainstem to the inner ear by shearing, but the effects may not be immediate or permanent. Other mechanisms are ischaemia caused by interruption of blood supply through the vertebral and basal arteries, or degeneration of the central auditory vestibular pathways. Damage of the inner ear itself may cause progressive sensorineural deafness (Makishima & Snow, 1976).

Head injury victims often arrive with external ears filled with blood from scalp wounds, and examination of the tympanic membranes may be delayed and forgotten. Temporal bone fracture should alert to potential problems, but other local trauma (perforation of tympanic membrane, disruption of ossicles, contracoup inner ear concussion) may pass undetected. An early opinion from an otolarygologist is indicated when there is uncertainty, and all cases of severe head injury should be assessed for hearing loss in the recovery period. There is a case for referring even children in coma to identify damage to middle ear function and auditory pathways, and the possible need for amplification to assist communication as they wake up. In practice, this is only likely to happen in prolonged coma when audiory evoked responses form part of the overall prognostic assessment.

The frequency spectrum widens with the severity of damage (Schuknecht *et al.*, 1951) but is usually between 4 and 8 kHz, i.e. in the higher end of the speech frequencies. Tinnitus, which is said to occur in one-third of adults irrespective of injury severity, is uncommon in children. Damage to central auditory processing may impair ability to hear in conditions of high background noise (e.g. school) and to localise sound (Katz, 1985).

Di Scala *et al.* (1992) found an instance of hearing impairment of 3.5% in a group of predominantly minor head injuries (probably normal background prevalence for conductive hearing loss), rising to 21.7% in the group containing mostly severe injuries.

Dizziness, a sensation of swaying or floating, is a common complaint in adults in the first weeks of recovery and represents a mismatch between the input from the labyrinth, eyes and proprioceptive apparatus. Benign positional vertigo is also common after mild head injury and may develop a few weeks later. It occurs in certain head positions accompanied by positional nystagmus whereas vestibular failure is associated with spontaneous nystagmus towards the normal side. Children seem to have vestibular symptoms as commonly as adults, but appear better able to compensate for them (Raglan, 1989).

Smell

The olfactory nerves are relatively vulnerable to injury, and anosmia was found in 72 of 1000 adults with severe head injury; 12 of these had perversion of smell perception (parosmia). Recovery took place in six, usually within 6 months of injury (Leigh, 1943).

There is no reason to suppose that children do not experience anosmia as frequently as adults, but they do not complain of it, and the sense of smell is rarely tested. Anosmia, and particularly parosmia, should be considered in children with loss of appetite after head injury.

Perception

Perceptive problems, e.g. hemiattention, visual or auditory neglect, hemianaesthesia or dysagnosia undoubtedly occur even in infancy, but are greatly underdiagnosed. Fortunately, many of them are transient, but a history of visual neglect behaviour in acute injury which is accompanied by evidence of residual hemiplegia should prompt follow-up for a persisting contralesional functional field defect (Crouchman, 1994). When unilateral neglect persists (usually as a result of right hemispheric damage) it has important implications for rehabilitation (Robertson et al., 1993).

Cognitive

When parents ask the question, 'Is he going to be able to lead a normal life again?' they are often asking whether their child will be left with cognitive impairment, resulting in learning difficulties. Post-traumatic cognitive impairment appears to have a more destructive effect on the family unit than does physical handicap (Bond & Brooks, 1976) and it is not surprising that this area of head injury research has received relatively more attention. The two main types of methodology used in research studies will inevitably give different quantitative and qualitative results. Group studies, where children are compared according to the severity of the injury with controls and with other severity groups, are more sensitive, but give little detail about patterns of deficit or recovery in the individual child. Descriptive accounts of small numbers of children followed over longer periods are highly informative for clinicians dealing with individual children, but do not give information about the epidemiology of injury and recovery.

Studies have shown that cognitive deficits are related to a number of factors. Severity of injury is predictably important, but methods of assessing it vary. Common measures used are length of coma, initial GCS, or length of PTA. A number of studies have concluded that length of coma is more strongly related to cognitive deficit than the initial GCS (Levin et al., 1988; Knights et al., 1991). In Brink & Garrett's retrospective series of very severely injured children and adolescents (Brink et al., 1970) only one-third of those children who were unconscious for longer than 1 week (mean 4 weeks) still had an IQ of 85 or above. Of the remainder, 14% were below 70 (5% of these had an average coma of 11 weeks). They demonstrated a direct relation to coma duration in the children under 8 years of age. This group, however, was in a rehabilitation unit and therefore excluded any who might have made a rapid recovery from severe injury (there are several documented cases, e.g. Knights *et al.* (1991), of children emerging from several weeks of coma with no persisting deficit). Klonoff & Low (1974) reported an average loss of 10 IQ points 1 year after injury. Lange-Cosack *et al.* (1979) followed up 50 children for 4–14 years and showed that residual cognitive deficit was directly related to duration of coma. The increased tendency to ventilate children with alteration of consciousness, particularly prior to transfer to a specialist unit, and the routine of morning extubation, makes accurate estimation of shorter periods of coma difficult.

Other studies have examined the relationship between length of PTA and subsequent cognitive deficits. Richardson (1963) looked retrospectively at ten children with a medium duration of coma of 28 days (7–47 days) and a medium duration of PTA of 49 days (25–65 days), followed up for at least 2 years. Each patient showed a larger range of variations in subtests than the normal population, all performed poorly on tests of rote memory, and there was an estimated loss of 10–30 IQ points. Chadwick *et al.* (1981) followed 60 children for 2.25 years, with a control group of orthopaedic admissions. Even transient cognitive deficits were rare after a PTA of less than 24 hours and they found no evidence of persistent cognitive damage in this group; however, PTA of 3 or more weeks was associated with persistent intellectual deficits. This study confirmed the findings of Levin & Eisenberg (1979) that permanent deficits were rare following a PTA of less than 3 weeks. Fay *et al.* (1993), in a study of mildly head injured children with controls individually matched for premorbid educational performance and behaviour, found no significant deficits at 1 year.

These studies appear to provide reassurance that mild head injury does not result in cognitive impairment, at least in children over the age of 5 years at injury. The follow-up was relatively short, certainly not long enough to exclude frontal effects. More subtle deficits may have been missed – a study of young adults with previous mild head injuries showed that although they were normal to testing at sea level, if placed in high altitude conditions cognitive impairments became apparent on the Paced Auditory Serial Addition Test (Ewing *et al.*, 1980). Children may appear to function normally until put under pressure. The performance items on the Wechsler Scale are timed, and therefore reveal problems with speeded performance in children with mild head injury who otherwise cope (Gulbrandsen, 1984). This probably explains the discrepancy often noted between Performance and Verbal IQ after head injury (Flach & Malmros, 1972). Bawden *et al.* (1985) found few differences between children with severe, moderate and mild head injury other than on tests of speeded performance. This may be due to slowing of motor responses, or of information processing, or both. A study such as Bawden's must inevitably exclude the very severely injured and may be overoptimistic about the prognosis at the severe end of the spectrum.

Recovery of cognitive deficits appears to continue for several years, but slows down after the first year (Klonoff *et al.*, 1977; Chadwick *et al.*, 1981; Jaffe *et al.*, 1995). In a 23-year follow-up, Klonoff *et al.* (1993) found intellectual sequelae which related significantly to the finding of lower IQs in 23% of the 90% classified as mild in the original 5-year study. There was a correlation between low IQ in the 17 subjects reporting emotional sequelae. Gaidolfi & Vignolo (1980) assessed 21 teenagers after childhood head injury and found four with IQs below 80. In the absence of good premorbid data such results are difficult to interpret and certainly are at odds with those of Levin & Isenberg (1979) who found that persistent intellectual deficits at the end of the first year were confined to children and adolescents in coma for longer than 24 hours.

Frontal lobe injury, behaviour and the dysexecutive syndrome

The frontal lobe may be damaged in direct impact injuries to the face (for example, when the head hits the windscreen) or by contrecoup in high-velocity accidents. Awareness of the subtle but devastating long-term effects of frontal injury (Kolb, 1989; Grattan & Eslinger, 1991) has been slow to develop since Kennard's early descriptions in monkeys. The frontal lobes are late to myelinate and this probably explains the lack of tools to assess them (Golden, 1981). It is really only in the last few years that the 'time bomb' nature of frontal damage during childhood has been recognised (Levin & Kraus, 1994). Black *et al.* (1971) showed no major increase in conduct problems until 4–5 years after head injury, and late-onset deterioration in behaviour can be wrongly attributed to the onset of adolescence. The term 'sleeper effect' has been coined to describe this quiescent period in frontally injured children.

The frontal lobes are responsible for attention control, planning and initiation of activity, and self-regulatory behaviour. Poor executive function as a result of damage can lead to lack of insight, facile, disinhibited behaviour, inability to understand abstractions, social nuances and inferences, and to change behaviour in response to feedback. Brown *et al.* (1981) describe 'undue outspokeness without regard to social convention, the frequent making of very personal remarks or asking of embarassing questions, or getting undressed in social situations where this would usually be regarded as unacceptble behaviour'. Children may show difficulty in shifting attention, managing and collating multiple sources of information, and in working memory. Perrott *et al.* (1991) used siblings as controls and found that although there were few differences on formal neuropsychological testing, including language, there were more behaviour problems, lower school performance, stress on child–parent relationship, and difficulty in adapting to daily living in the index children. Fletcher *et al.* (1990) found similar behaviour problems in children and adolescents after severe injury, and low correlation with cognitive scores.

Klonoff & Paris (1974), in a study of 231 children, found a high incidence of personality changes in both sexes and all age groups. The distinction between personality, mood and behaviour changes is difficult, and when parents refer to their child's changed personality they are often describing the manifestation of a 'dysexecutive syndrome' as described above. Lack of drive may be misinterpreted as depression, and lack of ability to follow extended conversations exacerbates social isolation. Changes in personality can occur at any age, but are more apparent in older children. Family and close friends are aware of changes which may pass unnoticed elsewhere, and will not necessarily mention them unless specifically asked. The problem is particularly associated with trauma to the frontal areas, and when manifested as social (often sexual) disinhibition can be extremely distressing to inexperienced staff as well as family.

This social disability increases with time (Ackerly, 1964; Thompsen, 1989; Eslinger *et al.*, 1992), partly because of changing expectations as the child grows up (Blau, 1936), but also because of the 'sleeper effect'. Chapman *et al.* (1992), studying children 1 year plus after injury, found they used fewer words and sentences, and had impaired narrative organisation (story retell task). Dennis & Barnes (1990) examined 33 children and adolescents on average 3 years after injury and found that most had problems with abstract verbal functioning (e.g. metaphors, irony, creating sentences from limited key information). Verbal intelligence did not predict ability to converse; comprehension of metaphor was not related to understanding of literal meaning. Such impairments can be isolated, and not detected by standard tests.

Behaviour may change dramatically after head injury, or the child may show exacerbation of premorbid conduct difficulties. There may be an increase in impulsivity and mood lability. Sometimes the child develops apathy and loss of drive, and a previously difficult child may be more acceptable to his family inspite of becoming shallow or bland in affect. Lack of motivation is less of a problem in the young child than in an adolescent who is expected to organise his own activities.

Episodic dyscontrol syndromes (EDS) may manifest after a long delay, and are seen in one-third of severe injuries at follow-up, which correlates with the MRI evidence of the commonest lesion being contusion of the anteromedial temporal lobes. Rapid mood swings, intermittent loss of impulse control or abberations of sexual behaviour may bring the adolescent into conflict with his family and the community. Episodes of explosively destructive behaviour, often sparked off by minor frustration, may respond to anticonvulsant drugs (Eames, 1989).

Severity of injury increases the risk of development of psychiatric disorder (Richardson, 1963; Klonoff & Low, 1974), but there are a number of other factors, including seizures, and stresses on family functioning, such as psychiatric disorder in a parent, marital discord, or four or more siblings (Rutter, 1981). Social disinhibition was identified as the only specific posthead injury psychiatric syndrome. Children of all ages appear to be equally vulnerable, but the manifestations appear to be developmentally related. Thus children injured under the age of 10 years exhibit hyperactivity, short attention span, impulsiveness and aggressive behaviour, whereas older children show poor judgement and affective disorders (Brink *et al.*, 1970); however, Taylor (1989) believes that the behaviour seen after head injury is not true Attention Deficit Disorder.

There is no correlation between mood and behaviour problems and damage to a particular hemisphere, but the prognosis is said to be poor when the brainstem is injured (Naughton, 1971; Klonoff & Low, 1974).

Memory

Most injured children retain a good memory for events prior to their injury, but this does not unfortunately preclude problems with short-term memory. In addition to direct damage to areas of the brain subserving memory (temporal lobe, diencephalon), verbal memory may be affected by lesions of the left (language) hemisphere and non-verbal memory by lesions of the right (spatial) hemisphere. Lesions of the frontal areas may produce problems with attention control and organisation of information in spite of normal memory function on direct testing.

Recovery of memory deficits can lag behind physical recovery (Fuld & Fisher, 1997), and may have devastating effects on social and educational rehabilitation. Impairment of long-term storage and retrieval of information is related to length of coma (Levin & Grossman, 1976; Levin *et al.*, 1979, 1982, 1988). Children who had been in coma for more than 7 days all showed memory deficits in spite of improvement in fine motor skills and adjustment to daily living (Richardson, 1963). Levin reported memory problems as the most common cognitive deficit found in adolescents.

These memory problems can unfortunately be persistent. Gaidolfi & Vignolo (1980) found that almost a quarter of their subjects had a verbal memory deficit 10 years after injury, but there have been no longer term studies of recovery of memory function after childhood head injury. The nature of the memory deficit tends to be predominantly a problem with verbal memory, with less effects on memory span for spatial location (Donders, 1993).

Ewing-Cobbs *et al.* (1990) showed that PTA was more predictive for verbal and non-verbal memory loss at 6 months and at 1 year, whereas the GCS was a better predictor of memory problems in the acute recovery phase.

Effects on family

The sudden transformation of a normal child into a disabled child devastates even the strongest families. Longer term follow-up often reveals marital difficulties or breakup and Brown *et al.* (1981) found such problems in one-fifth of the severely injured children in their study. Perrott *et al.* (1991) found that children with moderate to severe injury had reduced social competence and adaptive living skills, associated with a poorer relationship with their parents compared with that of their siblings. Gaidolfi & Vignolo (1980), in a study of 21 young adults who had had childhood head injury, found that parents were overprotective in more than half of the cases, particularly if the injury had been severe. It is hardly surprising that the constant physical and emotional demands on the carer (almost invariably the mother) may be associated with deterioration in her own health and emotional well-being.

Siblings also carry a heavy burden of fear and anxiety, and then sorrow at the loss of their normal childhood companion. Parents and siblings alike experience feelings of guilt (Pascucci, 1988) and of anger. The family grieves for their lost child, and the child grieves for his lost skills and lifestyle. The disabled child makes increased demands on their parents, but also on the siblings themselves, whose own needs may no longer be met at home. They may develop behaviour problems, psychosomatic symptoms, as well as educational underachievement. Embarrassment at the 'odd' behaviour or appearance of their brother or sister may lead to their own social isolation or reluctance to bring friends home, particularly during adolescence.

Parents may find it difficult to accept that their comatose child will not awake and be immediately normal again and they may often report seeing motor improvements in the child which cannot be substantiated (Romano, 1974; Rosin, 1977). This may result in families making unrealistic demands of the patient. Their anger at what has happened to their child may manifest in lack of cooperation and misinterpretation of information which can result in families claiming at a later stage that they were not adequately informed of the severity of the injury and prognosis. Nevertheless, the role of the family in promoting recovery cannot be underestimated (Gilchrist & Wilkinson, 1979).

Functioning at school

The importance of return to normal schooling after head injury is reflected in the number of studies using this as a measure of outcome. Caution must be used in interpreting this information, as we know that the educational system varies greatly from one part of the UK to another, and is not really comparable between countries either in Europe or the USA. The increased tendency for children with disabilities to be integrated into mainstreams schools, for example, makes assessment by type of school attended a very rough guide to outcome. Brink *et al.* (1970) reported that of 46 children surviving comas of more than 1 week, 12 were unable to return to school, 26 were in special schools, and eight were in normal schools; Flach & Malmros (1972) found that when the brainstem had been injured only one-half were making normal progress 8–10 years later; Heiskanen & Kaste (1974) found that children unconscious for more than 2 weeks were rarely able to make normal progress at school; and Klonoff *et al.* (1977) found that 74% of under 9 year olds and 66% of older children were making no real progress at school 5 years after the injury.

Rehabilitation

'An active process by which those disabled by injury achieve a full recovery, or if full recovery is not possible, realise their optimal physical, mental and social potential and are integrated into their most appropriate environment'. In the child this takes place through a process of recovery, adaptation and continuing development (Johnson, 1989), but requires intensive and specialised facilitation. Disruption of normal development means that children require even greater environmental enrichment than adults with a corresponding injury. A sound knowledge of normal child development and the response of the immature brain and musculoskeletal system to injury is essential to a realistic rehabilitation programme and the prevention of undesirable patterns of functioning.

There is evidence that disabilities continue to improve over many years and that children with severe head injury may benefit from months or years of intensive rehabilitation (Eames & Wood, 1985). Di Scala *et al.* (1992), in a study of 598 children aged 8–19 years, demonstrated a good correlation between the clinicians assessment of expected recovery time and the Functional Independence Measure (FIM). Time to recovery was also correlated with injury severity (GCS and ISS).

The basic principles of rehabilitation for children are the same as for adults, i.e. continuity of care, early engagement of the family, prevention of secondary damage, and realistic but optimistic forward planning in relation to housing, education and longer term prognosis. For the head injured child this process starts as soon as medical stabilisation has been achieved. Early involvement of a specialised multidisplinary rehabilitation team helps to prevent complications such as contractures, pressure areas and aspiration pneumonia, and provides support, information and continuity for parents and for staff during acute management. From the outcome perspective, this should lead to better initial information recording as well as improving the parents' perception of the quality of care offered to their child and themselves. The importance of the latter cannot be overstressed, as memories of these early days after injury may colour future relationships with health staff for many years to come.

Aims of rehabilitation

These are well described by Hoddy *et al.* (1996) and are summarised as:

1. To provide medical, social and environmental conditions which maximise natural recovery.
2. To provide conditions which prevent changes antagonistic to recovery.
3. To provide appropriate stimulation for the processes of recovery.
4. To assist the individual and the family to adjust emotionally to their change in circumstances.
5. To teach compensatory strategies and techniques.
6. To provide an environment in which the person can be as independent as possible.

The team required to carry out such a programme during the early and intermediate rehabilitation period is large and specifically trained in paediatric neurodisability (Table 14.1).

Each child has an individual written care-plan which is updated by weekly team meetings (Crouchman, 1990, 1994). Family members attend these meetings, and are encouraged to contribute to suitable areas of the child's management. The balance of the team input depends on the age of the child and the type and severity of the injury. In the longer term, identification of a keyworker is helpful to ensure that all the needs of the child and family are met consistently and without duplication. The parents' charter system proposed for children with cerebral palsy (Milner *et al.*, 1996) has great relevance to many areas of head injury management.

Services

Although adult rehabilitation services have much experience and expertise to share with paediatricians in this field, it has long been recognised that acquired disability in childhood is most appropriately managed by a specialised paediatric neurodevelopmental multidisciplinary team.

Rehabilitation services in the UK vary from one district to another and remain heavily dependent on individual enthusiasm and expertise. McMillan *et al.* (1987) carried out a postal survey of speech therapy in the UK and parts of the USA. She showed that parents reported more intensive treatment in hospitals with designated rehabilitation units, and that in the UK treatment methods tended to be the same for childhood stroke and for head injuries, whereas units in the USA differentiated between the two. In the UK a higher percentage of patients were discharged home and returned to school with special educational support as opposed to attending a rehabilitation unit. There was an increased tendency in the UK to return children to their

Table 14.1. *The team*

Physiotherapist
Speech and Language Therapist
Occupational Therapist
Neuropaediatrician
Specialist Nurse
Neuropsychologist
Psychiatrist
Dietician
Play Therapist
School Teacher
Social Worker

former schools both because community services and local education departments were unfamiliar with the needs of the head injured, and as a result of the policy to integrate those with special needs into mainstream education. Many assessments were geared towards children with developmental language problems because of a lack of suitable test material (Lees, 1989). This tendency to provide rehabilitation from a child development base often means that therapists are trained in neurodevelopmental techniques designed to be more suited to the treatment of cerebral palsy than for rapidly evolving acquired brain injury. Similar problems are inherent in school placements of head injured children (Middleton, 1989).

Residential rehabilitation units for children are very few in number and cannot accommodate all those who would benefit from them. Although the decision to send a very severely brain injured child to residential rehabilitation is relatively straightforward (compared with identifying the funding), the less overtly damaged child presents greater difficulties. The balance has to be weighed between the enormous advantages of an intensive specialised programme and the potential harm to the already stressed child and family from prolonged separation, often at great distances from home.

The increasing importance of rehabilitation in the UK is evident in the expansion of rehabilitation units and of medical training programmes. Services for children have lagged far behind, but the recent formation of a subgroup of the College of Paediatrics and Child Health will hopefully mean a greater recognition of this subspeciality.

Specific rehabilitation issues

Coma management

Coma is defined as the absence of eye opening, the inability to obey commands and no utterance of recognisable words. The theory of stimulation as a way of raising the level of awareness depends on the assumptions that changes in the normal sensory environment may lead to permanent physiological and behavioural abnormalities despite structural integrity (Layton *et al.*, 1978) and that skills aroused in this way can be generalised (not a true assumption in, for example, the rehabilitation of memory).

Social isolation in rats has been shown to reduce prefrontal dopamine activity (Kraemer, 1988); experimental occipital lobe lesions result in reduced weight and DNA content of other cortical areas (Will *et al.*, 1977); and an impoverished environment lowers brain acetylcholinesterases (Rosenzwieg *et al.*, 1969, 1972). In the head injured human, sensory deprivation results from the intensive care environment, but also from isolation, sedation, confinement to bed and lack of movement. Children nursed in isolation may resort to autostimulation, e.g. head rocking and thumb sucking, but the severely head injured child cannot control his physical activities in this way. "He cannot ask for food or changes in temperature or environment. As he emerges from this period of sensory deprivation he then becomes overstimulated, and may retreat from light, sound and people, leading to withdrawal and sometimes elective mutism" (Johnson, 1989). The balance between intensive and varied stimulation, and quiet periods for rest, can be difficult to achieve.

Persistent vegetative state (PVS)

PVS is a state of prolonged coma (at least 6 months) characterised by independent respiration, wakefulness without awareness, sleep/wake cycles, lack of purposeful movements, and abnormal motor responses in all extremities. The EEG may be normal.

PVS can usually be predicted in adults within 3 months of injury. Of 94 patients, only 10% regarded as vegetative at 3 months regained consciousness and all remained totally dependant (Jennet & Teasdale, 1981). PVS is unusual in children, and may carry a worse prognosis in the very young (Ashwal *et al.*, 1994). Fields *et al.* (1993) followed 20 children discharged home in PVS (not all due to traumatic brain injury) and found a 40% mortality after an average of 4.5 years. Twelve of the survivors were thought to have minimal awareness.

Spasticity

The initial response to injury of the motor cortex or pyramidal pathways is muscle flaccidity with absent tendon jerks. The longer the flaccid stage persists, the worse the prognosis. As tone returns, spasticity emerges. The pattern and extent of involvement of muscle groups will depend on the nature of the injury. The development of spasticity itself may be relatively unimportant compared with the disability resulting from postural disturbances and inability to stabilise trunk and head. Nociceptive stimuli, which promote synaptic sprouting, are known to promote the development of spasticity in the acute postinjury phase, particularly if there is damage to the spinal cord. Stimulation from the bladder, bowel or skin causes temporary increase in spasticity, and if this is frequently repeated may increase the eventual residual flexor spasticity. This needs to be explained to staff and to the family (especially younger siblings), as the natural response to an injured child is to stroke the limbs and to try to evoke a movement response. On the contrary, proprioceptive stimulation by normal position-ing of joints during this early phase may be helpful in maintaining normal extensor activity (Marsden, 1988).

Care must be taken to avoid wet, wrinkled sheets and tight dressings or manometer cuffs. For the same reason, the use of splints during the early recovery phase must be judicious, as any intervention which produces pain will be counterproductive. Unfor-tunately flexion contractures can develop within a matter of weeks, and although they can usually be reversed with intensive physiotherapy, this may take weeks or months of valuable rehabilitation time which could be better used for developing cognitive and daily living skills. For this reason attempts are often made to control spasticity with drugs. None is without problems. Baclofen, the most commonly used in children, has the disadvantage of being a sedative at effective doses, and may produce dizziness and nausea. At high doses it can result in confusion or seizures. Dantrolene, which directly inhibits muscle contraction by preventing the release of calcium ions, disturbs liver function in 10% of patients, and can cause gastrointestinal symptoms, as well as taking several weeks to build up to clinical efficacy. Benzodiazepines, although increasing synaptic inhibition, are not particularly effective in cerebral spasticity, but may be useful when anxiety or agitation is a dominant feature of the clinical picture.

The mainstay of treatment for spasticity remains regular physiotherapy. Stretching of individual muscle groups, sustained for several minutes, needs to be carried out at least once daily. Where this is not possible (for example, in the presence of other injuries) plaster casts may be used to hold the joint in an optimal position. Botulinum toxin injections into the muscle bulk weaken dynamic spasticity for up to 4 months and protect against contractures in this difficult management scenario. Botulinum is increasingly used in children with spasticity due to cerebral palsy as an alternative to surgical tendon release and is proving a useful adjunct to the management of acute spasticity after acquired brain injury in children.

Tremor may be persistent and inhibiting to the rehabilitation process. Unfortunate-ly, drug treatment has limited success.

Heterotopic ossification

New bone formation, resulting in pain and restriction of joints movements, is a common complication of severe head injuries in adults. It is relatively unusual in adolescents (occurring in 14%), and rarely, if ever, a problem in prepubertal children. There is an association with coma length and poor functional outcome, and the condition is probably more common in the presence of multiple long bone fractures. Treatment is with etidronate, or non-steroidal anti-inflammatory drugs (Hurvitz *et al.*, 1992).

Care of the skin

Robertson *et al.* (1980) showed that normal adults make 14–48 weight-relieving movements every hour during sleep in a supine position. Children are almost certainly more restless even than adults, which is perhaps one reason why they do not develop deep vein thrombosis. Prolonged immobility during coma or ventilation following severe head injury leads to an increase in local skin temperature and tissue metabolic changes which may result in pressure sores. Although large areas of tissue breakdown are uncommon in young children, small pressure sores on the heels and on the occiput can appear within hours. Traditionally, head injured patients at risk of raised intracranial pressure are nursed supine without normal turning. This is not the optimal management for skin, spasticity or lung function, and there is a strong case for placing the child in a lateral position if the intracranial pressure allows.

Nutrition

Nutrition plays an important role in maintaining skin integrity and preventing infection after head injury, but there is evidence for an even more important role in cerebral metabolism. Neurotransmitter metabolism is known to be affected by both tissue damage and nutritional insufficiency. Vitamins needed for the production of neurotransmitters include C, B2, B6, folic acid and iron.

Although a major concern is to prevent protein energy malnutrition, total carbohydrate and calorie intake must be adequate for the increased demands and to maintain the production of neurotransmitters (acetylcholine, noradrenaline, dopamine, 5-hydroxytryptamine, GABA, aminobytyric acid, glutamic acid, aspartic acid and glycine). Tryptophan, the precursor of 5-hydroxytryptamine, exists in small amounts in body stores and in the diet. Carbohydrate intake stimulates secretion of insulin which facilitates the passage of tryptophan into the brain by altering the plasma concentrations of other competing amino acids. In contrast, a protein rich low carbohydrate diet, by raising the level of competing amino acids, reduces tryptophan passage into the brain. The normal diurnal rhythm of plasma tryoptophan levels may be disrupted by head injury (Fernstrom & Wurtman, 1974). A similar mechanism exists for tyrosine and phenylalanine, which influences brain catecholamine activity. Choline, another neurotransmitter, is found in the diet in the form of lecithin. Future management of head injury will involve ways of protecting the brain from excessive release of these neurotransmitters while ensuring adequate continuing production (Eames, 1989).

There are no good studies looking at the effects of nutrition on survival or long-term outcome after brain injury, and management has to be based on what is known about nutrition and cerebral metabolism in children. Blood flow through the various parts of the brain is proportional to the local metabolic rate. The highest rate is found in the white matter during myelination and malnutrition impairs brain growth and normal development in young children. By the age of 6 years the brain has achieved 90% of adult size and cerebral blood flow and oxygen consumption reach peak values. The curve of percentage of basal metabolic energy needed for cerebral metabolism ranges from two-thirds for a 5 kg baby, 40% for a 20 kg child, to one-quarter in adulthood (Heird et al., 1972). The brain contains negligible amounts of glycogen and fat and is therefore dependent upon glucose derived from the diet. It does not have priority at times of dietary insufficiency, but can use ketones as a source of energy. This facility is particularly efficient in babies.

Severe hypercatabolism, nitrogen loss, and glucose intolerance (and hence nutritional requirements) are related to the severity of the brain injury (Rapp et al., 1983). The circulating levels of noradrenaline after severe head injury are those seen during vigorous exercise (Clifton et al., 1981). Glucocorticoid release in response to trauma stress may compromise the capacity of neurons to survive metabolic insults (Sapolsky, 1987). The general metabolic response to severe trauma is considered elsewhere in this book.

Acute malnutrition occurs after head injury in the first few days of coma or PTA. The child is usually well-nourished on arrival in intensive care, and nutritional needs may not be perceived as a priority. Nasogastric feeding is suspended for several hours prior to attempted extubation, and even when parenteral feeding has been instituted for prolonged coma, this is frequently interrupted for radiography, physiotherapy, scanning or drug infusions. Early conversion to gastrostomy feeding solves some of these problems, and makes later speech and language therapy easier. When the child is very confused and pulling at lines it may be impossible to maintain any form of nutritional intake (and sometimes even fluid) for worrying long periods.

The resumption of oral feeding is an important milestone in recovery, and allows the family to take an active role. A head injured child may have difficulty expressing hunger or craving, and at least one severely spastic quadriplegic child has been seen to snatch food from passing food trolleys, and avidly consume hamburgers in spite of considerable swallowing difficulties. Parents may also feed the child unknown to staff. At a later stage appetite may be disturbed, with hyperphagia (Rutter et al., 1984), or loss of interest in food, or failure to recognise food from non-food items. In the author's experience, mild hyperphagia is common in the first few months of recovery, but usually resolves spontaneously without excessive weight gain. True hyperphagia may be associated with the treatment of agitation with chlorpromazine, haloperidol or thioridazine. It may also be a manifestation of disinhibition, in which case it is difficult to treat, particularly in adolescence. Rarely, it may represent structural damage to the appetite centres.

Dickerson *et al.* (1982) have expressed concern that the poor socioeconomic status of many head injury victims, and the additional stress to the family, may result in the damaging combination of long-term malnutrition and understimulation.

Drugs

Doctors should think twice before prescribing even routine drugs to a child recovering from head injury (Eames, 1989). Antihistamines for hayfever can intensify attention and arousal deficits, induce or exacerbate agitation and are potentially epileptogenic. Prochlorperazine, used for nausea and vomiting, is also epileptogenic, and both it and haloperidol (prescribed for sedation) can cause extrapyramidal side-effects at quite low doses.

Drugs which assist in early rehabilitation by reducing spasticity should be introduced cautiously but early (see Spasticity above) to prevent permanent secondary damage. Most drugs acting on the central nervous system initially produce sedation. This is believed to be caused by the tendency for sprouting to occur when existing receptors are blocked for any length of time. These mechanisms mean that initial and long-term effects of drugs may not be the same.

Measuring recovery

There is no doubt that early rehabilitation prevents secondary damage following head injury, and is therefore essential on grounds of cost-benefit as well as compassion. It is important, nonetheless, to attempt to measure the child's progress and to relate it to the nature and severity of the trauma. There are a large number of validated assessment scales suitable for use in older adolescents and adults with brain injury (Wade, 1992). For example, the Glasgow Outcome Scale (Jennett & Bond, 1975) gives eight categories of outcome, but is a very 'broad brush' approach designed for epidemiological studies rather that individuals. The Vineland Adaptive Behavioural Scale is a more detailed and meaningful research tool for assessment of the child's 'real-life' functioning (Sparrow *et al.*, 1984). In practice, progress is measured by regularly setting goals in each of the important areas (mobility, self-help, behaviour, communication) and documenting their achievement.

There is less certainty about the efficacy of longer term intensive rehabilitation in children, whose natural recovery differs from that of adults, and more studies are needed. What is unfortunately very clear from talking to head injured adolescents and their families, is the paucity of educational and social support once the young person becomes an adult (Thomas *et al.*, 1989). Those of us who are involved at any stage of their care should be concerned about the lack of long-term provision for the young disabled. We should also press for a realistic accident prevention programme in our local communites to try to stem the relentless tide of injured children.

References

Ackerly, S. S. (1964). A case of perinatal bilateral frontal lobe defects observed for 30 years. *The Frontal Granular Cortex & Behaviour*, eds. Warren, J. M. & Ackert, A., pp. 192–219. New York, McGraw-Hill.

Annegers, J. F., Grabow, J. D., Kurland, L. T. & Laws, E. R. (1980). The incidence, causes, and secular trends of head trauma in Olmsted County, Minnesota. *Neurology*, 30, 912–19.

Aram, D. (1988). Language sequelae of unilateral brain lesions in children. In *Language Communication and the Brain*, ed. Plum, F., New York, Raven Press.

Ashwal, S., Eyman, R. K. & Call, T. L. (1994). Life expectancy of children in a persistent vegetative state. *Pediatric Neurology*, 10, 27–33.

Bawden, H. N., Knights, R. M. & Winogren, H. W. (1985). Speeded performance following head injury in children. *Journal of Clinical and Experimental Neuropsychology*, 7, 39–54.

Black, P., Blumer, D., Wellner, A. M. & Walker, A. E. (1971). The head injured child: time course of recovery with implications for rehabilitation in head injury. *Proceedings of an International Symposium*. Edinburgh, Churchill Livingstone.

Blau, A. (1936). Mental changes following head trauma in children. *Archives Neurology and Psychiatry*, 35, 723–69.

Bond, M. R. & Brooks, D. N. (1976). Understanding the process of recovery as the basis for the investigation of rehabilitation for the brain injured. *Scandinavian Journal of Rehabilitation Medicine*, 8, 127–33.

Brink, J. D., Garrett, A. L., Hale, W. R., Woo-Sam, J. & Nickel, V. L. (1970). Recovery of motor and intellectual functioning in children sustaining severe head injuries. *Developmental Medicine and Child Neurology*, 12, 565–71.

Brink, J. D., Imbus, C. & Woo-Sam, J. (1980). Physical recovery after severe closed head trauma in children and adolescents. *Journal of Pediatrics*, 87, 721–7.

Bruce, D. A., Raphaely, R. C., Goldberg, A. I., Zimmerman, R. A., Bilaniuk, L. T., Schut, L. & Kuhl, D. E. (1979). Pathophysiology, treatment and outcome following severe head injury in children. *Child's Brain*, 5, 174–91.

Brown, G., Chadwick, O., Shaffer, D., Rutter, M. & Traub, M. (1981). A prospective study of children with head injuries. III. Psychiatric sequelae. *Psychological Medicine*, 11, 63–78.

Caffey, J. (1972). The whiplash shaken infant syndrome. *Paediatrics*, 55, 306–403.

Caveness, W. F., Meirowsky, A. M., Rish, B. L., Mohr, J. P., Kistler, J. P., Dillon, J. D. & Weiss, G. H. (1979). The nature of post-traumatic epilepsy. *Journal of Neurosurgery*, 50, 545–53.

Chadwick, O., Rutter, M., Brown, G., Shaffer, D. & Traub, M. (1981). A prospective study of children with head injury. II. Cognitive sequelae. *Psychological Medicine*, 11, 49–62.

Chapman, S. B., Culhane, K. A., Levin, H. S., Harward, H., Mendlesohn, D., Ewing-Cobbs, L., Fletcher, J. M. & Bruce, D. (1992). Narrative discourse after closed head injury in children and adolescence. *Brain and Language*, 43, 42–65.

Clifton, G. L., Ziegler, M. G. & Grossman, R. G. (1981). Circulating catecholamines and sympathetic activity after head injury. *Journal of Neurosurgery*, **8**, 10–14.

Cooper, J. A. & Flowers, C. R. (1987). Children with a history of acquired aphasia: residual language and academic impairments. *Journal of Speech and Hearing Disorders*, **52**, 251–62.

Cowan, W. M., Fawcett, J. W., O'Leary, D. D. M. & Stanfield, B. B. (1984). Regressive events in neurogenesis. *Science*, **225**, 1258–65.

Crouchman, M. R. (1994). The rehabilitation of head injuries. *Maternal and Child Health*, **19**, 144–50.

Crouchman, M. R. (1987). The health of inner-city 12 year olds. *Presented at Meeting on Health and Disease: Educating Children and Parents*. Association of Paediatric Education in Europe, The Hague.

Crouchman, M. R. (1990). Head injuries: how community paediatricians can help. *Archives of Disease of the Child*, **65**, 1286–7.

Cummins, B. H. & Potter, J. M. (1970). Head injury due to falls from heights. *Injury*, **2**, 61.

Dennis, M. & Barnes, M. A. (1990). Knowing the meaning, getting the point, bridging the gap, and carrying the message. Aspects of discourse following closed head injury in childhood and adolescence. *Brain and Language*, **39**, 428–46.

Dickerson, J. W. T., Merat, A. & Yusuf, H. K. M. (1982). Effects of malnutrition on brain growth and development. *Brain and Behavioural Development*, ed. Dickerson, J. W. T. and McGurk, H. Glasgow, Surrey University Press.

Di Scala, C., Grant, C. C., Brooke, M. M. & Gans, B. M. (1992). Functional outcome in children with traumatic brain injury. Agreement between clinical judgement and the Functional Independence of Measure. *American Journal of Physical Medicine and Rehabilitation*, June **71**(3), 145–8.

Donders, J. (1993). Memory function after traumatic brain injury in children. *Brain Injury*, **7**, 431–7.

Duhaime, A. C., Gennarelli, T. A., Thibauld, L. E., Bruce, D. A., Marguilies, S. S. & Wiser, R. (1987). The shaken baby syndrome, a clinical, pathological, and biomechanical study. *Journal of Neurosurgery*, **66**, 409–15.

Eames, P. (1989). Rational drug interventions. In *Childrens Head Injury Who Cares?* ed. Johnson, D. A., Uttley, D. & Wyke, M., pp. 40–54. London: Taylor Francis.

Eames, P. & Wood, R. (1985). Rehabilitation after severe brain injury. A follow up study of a behaviour modification approach. *Journal of Neurology, Neurosurgery and Psychiatry*, **48**, 613–19.

Eslinger, P. J., Grattan, L. M., Damasio, H. & Damasio, A. R. (1992). Developmental consequences of childhood frontal lobe damage. *Archives of Neurology*, **49**, 764–9.

Ewing, R., McCarthy, D., Gronwall, D. & Wrightson, P. (1980). Persisting effects of minor head injury observable during hypoxic stress. *Journal of Clinical Neuropsychology*, **2**, 147–55.

Ewing-Cobbs, L., Levin, H. S., Eisenberg, H. M. & Fletcher, J. M. (1987). Language functions following closed head injury in children and adolescence. *Journal of Clinical and Experimental Neuropsychology*, **9**, 575–92.

Ewing-Cobbs, L., Fletcher, J. M. & Levin, H. S. (1985). Neuropsychological sequelae following paediatric head injury. *Head Injury Rehabilitation: Children and Adolescents*, ed. Ylvisaker, pp. 71–9. Austin TX, Pro-ed.

Ewing-Cobbs, L., Levin, H. S., Fletcher, J. M., McLochlin, E. J., McNeily, D. J., Ewitt, J. & Francis, D. (1984). Assessment of post-traumatic amnesia in head injury children. *Presented to Neuropsychological Society*.

Ewing-Cobbs, L., Levin, H. S., Fletcher, J. M., Miner, M. E. & Eisenberg, A. M. (1990). The Children's Orientation and Amnesia Test: relationship to severity of acute head injury and to recovery of memory. *Neurosurgery*, **27**, 683–91.

Ewing-Cobbs, L., Miner, M., Fletcher, J. M. & Levin, H. S. (1989). Intellectual, motor, and language sequelae following closed head injury in infants and pre-schoolers. *Journal of Paediatric Psychology*, **14**, 531–44.

Fay, G. C., Jaffe, K. M., Polissar, N. L., Liao, S., Martin, K. M., Shurtleff, H. A., Rivara, J. B. & Winn, R. (1993). Mild pediatric traumatic brain injury: a cohort study. *Archives of Physical Medicine and Rehabilitation*, **74**, 895–901.

Fernstrom, J. D. & Wurtman, R. J. (1974). Nutrition and the brain. *Scientific American*, **230**, 84–91.

Field, J. H. (1976). *Epidemiology of Head Injury in England and Wales: with Particular Application to Rehabilitation*. Leicester, Printed for HMSO by Willsons.

Fields, A. I., Coble, D. H., Pollack, M. M., Cuerdon, T. T. & Kalfman, J. (1993). Outcomes of children in a persistent vegetative state. *Critical Care Medicine*, **21**, 1890–4.

Finger, S. & Stein, D. G. (1982). *Brain Damage and Recovery. Research and Clinical Perspectives*. New York, Academic Press.

Finger, S., Jonowsky, J. S. & Finlay, B. L. (1986). The outcome of perinatal brain damage: the role of neuronal loss and axonal retraction. *Developmental Medicine and Child Neurology*, **28**, 375–89.

Fletcher, J. M., Ewing-Cobbs, L., Miner, M. & Levin, H. S. (1990). Behavioural changes after closed head injury in children. *Journal of Consulting and Clinical Psychology*, **58**, 93–8.

Flach, J. & Malmros, R. (1972). A long-term follow up study with severe head injury. *Scandinavian Journal of Rehabilitation and Medicine*, **4**, 9–15.

Foa, B., Steckatee, G. & Olasov-Rothbaum, B. O. (1989). Behavioural cognitive conceptualisations of post-traumatic stress disorder. *Behaviour Research and Therapy*, **20**, 155–76.

Frowein, R. A., Terhaag, D., auf der Haar, K., Richard, K. E. & Firsching, R. (1992). Rehabilitation after severe injury. *Acta Neurochirurgica*, **55** (Suppl), 72–4.

Fuld, P. A. & Fisher, P. (1997). Recovery of intellectual ability after closed head injury. *Developmental Medicine and Child Neurology*, **19**, 495–502.

Gaidolfi, E. & Vignolo, L. A. (1980). Closed head injuries of school aged children: neuropsychological sequelae in early adulthood. *Italian Journal of Neurological Science*, **1**, 65–73.

Gennarelli, T. A. (1992). Biomechanics of head injury. *Presented at Meeting held at the Institution of Mechanical Engineers*, London.

Gennarelli, T. A. & Thibault, L. E. (1985). Biological models of head injuries. *Central Nervous System Trauma Status Report*, ed. Becker, D. P. and Povlishock, J. T., Maryland, NIH.

Gilchrist, E. & Wilkinson, M. (1979). Some factors determining prognosis in young people with severe head injuries. *Archives of Neurology*, **36**, 355–8.

Golden, C. J. (1981). The Luria-Nebraska Children's Battery: theory and formulation. In *Neuropsychological Assessment and the School Aged Child*, ed. Hynd, G. W. and Obrzut, J. E., pp. 277–302. New York, Grune & Stratton.

Goodman, R. (1989). Limits to cerebral plasticity. In *Childrens Head Injury Who Cares?*, ed. Johnson, D. A., Uttley, D. and Wyke, M., pp. 12–22.

Granholm, L. & Srendgaard, N. (1972). Hydrocephalus following traumatic head injuries. *Scandinavian Journal of Rehabilitation and Medicine*, **4**, 31–4.

Grattan, L. M. & Eslinger, P. G. (1991). Frontal lobe damage in children and adults: a comparative review. *Developmental Neuropsychology*, **7**, 283–326.

Greenspan, A. I. (1996). Functional recovery following head injury in children. *Current Problems in Paediatrics*, **26**, 170–7.

Gronwall, W. (1980). Duration of post-traumatic amnesia after mild head injury. *Journal of Clinical Neuropsychology*, **2**, 51–60.

Gulbrandsen, G. B. (1984). Neuropsychological sequelae of light head injuries in old children six months after trauma. *Journal of Clinical Neuropsychology*, **6**, 257–68.

Gurdjian, E. S. & Webster, J. E. (1958). *Head Injuries: Mechanisms, Diagnosis, and Management*, Boston, Little, Brown & Co.

Hawthorne, V. M. (1978). Epidemiology of head injuries. *Scottish Medical Journal*, **23**, 92.

Hebb, D. O. (1942). The effect of early and late brain injury upon test scores, and the nature of normal adult intelligence. *Proceedings of the American Philosophical Society*, **85**, 275–92.

Hecaen, H. (1976). Acquired aphasia in children and the ontogenesis of hemispheric specialisation. *Brain and Language*, **3**, 114–34.

Heird, W. C., Driscoll, J. M., Schullinger, J. N., Grebin, B. & Winters, R. W. (1972). Intravenous alimentation in paediatric patients. *Journal of Paediatrics*, **8**, 351–72.

Heiskanen, O. & Kaste, M. (1974). Late prognosis of severe brain injury in children. *Developmental Medicine and Child Neurology*, **16**, 11–14.

Hoddy, M., Yoemans, J., Smith, H. & Johnson, J. (1996). In *Brain Injury and After: Towards Improved Outcome*, ed. Rose, F. D. and Johnson, D. A. Chichester, John Wiley.

Horowitz, M. J. (1976). Stress response syndromes. *American Psychological Association*. New York, Jason Aronson.

Hurvitz, E. A., Mandac, B. R., Davidoff, G., Johnson, J. H. & Nelson, V. S. (1992). Risk factors for heterotopic ossification in children and adolescents with severe traumatic brain injury. *Archives of Physical Medicine and Rehabilitation*, **73**, 459–62.

Janowsky, J. S. & Finlay, B. L. (1986). The outcome of perinatal brain-damage: the role of normal neuronal loss and axonal retraction. *Developmental Medicine and Child Neurology*, **28**, 375–89.

Jaffe, K. M., Polissar, N. L., Fay, G. C. & Liao, S. (1995). Recovery trends over 3 years following paediatric traumatic brain injury. *Archives of Physical Medicine and Rehabilitation*, **76**, 17–26.

Jennett, B. (1976). Assessment of severity of head injury. *Journal of Neurology, Neurosurgery and Psychiatry*, **39**, 647–55.

Jennett, B. & Bond, M. (1975). Assessment of outcome after severe brain damage. A practical scale. *Lancet*, **1**, 480–4.

Jennett, B. & Teasdale, G. (1981). *Management of Head Injuries*. Philadelphia, F. A. Davis.

Johnson, D. A. (1989). Early recovery, can we help? In *Childrens Head Injury Who Cares?* ed. Johnson, D. A., Uttley, D. & Wyke, M., pp. 23–39.

Katz, M. (1985). *Handbook of Clinical Audiology*, 3rd edn. Baltimore, Williams and Wilkins.

Kennard, M. A. (1938). Reorganisation of motor function in the cerebral cortex of monkeys deprived of motor and premotor areas in infancy. *Journal of Neurophysiology*, **1**, 477–96.

Kolb, B. (1989). Brain development, plasticity, and behaviour. *American Psychologist*, **44**, 1203–12.

Klonoff, H. & Low, M. (1974). Disordered brain function in young children and early adolescence: neuropsychological and electroencephalographic correlates. *Clinical Neuropsychology: Current Status and Applications*, ed. Reightan, R. M. & Davison, L. A., New York, John Wiley.

Klonoff, H. & Paris, R. (1974). Immediate, short-term and residual effects of acute head injuries in children: neuropsychological and neurological correlates. *Clinical Neuropsychology: Current Status and Applications*, ed. Reightan, R. M. & Davison, L. A., pp. 179–210. New York, John Wiley.

Klonoff, H., Clark, C. & Klonnoff, P. S. (1993). Long-term outcome of head injuries: a 23 year follow up study of children with head injuries. *Journal of Neurology, Neurosurgery and Psychiatry*, **56**, 410–15.

Klonoff, H., Low, M. D. & Clark, C. (1977). Head injuries in children: a prospective 5 year follow up. *Journal of Neurology, Neurosurgery and Psychiatry*, **40**, 1211–19.

Knights, R. M., Ivan, L. P., Venturey, E. C. G., Bentivoglio, C., Stoddard, T., Winogron, W. & Bawden, H. N. (1991). The effects of head injury in neuropsychological and behavioural functioning. *Brain Injury*, **54**, 339–51.

Kraemer, G. W. (1988). The primate social environment, brain neurochemical changes and psychopathology. *Trends in Neuroscience*, **8**, 339–40.

Kraus, J. F., Fife, D., Cox, P., Ramstein, K. & Conroy, C. (1986). Incidence, severity, and external causes of paediatric brain injury. *American Journal of Diseases of Children*, **140**, 687–93.

Lange-Cosack, H., Wider, B., Schlesner, H. J., Frumme, T. & Kupicki, S. (1979). Prognosis of brain injuries in young children (1 until 5 years of age). *Neuropaediatrie*, **10**, 105–27.

Layton, B. S., Corrick, G. E. & Toga, A. W. (1978). Sensory restriction and recovery of function. In *Recovery from Brain Damage*, ed. Finger, S., New York, Plenum Press.

Lees, J. A. (1989). Recovery of speech and language deficits after head injury in children. *Childrens Head Injury Who Cares?* ed. Johnson, D. A., Uttley, D. & Wyke, M., pp. 80–95.

Leigh, A. D. (1943). Defects of smell after head injury. *Lancet*, **1**, 38–40.

Levin, H. S., Aldrich, E. F., Saydjari, C., Eisenberg, H. M., Foulkes, M. A., Bellefleur, M. (1992). Severe head injury in children: experience of the traumatic coma data banks. *Neurosurgery*, **31**, 435–44.

Levin, H. S., Eisenberg, H. M., Wigg, N. R. & Kobayashai, K. (1982). Memory and intellectual ability after head injury in children and adolescence. *Neurosurgery*, **11**, 668–73.

Levin, H. S., Eisenberg, H. M. & Miner, M. E. (1983). Neuropsychological findings in head injured children. *Paediatric Head Trauma*, ed. Shapiro, K., pp. 223–40. Mount Kisco, New York, Futura Publishing.

Levin, H. S. & Grossman, R. G. (1976). Effects of closed head injury on storage and retrieval in memory and learning of adolescence. *Journal of Paediatrics and Psychology*, **1**, 38–42.

Levin, H. S., Grossman, R. G., Rose, J. E. & Teasdale, G. (1979). Long-term neuropsychological outcome of closed head injury. *Journal of Neurosurgery*, **50**, 601–6.

Levin, H. S., High, W. M., Ewing-Cobbs, L., Fletcher, J., Eisenberg, H. M., Miner, M. E. & Goldstein, F. C. (1988). Memory functioning during the first year after closed head injury in children and adolescents. *Neurosurgery*, **22**, 1043–52.

Levin, H. S. & Isenberg, H. M. (1979). Neuropsychological outcome of cloned head injury. *Child's Brain*, **5**, 281–292.

Levin, H. S. & Kraus, M. F. (1994). The frontal lobes and traumatic brain injury. *Journal of Neurology, Psychology, Clinical Neurological Sciences*, **6**, 443–54.

Lonigan, C. J., Shannon, M. P., Finch, A. J., Daugherty, T. K. & Taylor, C. M. (1991). Children's reaction to a natural disaster: symptom severity and degree of exposure. *Advances in Behavioural Research Therapy*, **13**, 135–54.

Mahoney, W. J., De-Souza, E. J., Haller, J. A., Rogers, M. C., Epstein, M. M. & Freeman, J. M.

(1983). Long-term outcome of children with severe head trauma and prolonged coma. *Paediatrics*, **71**, 756–61.

Makishima, K. & Snow, J. B. (1976). Histopathological correlates of neurological manifestations following head trauma. *The Laryngoscope*, February, 1303–14.

Marsden, D. (1988). *Spasticity in Rehabilitation of the Physically Disabled Adult*, ed. Goodwill, C. J. & Chamberlain, M. A. London, Croomhelm.

McClelland, C. Q., Rekate, H., Kaufman, B. & Bersse, L. (1980). Cerebral injury in child abuse: a changing profile. *Child's Brain*, **7**, 225–35.

McDonald, C. M., Jaffe, K. M., Fay, G., Polissar, N. L., Martin, K. M., Leiau, S. & Rivara, J. B. (1994). Comparison of indices of traumatic brain injury severity as predictors of neurobehavioural outcome in children. *Archives of Physical Medicine and Rehabilitation*, **75**, 328–37.

McMillan, M. E., Mule, L. N. & Lees, J. A. (1987). Acquired neurological insult in children; current management issues – USA/UK. *Presented at the 8th annual traumatic head injury programme*, Braintree, Massachusettes. Quoted in *Recovery of Speech and Language deficits after head injury in children*, Lees, J. A., 1989, *Children's Head Injury, Who Cares?*, ed. D. A. Johnson, D. Uttley & M. Wyke. London: Taylor Francis.

McMillan, T. M. (1991). Post-traumatic stress disorder and severe head injury. *British Journal of Psychiatry*, **159**, 431–3.

Michaud, L. J., Rivara, F. P., Grady, M. S. & Reay, D. T. (1992). Predictors of survival and severity of disability after severe brain injury in children. *Neurosurgery*, **31**, 254–64.

Middleton, J. (1989). Thinking about head injuries in children. *Journal of Child Psychology and Psychiatry*, **30**, 663–70.

Milner, J., Bungay, C., Jellinek, D. & Hall, D. M. B. (1996). Needs of disabled children and their families. *Archives of Diseases of Children*, **75**, 399–404.

Naughton, J. A. L. (1971). The effects of severe head injuries in children. Psychological aspects. *Proceedings of an international symposium on head injury*. Edinburgh, Churchill Livingstone, pp. 106–10.

Oddy, M., Yoeman, J., Smith, H. & Johnson, J. (1996). Rehabilitation. In *Brain Injury and After*, ed. Rose, F. D. & Johnson, D. A. Chichester, John Wiley.

Oppenheimer, D. R. (1968). Microscopic lesions in the brain following head injury. *Journal of Neurology, Neurosurgery and Psychiatry*, **31**, 299–306.

Pascucci, R. C. (1988). Head trauma in the child. *Intensive Care Medicine*, **14**, 185–95.

Perrott, S. B., Taylor, H. G. & Montes, J. L. (1991). Neuropsychological sequelae, familial stress, and environmental adaptation following paediatric head injury. *Developmental Neuropsychology*, **7**, 69–86.

Pfurtscheller, G., Schwarz, G. & List, W. (1986). Long lasting EEG reactions in comatose patients after repetitive stimulation. *Electroencephalography and Neurology*, **64**, 402–10.

Raimondi, A. J. & Hirschauer, J. (1984). Head injury in the infant and toddler. *Child's Brain*, **11**, 12–35.

Raglan, E. (1989). Disorders of hearing and balance. In: *Head Injury: Who Cares?* ed. Johnson, D. A., Uttley, D. & Wyke, M. London: Taylor Francis.

Rapp, R. P., Young, B., Twyman, D., Bivins, B. A., Haack, D., Tibbs, P. A. & Bean, J. R. (1983). The favourable effect of early parenteral feeding on survival in head injured patients. *Journal of Neurosurgery*, **58**, 906–12.

Rappaport, M., Hall, K., Hopkins, K., Belleza, T., Berrol, S. & Reynolds, G. (1977). Evoked brain potentials and disability in brain damaged patients. *Archives of Physical Medicine and Rehabilitation*, **58**, 333–8.

Rappaport, M., Hopkins, K., Hall, K. Belleza, T. & Berrol, S. (1978). Brain evoked potential use in a physical medicine and rehabilitation setting. *Scanned Journal of Rehabilitation and Medicine*, **10**, 27–32.

Richardson, F. (1963). Some effects of severe head injury. A follow up study of children and adolescents after protracted coma. *Developmental Medicine and Child Neurology*, **5**, 471–82.

Robertson, J. C., Shah, J. & Amos, H. (1980). An interface pressure sensor for routine clinical use. *England Medicine*, **9**, 151–66.

Robertson, I. H., Halligan, I. N., Peter, W. & Marshall, J. C. (1993). *Prospects for the Rehabilitation of Unilateral Neglect: Clinical and Experperimental Studies*, ed. Robertson, I. H. & Marshall, J. C., pp. 279–92. UK, Lawrence Erlbaum Associates.

Romano, M. D. (1974). Family response to traumatic head injury. *Scandinavian Journal of Rehabilitation and Medicine*, **6**, 1–4.

Rosenzweig, M. R., Bennett, E. L. & Diamond, M. C. (1972). Brain changes in response to experience. *Scientific American*, **226**, 26–9.

Rosenzweig, M. R., Bennett, E. L., Diamond, M. C., Wu, S.-Y., Slagler, W. & Saffran, E. (1969). Influences of environmental complexity and visual stimulation on development of occipital cortex in the rat. *Brain Research*, **14**, 427–45.

Rosein, A. J. (1977). Reactions of families of brain injured patients who remain in a vegetative state. *Scandinavian Journal of Rehabilitation and Medicine*, **9**, 1–5.

Ruijs, M. B., Keyser, A. & Gabreels, F. J. (1992). Assessment of post-traumatic amnesia in young children. *Developmental Medicine and Child Neurology*, **34**, 855–92.

Ruijs, M. B., Keyser, A. & Gabreels, F. J. (1994). Clinical neurological trauma parameters as predictors for neuropsychological recovery and long-term outcome in paediatric closed head injury: a review of the literature. *Clinical Neurology and Neurosurgery*, **96**, 273–83.

Rune, V. (1970). Acute head injuries in children. *Acta Paediatrica Scandinavica* (Suppl. 209).

Rutter, M. (1981). Psychological sequelae of brain damage in children. *American Journal of Psychiatry*, **138**, 1533–44.

Rutter, M., Chadwick, O. & Shaffer, D. (1984). Head Injury. ed. Rutter, M. *Developmental Neuropsychology*, Edinburgh, Churchill Livingston.

Sapolsky, R. M. (1987). Glucocorticoids and hippocampal damage. *Trends in Neuroscience*, **10**, 346–9.

Sbordone, R. J. & Liter, J. C. (1995). Mild traumatic brain injury does not produce post-traumatic stress disorder. *Brain Injury*, **9**, 405–12.

Schuknecht, H. F., Neff, W. D. & Perlmann, H. B. (1951). An experimental study of auditory damage following blows to the head. *Annals of Otology, Rhinology and Laryngology*, **60**, 273–90.

Sekino, H., Nakamura, N., Yuki, K., Satch, J., Kikuchi, H. & Sanada, S. (1981). Brain lesions detected by CT scans in cases of minor head injury. *Neurologica Medica Chirurgica*, **21**, 677–83.

Sparrow, S. S., Balla, D. A. & Cichetti, D. V. (1984). *Vineland Adaptive Behaviour Scales*. (Interview Ed., Survey Form.) Circle Pines MN, American Guidance Service.

Stirling-Meyer, J., Hata, T. & Imai, A. (1987). Clinical and external studies of diaschisis. *Cerebral Bloodflow: Physiologic and Clinical Aspects*, ed. Wood, J. H., New York, McGraw-Hill.

Takahashi, H. & Nakazawa, S. (1980). Specific type of head injury in children. Report of 5 cases. *Child's Brain*, **7**, 124–31.

Taylor, E. (1989). Disorders of self-regulation in head injured children. In *Children's Head*

Injury Who Cares? ed. Johnson, D. A., Uttley, D. & Wyke, M. London: Taylor Francis.

Teuber, H. L. (1975). Recovery of functions after brain injury in man. In *Outcome of Severe Damage to the Central Nervous System*. Ciba Foundation Symposium 34, Amsterdam, Elsevier.

Thatcher, R. W., Cantor, D. S., McAlister, R., Geisler, F. & Krause, P. (1991). Comprehensive predictions of outcome in closed head injured patients. *Annals New York Academy of Sciences*, **620**, 82–101.

Thomas, A. P., Bax, M. C. O. & Smyth, D. P. L. (1989). *The Health and Social Needs of Young Adults with Physical Disabilities*. MacKeith Press.

Thompsen, I. V. (1989). Do young patients have worse outcomes after severe head trauma? *Brain Injury*, **3**, 157–62.

Todorow, S. & Heiss, E. (1978). The 'fall asleep' syndrome, a kind of secondary disturbance of consciousness after head injury. In *Head Injuries: Tumours of the Cerebral Region*, ed. Frowein, R. A., Karimi-Nejad, O., Brock, M. & Klinger, M. New York, Springer-Berlag.

Tsui, E. P. (1990). *The Jupiter sinking disaster: effects on teenagers' school performance*. MSc dissertation University of London, Inst. Psycho. quoted in Yule 1994.

Van Dongen, K. J. & Loonen, M. C. B. (1977). Factors related to prognosis of acquired aphasia in children. *Cortex*, **13**, 131–6.

Vargha-Khadem, F. & Polkey, C. E. (1992). A review of cognitive outcome after hemidecortication in humans. *Recovery from Brain Damage, Reflections and Directions*, ed. Rosen, F. D. & Johnson, D. A., pp. 137–51. New York, Plenum Press.

Wade, D. T. (1992). *Measurement in Neurobiological Rehabilitation*. Oxford, Oxford University Press.

Wall, P. D. (1977). The presence of ineffective synapses and the circumstances which unmask them. *Philosophical Transactions of the Royal Society of London, Series B*, **278**, 361–72.

Will, B. E., Rosenzweig, M. R., Bennett, E. L., Herbert, M. & Morimoto, H. (1977). Relatively brief environment enrichment aids recovery of learning capacity and alters brain measures after postweaning brain lesions in rats. *Journal of Comparative Physiology*, **19**, 35–50.

Wilson, P. J. E. (1970). Cerebral hemispherectomy for infantile hemiplegia. A report of 50 cases. *Brain*, **93**, 147–80.

Winogron, H. W., Knights, R. M. & Bawden, H. N. (1984). Neuropsychological deficits following head injury in children. *Journal of Clinical Neuropsychology*, **6**, 269–86.

Wo, S., Zimmerman, T. L., Brink, J. D., Uyehara, K. & Miller, A. R. (1970). Socioeconomic status and post-trauma intelligence in children with severe head injury. *Psychological Report*, **27**, 147–53.

Woods, B. T. & Carey, S. (1979). Language deficits after apparent clinical recovery from childhood aphasia. *Annals of Neurology*, **6**, 405–9.

Ylvisaker, M. (1993). Communication outcome in children and adolescents with traumatic brain injury. *Neuropsychology Rehabilitation*, **3**, 367–87.

Yule, W. (1994). *Post-traumatic Stress Disorder in Child and Adolescent Psychiatry*, 3rd edn, ed. Rutter, M., Herzog, L. & Taylor, E., pp. 392–406. Blackwell Scientific Publications.

Yule, W. & Williams, R. (1990). Post-traumatic stress reaction in children. *Journal of Traumatic Stress*, **3**, 279–95.

Zimmermann, R. A., Bilaniuk, L. T., Bruce, D., Dolinskas, C., Obrist, W. & Kuhl, D. (1978). Computed tomography of paediatric head trauma: acute general cerebral swelling. *Radiology*, **126**, 403–8.

15
Children's rights and child protection

J. HARRIS

Introduction

Despite an avalanche of interest in and legislation concerning children's rights in the last decade and an increase in, and in the incidence of, child abuse, little of value has emerged concerning the acute problem of how to reconcile the increasing emphasis on and respect for children's rights with the increasing need to protect children from abuse.

There is the hint of a paradox here. For rights and protection are often incompatible. In so far as I have a right to do something, you are not entitled to prevent me from doing it or to protect me, against my will, from its harmful effects. Rights protect liberties. The two classic antilibertarian approaches to morality are essentially protectionist in character. They are paternalism and moralism. Paternalism claims the right to control the behaviour of another for that other's own good while moralism asserts that right to protect others from wickedness. The characteristic call of the paternalist is: 'don't do that, it will harm you!', that of the moralist is: 'don't do that, its wicked!'.

If we are concerned about children's rights and hence concerned not only to protect children from abuse, but more importantly to deal justly and appropriately with them when their vulnerability is increased by the need for some form of health care, then we cannot ignore the question of whether they have a right to choose to refuse treatment which might, objectively considered, be clearly in their interests.

In the brief space available here I attempt to do four things. They are, first to articulate, although not defend,[1] a principle of respect for persons which expresses children's rights in their strongest form. Then I show how, at least in principle, this is not incompatible with a principle of protection. Third, I set out some general principles about the nature of autonomy and the scope and limits of paternalism and finally I address briefly the question of the legitimacy of consents to treatment offered by others on behalf of children allegedly incompetent to consent.

Children's rights and respect for persons

If, as I believe, children's rights can only be coherently defended as a dimension of human rights, i.e. as part of a general theory of the rights of persons, then certain interesting and alarming consequences flow.

No one in the history of political theory has succeeded in answering the puzzling question as to where rights come from; however, we can say something about those on whom they fall, about the possessors of rights.

I believe there are really only two alternatives here: either rights are possessed in virtue of the type of being in question, a human say, or they are possessed in virtue of the capacities possessed by that being. In either case we have big problems. Let me explain.

Rights are possessed by natural kinds

If rights are possessed by types of beings, then there are two types possible: either they are possessed by natural kinds of beings, like humans, or they are possessed by beings defined in terms of their properties. For example the category persons, is often defined in terms, not of species membership but, following the English seventeenth century philosopher John Locke, in terms of the possession of properties like self-consciousness and rationality. These are, of course, possessed not in virtue of an individual's identity as a particular kind of being per se but in virtue of that being's capacities – our second type.

Now, if rights are possessed by 'natural kinds' of creatures simply in virtue of their being a particular kind of natural kind, they are certainly possessed by humans. It is not possible (despite the best endeavours of some) to deny that children are humans and so children have whatever rights are distinctively human rights.

I refer you to the Universal Declaration of Human Rights and the European Convention on Human Rights for further (if bizarre) insights as to what these might be in fact.

From this it follows that all children, and almost certainly fetuses as well in so far as they are in being and human, have full human rights.

Rights are possessed by beings with certain capacities

This view which I believe, for reasons I do not have space to detail here,[2] to be the right one, yields conclusions almost equally complicated from the perspective of the paternalistic control and protection of children. For if rights are possessed by beings with certain capacities, then it follows that those who possess the capacities have the rights.

On any analysis of the way rights, either generally or particularly, may be linked to capacities, this is a disaster. For many adults will lack the relevant capacities and have to be deprived of substantial rights; and many children will possess the capacities which confer the most powerful of rights. We cannot in consistency be selective; either we must deny many adults substantial rights and be selective; either we must deny many adults substantial rights and freedoms in order to preserve the right to paternalist control and protection of children, or, we will have to grant substantial rights to many children and full rights, including the franchise, to all children who have capacities relevantly comparable to any adults also granted the franchise and other rights.

Either model of rights I believe implies a revolution in our thinking about children we might well call Children's Liberation on the model of women's liberation.[3] Both imply that children have in most cases the same moral and political status as most adults. Moreover, from the perspective of rights, they are entitled not only to the same concern, respect and protection as is accorded to any other member of the community, no more and no less, but also are entitled to the same freedoms and self-determination.

Does Children's Liberation imply loss of protection?

One very important and persuasive argument seems poised to undermine the conclusions so far reached. It achieved perhaps its clearest and most powerful articulation in the work of the famous nineteenth century jurist James Fitzjames Stephen who argued that 'if children were regarded as the equal of adults ... it would involve a degree of cruelty to the young which can hardly be realised even in imagination'. The spectre raised by Stephen of cruelty to and perhaps exploitation of young children on a new, vast and unprecedented scale must be taken very seriously. He had in mind things like the exploitation of children in the labour market, sending them down mines, up chimneys; low pay, long hours and so on. He would also doubtless have been aware of the then huge problem of child prostitution which today would perhaps be regarded simply as one dimension of the problem of child abuse. If these were to be the consequences of the emancipation of children, then the price would be one no civilised society should be prepared to pay; but is this where my suggestions have been leading?

If Stephen is taken to mean that unless children are protected from predatory and exploitative adults they will be cruelly used, this might well be true, but it need not concern us. For my suggestion is simply that the only defensible views as to which sorts of creatures possess rights involves the idea that all persons, adult or child, are entitled to equal concern, respect and protection, including equality before the law and other civil rights. But any principle of equality worthy of the name and ceertainly the idea towards which we have been arguing, is itself a principle of protection. If children are genuinely regarded as the equals of adults, then they are regarded as being entitled, among other things, to equal protection. To regard people as equals is to recognise that they may well not be equally able to protect themselves and their interests. It is rather to recognise that their wishes and interests matter as much as anyone else's regardless of their ability to protect them or further them unaided. It is when people are not regarded as the equals of others that they are in danger of arbitrary or ill usage, tyranny and exploitation.

To regard people as the equals one of another is to take a stand on how they are entitled to be treated, not to make a remark about their capacity to obtain that treatment by their unaided efforts. It is to recognise that there is something about them in virtue of which they are justified in claiming and receiving the same political status as others irrespective of their ability to achieve that status for themselves.

Indeed, if the point of Stephen's argument is well taken, it might be argued against his conclusion that it is precisely because children have been treated as children and not as equals that they have been fair game for adults: exploited, abused, and even tortured and arbitrarily done to death. Perhaps irrespective of the merits of the case for their being accorded equality with adults, we should grant this status merely out of paternalistic concern for their welfare.

The recognition of full rights for children does not then necessarily imply a cruel disregard of their needs and interests. It is rather a claim that they are entitled to the same concern, respect and protection as are adults and in particular, and this is crucial, that any claim that a certain child cannot make his or her own choices and assert and demand aid in protecting his or her own rights, in short any claim that a particular child is not competent, must be established in the same way that it would have to be for an adult about whom similar claims were made.

The status of children

What we might call the status of children, the way they are treated and the freedoms or privileges they enjoy, in all societies reflects the almost universally held belief that children are incompetent to exercise the responsibilities and discharge the obligations of full citizenship.

In consequence of this supposed incompetence adults have felt entitled to place children in what amounts to protective custody. In addition to the comprehensive list of legal disabilities imposed on children: inability to vote, to initiate or defend legal proceedings on their own account, consent to sexual relations, see and read uncensored material and so on, they find their lives positively controlled by the preferences of adults. This control finds dramatic and public expression and reinforcement in the system of compulsory attendance at and obedience in schools.

While the supposed incompetence of children is the ground for the imposition of political and legal disabilities, protective custody is justified both on the grounds of the incompetence of children and also as the measure required most effectively to remove that incompetence and to allow children to proceed, without danger or mishap, to the stage where they will shed their incompetence and be sufficiently autonomous to join the community of self-determining adults.

Now, if it is supposed that it is the comprehensive possession by adults of capacities lacked equally comprehensively by children that sustains and justifies the disabling of children and their control by adults, then the supposition is quite clearly and obviously false. False because we all know that there are numerous children whom it would be implausible to regard as incompetent, and numerous adults whom it would be implausible to regard as anything but incompetent. So that if we really care about protecting the incompetent we would have to take many adults into protective custody. And, if we believe that those individuals who possess whatever range of capacities it is believed that most normal adults possess, should be 'licensed' fully to participate in decision making and should enjoy whatever freedoms are granted to full citizens then, we would have to enfranchise and grant adult freedoms to very many children.

The idea of taking many adults (or many more adults)[4] into protective custody is as abhorrent to most people as is the idea of enfranchising millions of children. To know whether either or both of these 'horrors' should be supported we need to be clearer about just what it is that entitles adults to determine their own fates and to take upon themselves the determination of the fate of their children and of children generally. The umbrella under which that 'something' or range of 'somethings' that it is believed adults comprehensively[5] possess and children equally comprehensively lack, all shelter, is the idea of autonomy. Equally it is the idea that many children are obviously autonomous and many adults obviously are not, that seems to require that in consistency we should enfranchise many children and take into protective custody many adults. Clearly it is time to be clearer about what we mean by autonomy.

I have talked here about the franchise to dramatise a point about competence. It is that when considering the question of whether a particular child is competent to consent to treatment, we should not employ assumptions or use criteria which, if applied to adult patients, would leave many subject to paternalist control.

Autonomy

I have set out elsewhere[6] an account of the defects that can occur in an individual's autonomy and what follows is an abbreviated but importantly modified and I hope improved account of these defects. Of course when we are clear or at least clearer about what tends to undermine an individual's autonomy, we will also be clearer about what autonomy is.

While the list of possible defects in autonomy is not intended to be exhaustive it is useful to think of the ways in which autonomy can be undermined under four general headings.

There are:

1. Control: The individual may not be in control or in complete control of either her desires or her actions or both.
2. Reasoning: This ability may be impaired in many ways which affect the individual's capacity to make genuine decisions.
3. Information: This may be defective in many ways which affect decision making.
4. Stability: An individual's preferences may change over time and 'mature' in various important ways which seem to affect the reality of her choices.

If we look at each of these in turn we will see how they each bear upon the question of whether the individual can be said to be in autonomous control of herself.

Defects in control

We are all familiar with the idea that people literally lose control of themselves and that when this genuinely occurs they may not be responsible for what they 'do' while out of control. Such loss of control may afford a defence in law as in the case of 'guilty but insane' or 'diminished responsibility' verdicts in trials. Mental illness of various kinds is often thought to be a source of such loss of control. Another important case occurs where the individual finds his behaviour controlled by desires he does not wish to have. The classic case here is that of addiction where the addict desires to take drugs but wishes he didn't. The loss of control involves the first order desire for a fix controlling the second order desire not to be an addict. With something like heroin addiction we are accustomed to thinking of the addict as literally controlled by his habit, but whether even this is true may be doubtful. Addiction is a much abused term. Someone who wishes to lose weight but who cannot resist another cake may be said to have their first-order desire to lose weight controlled by their second order desire for another delicious mouthful. There is some ambivalence here and it is unclear that many people who seem to lack self-control in cases like this have really worked out where the balance in the priority of their desires lies. The issue is further complicated by the fact that addiction itself is not destructive of autonomy. We are all addicted to lots of things fully voluntarily. When I choose to play squash or study philosophy, my autonomous choice is in no way defective because, although I am conscious that I cannot give these activities up, or at least that it would be extraordinarily difficult for me to do so, I have no desire at all to do so.

Children are thought to be particularly prone to being controlled by desires that either they do not wish to have or, more commonly, desires it is thought that they would not wish to have if their reasoning or information were better. We will postpone discussion of the plausibility of such claims until we have considered these other supposed defects in autonomy.

Defects of reasoning

This is a broad category which subsumes many ways in which an individual's autonomy may be vitiated or weakened by defects in her ability to reason or be 'rational'. Some examples will help to make clear what is involved here. Someone who could not draw inferences or appreciates the connection between cause and effects would have substantial difficulties in making autonomous choices. If they failed to see that smoking was dangerous, or that alcohol impaired their ability to drive safely, they would end up by doing things that they didn't want to do: like endangering their own lives and those of others.

Similarly where people allow received opinion or an emotional reaction to form the basis of their values or when they make judgements based on manifestly implausible 'facts', their autonomy is undermined. As it is when through something like 'bad faith' they refuse to admit or recognise something they know to be true.

Defects in information

Where someone's beliefs or choices are made on the basis of false or incomplete information they will to that extent be less autonomous simply because they will be in danger of doing something they wouldn't do if their information were better or more complete. Under this heading comes also the sort of 'information' which it is very hard to categorise. This is like a cross between reasoning and information. I have in mind that elusive thing called experience. Those who have what is called the relevant experience will be less in danger of making non-autonomous choices than those who lack such experience – or so experience tells us.

Defects in stability

This may be an unfamiliar category to many but the problem it highlights will not be. It is simply that our particular preferences, and indeed often our whole pattern of preferences, tend to change over time so that the choices I made when 12 or 14 years old say, may come to seem absurd, and even absurdly misjudged, when I look back on them in my forties. Some of them may even be bitterly regretted for they have shaped my life and if I had my time over again I would behave differently. This instability in our preferences is often cited as a justification for paternalism. 'I'm only doing this for your own good and one day you'll be grateful'. Since we all change not only our minds but our personalities over time, it is hardly surprising that there is a sort of inbuilt instability in our preferences. The sort of people we are and the things we choose will change over time as the things we choose modifies the sort of person we are. If the very confident prediction that we will later regret what we now choose to do were to be a justification for paternalism and a reason to believe that our present decisions were somehow less than fully autonomous, then full autonomy would only be achieved (if ever) in extreme old age. Apart from the absurdity of this it reveals a fundamental mistake about the nature of autonomy. An autonomous individual is one who governs herself, who runs her life the way she pleases. If what pleases her changes over time this provides no evidence at all that there was something spurious about her earlier preferences. They were not less genuinely hers, just different.

Autonomous persons

Now that we have reviewed the various types of defects which may count against the autonomy of an individual's decision we are in a position to draw some conclusions. We should note to start with that the four apparent categories of defect in the autonomy of our decision-making have been reduced to three. The last category considered, that of the instability of our preferences, was found on inspection to provide no grounds for supposing that a decision was defective from the point of view of autonomy merely because the individual might (or even would certainly) regret it later. This is a risk of all decision-making.

Conclusion

We may (and should) conclude that where children's decisions or preferences cannot be shown to suffer from any of the defects that render decisions non-autonomous, they should be given absolute control over their own destiny, exactly as are adults, and for the same reasons.

Where it is claimed that control of children is justified because they necessarily fail, or fail fully to comprehend, the dangers that may face them we again usually fail to make a relevant distinction between adults and children. What is it to fail, or fail fully, to comprehend a danger? What counts as a remedy for the defects in autonomy that generate such lack of comprehension?

Think for a moment of some fairly standard adult actions and choices. Think of the woman who smokes cigarettes or the man who eats a high cholesterol diet, or those who refuse to give up alcohol when its abuse is killing them and endangering others. Can such people be said to comprehend, or comprehend fully, the danger they are in? Whether or not they comprehend the danger, what follows? Are we entitled or obliged to impose abstinence or a modified diet upon them?

Certainly we are obliged to point out, and to do so quite unequivocally, the dangers. This is simply because to fail to do so would be to partake in the responsibility for their coming to grief. Where the individual knows the dangers (or at least knows the consensus of informed opinion is that there are dangers) and both wishes to persist in the life-threatening practice and wants to have a long and a happy life, then clearly their decision-making is defective.

Obviously the decision-making of very many adults indeed is defective in precisely this way and yet it is seldom suggested that this fact constitutes grounds for paternalistic control. If the very same grounds were thought of as justifying the control of children then we require some additional argument which would distinguish the two cases. One way out of this problem is shown by remembering that it is possible autonomously to accept certain defects in autonomy, but the consequences of bearing this in mind are far from providing the necessary distinguishing argument.

The autonomous acceptance of defects in autonomy

In the circumstances we have described, an individual can autonomously decide to live with some defects in the autonomy of her decision making. And it is clearly better, from the point of view of autonomy, for the individual to do this than live subject to the paternalist control of others. Where the individual has so chosen, the paternalist cannot claim to be acting in the interests of the individual's autonomy when she claims the moral right to control that person's behaviour for her own good.

If this were right, it is precisely the same for adults as for children and the only question is simply whether the individual in question, adult or child, has autonomously chosen to live with some defects in autonomy. Whether they are capable of such autonomous choice will be a question of fact in each case.

That it is a matter of fact, or at least a matter of judgement, in each case as to whether an individual is capable of autonomous choice, provides a framework for dealing with the consequences of recognising the ageism of the accepted approach to the treatment of children. I cannot elaborate that framework now but its outlines will surely be clear. They are that it is decisions which are autonomous not people. Autonomy is not an existential state – a state of being. Rather persons make decisions which either are, or are not, autonomous. Those who respect persons will respect their autonomous decisions at whatever age such decisions are made and will not assume, or be permitted to act on the assumption, that a decision is not autonomous because of the chronological age of the decider.[7]

The tenor of what I have said here is in line with recent legal thinking on the decision-making of children, although it is fair to say it takes that line a lot further than the courts have so far been prepared to do.[8]

Before completing this discussion of the position of children with respect to their control over their destiny as far as health care provision goes, we should look at the issue of consent by others to the treatment of children.

Proxy or assumed consent

There are a number of instances in health care where the patients' consent is appealed to and used, where her actual consent is unobtainable. These are circumstances in which the patient is either unconscious or unable to process the information required to give a valid consent, or is temporarily or permanently lacking the relevant capacity to consent. Children, as we have seen, are often thought to combine a number of these disabilities.

In such cases terms like 'proxy consent', 'substituted judgement', 'presumed consent' or even 'retrospective consent' are used to justify treating a patient. Not only are these all fictions, but they totally fail to be justifications for treating the patient in particular ways. Where parental consent is substituted for the consent of the child it is a form of proxy consent.

In all these cases, and in particular where parents or others consent on behalf of children, the reason why it is right to do what presumed consent or substituted judgement seems to suggest in these cases, is simply because treating the patient in the proposed ways is in his or her best interests, and to fail to treat the patient would be deliberately to harm him. It is the principle that we should do no harm that justifies treating the patient in particular ways. The justification for treatment is not that the patient did consent (which he didn't) nor that he would have, nor that it is safe to presume that he would have, nor that he will when he acquires the relevant comptence, but simply that it is the right thing to do, and it is right precisely because it is in his best interests and, by hypothesis, the patient is herself unable to consent. That it is the 'best interests' test that is operative is shown by the fact that we do not presume consent to things that are not in the patient's best interests, even where it is clear that he would have consented. We do not infuse known heavy smokers with cigarette smoke while they are unconscious even where it is reasonable to suppose they would have consented; nor do we usually give patients in hospital alcoholic beverages or cigarettes, even when they specifically request them.

Of course we do not give beneficial treatment to patients who have refused them, say by advanced directive, because to do so would constitute an assault and a violation of their will. It is not a violation of someone's will or an assault to give a treatment they have not refused, the withholding of which would constitute an injury. The reason that it is not a violation, is not because they have consented in some notional or fictional sense, but because it is the right thing to do, and the reason it is the right thing to do is that to fail or omit to do it would injure the patient. It is the infliction of that injury, by act or omission,[9] that would constitute the violation or assault, and because we not only should not harm people who do not want to be harmed, we also should not harm even those who do want to be harmed, this is sufficient reason not to withhold treatment the absence of which would harm. Not only do we not need the concept of implied or assumed or proxy consent, because it literally does not work, we do not need it because it misleads us as to the character and meaning of our actions.

So parental consent to the treatment of their children is no consent at all. If we accept such consent, it is because we presume that the parents are the best judges of the best interests of their own children and not because they have any special ethical right or ability to consent on behalf of their children. Again, that this is so can be seen by our attitude to parents' consent which is clearly not in the best interests of their child. Here we rightly ignore their preferences and protect the children from harm.

Acknowledgement

I am grateful to my colleague Charles Erin for many helpful suggestions in the preparation of this chapter.

Notes

1 There won't be time.
2 See my *The Value of Life*, Routledge, London, 1985 and 1992.
3 Indeed there are many interesting parallels with women's liberation, particularly, the arguments that have been used to deny women's rights are remarkably similar to those which have been used to deny children's rights. See my 'The Political Status of Children' in *Contemporary Political Philosophy*, ed. Keith Graham. Cambridge University Press, Cambridge, 1983.
4 I say 'many more' since substantial numbers of adult people are compulsorily detained under various sections of The Mental Health Acts.
5 With the exception noted above.
6 In my *The Value of Life*, Routledge, 1985, Chapter 10.
7 For more on respect for persons see my 'Euthanasia and the value of life' in *Examining Euthanasia: Ethical, Legal and Clinical Perspectives*, ed. John Keown. Cambridge University Press, Cambridge, 1996.
8 See for example the landmark case of Gillick v. West Norfolk and Wisbech AHA [1985] 3

All ER 402, and Margaret Brazier's illuminating discussion of the issues it raises in her *Medicine, Patient's and The Law*, Penguin Books, London, 1992.

9 I argued against the relevance of the moral distinction between acts and omissions in my *Violence and Responsibility*, Routledge & Kegan Paul, 1980. This irrelevance has recently and belatedly been recognised by the highest court in the United Kingdom. See Lord Mustil's judgement in Airedale NHS Trust v. Bland, [1993] 1 All England Rep. 821 H.L.

Index